AF725518

Diagnosis and Treatment of Ischemic Stroke

Diagnosis and Treatment of Ischemic Stroke

Edited by Lenny Cowan

AMERICAN
MEDICAL PUBLISHERS
www.americanmedicalpublishers.com

American Medical Publishers,
41 Flatbush Avenue,
1st Floor, New York,
NY 11217, USA

Visit us on the World Wide Web at:
www.americanmedicalpublishers.com

© American Medical Publishers, 2022

This book contains information obtained from authentic and highly regarded sources. Copyright for all individual chapters remain with the respective authors as indicated. All chapters are published with permission under the Creative Commons Attribution License or equivalent. A wide variety of references are listed. Permission and sources are indicated; for detailed attributions, please refer to the permissions page and list of contributors. Reasonable efforts have been made to publish reliable data and information, but the authors, editors and publisher cannot assume any responsibility for the validity of all materials or the consequences of their use.

ISBN: 978-1-63927-289-1

Trademark Notice: Registered trademark of products or corporate names are used only for explanation and identification without intent to infringe.

Cataloging-in-Publication Data

Diagnosis and treatment of ischemic stroke / edited by Lenny Cowan.
p. cm.
Includes bibliographical references and index.
ISBN 978-1-63927-289-1
1. Cerebrovascular disease. 2. Cerebral ischemia. 3. Cerebrovascular disease--Diagnosis.
4. Cerebrovascular disease--Treatment. I. Cowan, Lenny.
RC388.5 .D53 2022
616.81--dc23

Table of Contents

Preface

The condition of stroke arises due to the insufficient flow of blood towards the brain that causes cell death. There are two types of strokes, namely, ischemic stroke and hemorrhagic stroke. The ischemic stroke occurs when the blood flowing towards the brain is insufficient to meet its metabolic demands. This leads to the condition of poor oxygen supply called as cerebral hypoxia and death of the brain tissue known as infarction. The depletion of oxygen and glucose in ischemic brain tissue forces the brain to resort to anaerobic metabolism. During anaerobic metabolism, lactic acid is produced as a by-product. Lactic acid kills cells and disturbs the normal acid-base balance in the brain. The causes of ischemic stroke include anemia and tumors. A few of its symptoms are blindness in one eye, weakness in one limb or weakness in one whole side of the body. This book contains some path-breaking studies in the field of ischemic stroke. It presents researches and studies performed by experts across the globe. It will serve as a valuable source of reference for graduate and post graduate students.

Significant researches are present in this book. Intensive efforts have been employed by authors to make this book an outstanding discourse. This book contains the enlightening chapters which have been written on the basis of significant researches done by the experts.

Finally, I would also like to thank all the members involved in this book for being a team and meeting all the deadlines for the submission of their respective works. I would also like to thank my friends and family for being supportive in my efforts.

Editor

Preface

Randomized controlled trial of a coordinated care intervention to improve risk factor control after stroke or transient ischemic attack in the safety net: Secondary stroke prevention by Uniting Community and Chronic care model teams Early to End Disparities (SUCCEED)

Amytis Towfighi[1,2,3*], Eric M. Cheng[4], Monica Ayala-Rivera[3,4], Heather McCreath[4], Nerses Sanossian[2,5], Tara Dutta[3,6], Bijal Mehta[4,7], Robert Bryg[4,8], Neal Rao[4,8], Shlee Song[9], Ali Razmara[3,10], Magaly Ramirez[11], Theresa Sivers-Teixeira[2,3], Jamie Tran[7], Elizabeth Mojarro-Huang[3,5], Ana Montoya[3,7,8], Marilyn Corrales[1,3], Beatrice Martinez[3,7], Phyllis Willis[12], Mireya Macias[13], Nancy Ibrahim[14], Shinyi Wu[15,16], Jeremy Wacksman[17], Hilary Haber[17], Adam Richards[4], Frances Barry[4], Valerie Hill[3], Brian Mittman[18], William Cunningham[4], Honghu Liu[4], David A. Ganz[4,16,18], Diane Factor[13] and Barbara G. Vickrey[4,19]

Abstract

Background: Recurrent strokes are preventable through awareness and control of risk factors such as hypertension, and through lifestyle changes such as healthier diets, greater physical activity, and smoking cessation. However, vascular risk factor control is frequently poor among stroke survivors, particularly among socio-economically disadvantaged blacks, Latinos and other people of color. The Chronic Care Model (CCM) is an effective framework for multi-component interventions aimed at improving care processes and outcomes for individuals with chronic disease. In addition, community health workers (CHWs) have played an integral role in reducing health disparities; however, their effectiveness in reducing vascular risk among stroke survivors remains unknown. Our objectives are to develop, test, and assess the economic value of a CCM-based intervention using an Advanced Practice Clinician (APC)-CHW team to improve risk factor control after stroke in an under-resourced, racially/ethnically diverse population.

(Continued on next page)

* Correspondence: towfighi@usc.edu
[1]Los Angeles County Department of Health Services, Los Angeles, California, USA
[2]University of Southern California, Los Angeles, California, USA
Full list of author information is available at the end of the article

(Continued from previous page)

Methods/design: In this single-blind randomized controlled trial, 516 adults (≥40 years) with an ischemic stroke, transient ischemic attack or intracerebral hemorrhage within the prior 90 days are being enrolled at five sites within the Los Angeles County safety-net setting and randomized 1:1 to intervention vs usual care. Participants are excluded if they do not speak English, Spanish, Cantonese, Mandarin, or Korean or if they are unable to consent. The intervention includes a minimum of three clinic visits in the healthcare setting, three home visits, and Chronic Disease Self-Management Program group workshops in community venues. The primary outcome is blood pressure (BP) control (systolic BP <130 mmHg) at 1 year. Secondary outcomes include: (1) mean change in systolic BP; (2) control of other vascular risk factors including lipids and hemoglobin A1c, (3) inflammation (C reactive protein [CRP]), (4) medication adherence, (5) lifestyle factors (smoking, diet, and physical activity), (6) estimated relative reduction in risk for recurrent stroke or myocardial infarction (MI), and (7) cost-effectiveness of the intervention versus usual care.

Discussion: If this multi-component interdisciplinary intervention is shown to be effective in improving risk factor control after stroke, it may serve as a model that can be used internationally to reduce race/ethnic and socioeconomic disparities in stroke in resource-constrained settings.

Keywords: Community health worker, Stroke, Transient ischemic attack, Intracerebral hemorrhage, Vascular risk, Blood pressure, Coordinated care, Disparities, NINDS Common Data Elements, Biomarkers

Background

Background and rationale

A small group of individuals with multiple comorbidities account for a disproportionate share of health care costs; in the United States, 10% of patients account for 70% of total health care expenditures [1]. These individuals have multiple chronic conditions, frequent hospitalizations, and often have limited ability to perform basic daily functions due to physical, mental, or psychosocial challenges. In recent years, coordinated care management models targeting these high-cost, high-need patients have been proposed to improve quality, reduce disparities, and minimize unnecessary healthcare spending [2–5].

Individuals with stroke or transient ischemic attack (TIA) are an important example of those high utilizers given their complex needs, including disability, multiple medical comorbidities, and highly prevalent concomitant depression. They have high rates of recurrent strokes and other future cardiovascular events. In fact, a prior stroke or TIA is the strongest predictor of a subsequent stroke, and the cumulative 5-year risk of recurrent stroke ranges from 15 to 25% [6]. Furthermore, the overwhelming majority of strokes each year could be prevented through awareness and optimal management of hypertension, and through lifestyle changes to healthier diets, greater physical activity, and smoking cessation [7, 8]. These four factors plus abdominal obesity account for 82 and 90% of the population-attributable risk for ischemic stroke and for hemorrhagic stroke, respectively [9]. Hypertension is the most important modifiable risk factor for stroke worldwide and is responsible for approximately two-thirds of cerebrovascular disease burden [10]. Although recurrent stroke risk can be substantially reduced by controlling modifiable vascular risk factors, these risk factors are optimally controlled in only a small proportion of stroke survivors [11–13]. Under-resourced blacks and Latinos in particular, have well-documented and substantial disparities in risk factor control as well as quality of care, and outcomes after stroke [14, 15].

To redress disparities in risk factor control after stroke or TIA, it is critical to enhance access to high quality health care services and to use patient-centered, culturally- and individually-tailored methods to improve lifestyle habits, health literacy, self-management skills, and medication adherence. The Chronic Care Model (CCM), advocated as a guide for developing care improvement interventions for patients with chronic disease, has been an effective framework for multi-component intervention programs aimed at improving care processes and outcomes while reducing costs for various chronic conditions, including diabetes and hypertension [16, 17]. The six components of this model are self-management support, clinical information systems, delivery system redesign, decision support for application of evidence-based care guidelines, health care organization championship and leadership support, and community resources. We recently completed a different randomized controlled trial (RCT) of a CCM-based intervention for secondary stroke prevention, Systemic Use of STroke Averting INterventions (SUSTAIN) [18]. This experience highlighted our need for a strong community-based component to intensively address behavioral risk factors by accounting for social determinants of health, such as the social and community context, living situation, physical environment, education, and access to healthcare.

CHWs – trained lay members of the community who serve as patient and community advocates, or "coaches" for disease management– have been engaged in the healthcare workforce for decades in low-income countries. CHWs are now also receiving heightened attention in high-income countries as healthcare is evolving to recognize and reimburse for a broader range of potential providers than physicians, physician assistants, and nurse practitioners, and to incorporate cultural competency in interventions targeting disparities in health. CHW interventions have been successful in various US populations with chronic conditions such as hypertension and diabetes, demonstrating significant improvements in health literacy, risk factor control, self-management skills, lifestyle habits, and a decrease in inappropriate health care utilization [19–27]. Few studies have evaluated the effectiveness of CHW interventions among stroke survivors, [28, 29] but none have evaluated such interventions in conjunction with a broader CCM-based healthcare system re-design.

Objectives

Our objectives are to develop, test, and evaluate the effectiveness and assess the economic value of CCM-based intervention, Secondary stroke prevention by Uniting Community and Chronic care model teams Early to End Disparities (SUCCEED), to improve risk factor control after stroke in an under-resourced, racially and ethnically diverse population. The intervention consists of care from a team consisting of an Advanced Practice Clinician (APC) who is either a Nurse Practitioner (NP) or Physician Assistant (PA) and a CHW providing care in the healthcare setting (via clinic visits) and the community (through home visits and self-management group workshops held in community venues). The APCs and CHWs use mobile technology to communicate with each other, manage patient panels, reinforce self-management skills, employ culturally-, language-, and education level-appropriate patient education tools, and follow protocols of care, with decision support. We hypothesize that by promoting health care access, evidence-based care, care coordination, health literacy, self-management skills, a healthy lifestyle, and medication adherence; recognizing and treating depression, and minimizing social isolation, we can improve vascular risk factor control - particularly blood pressure (BP) - among a vulnerable population of stroke survivors (Fig. 1).

Trial design

SUCCEED is an RCT, randomizing participants in a 1:1 fashion to usual care vs. intervention, stratified by site,

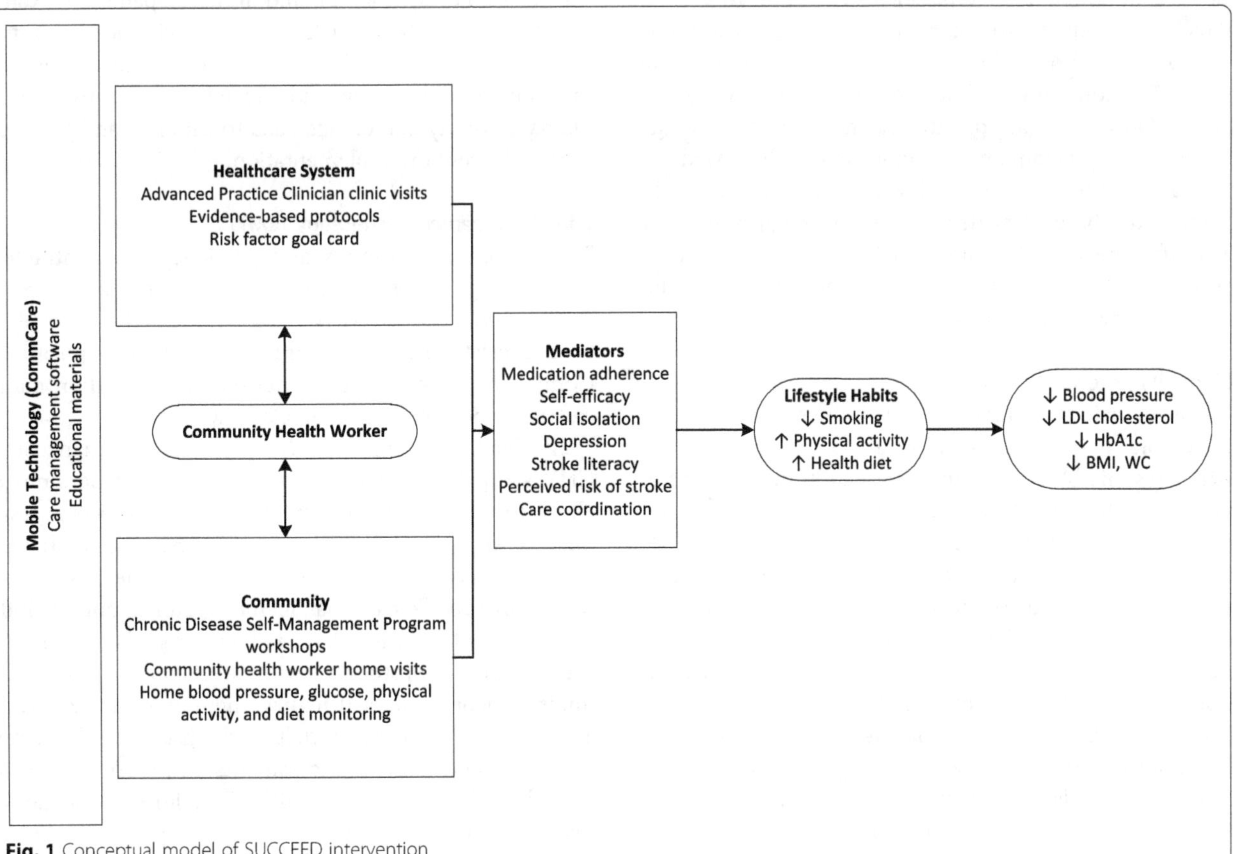

Fig. 1 Conceptual model of SUCCEED intervention

language (English, Spanish, or other [Mandarin/Cantonese and Korean]), and type of stroke (ischemic vs. hemorrhagic).

Methods: participants, interventions, and outcomes

Study setting

Patients are enrolled from the four safety-net public Los Angeles County-Department of Health Services (LAC-DHS) medical centers and one private medical center that serves the indigent. The four hospitals that anchor care for patients in the LAC-DHS system are Los Angeles County-University of Southern California Medical Center, Harbor-UCLA Medical Center, Olive View Medical Center, and Rancho Los Amigos National Rehabilitation Hospital (composed of an acute care hospital and an acute rehabilitation hospital). This system serves the largest, most ethnically diverse county in the United States. LAC-DHS provides healthcare to 700,000 people each year and treats more than 300,000 emergency and trauma victims annually. Through an integrated network of hospitals, health centers and clinics, the LAC-DHS system makes medical and preventive care services accessible in communities across the county. Over 90% of individuals who utilize this system are from socioeconomically disadvantaged minority groups and the majority are Latino. A retrospective review of all stroke/TIA admissions from 2007 to 2012 at Rancho Los Amigos revealed the following racial/ethnic distribution: 58% Latino, 20% Asian, 13% non-Latino black, 7% non-Latino white, and 2% Native American/other. Only 3% had private insurance and 10% had Medicare; the remainder were uninsured or had Medicaid insurance [30]. According to Los Angeles County administrative databases, less than 50% speak English at home. The fifth site is Cedars-Sinai Medical Center; we limited enrollment to individuals residing in the Centinela Valley, an underserved area of Los Angeles County.

Eligibility criteria

Inclusion criteria include (1) TIA, ischemic stroke or intracerebral hemorrhage within the prior 90 days and (2) either systolic blood pressure (SBP) ≥130 mmHg, or SBP between 120 and 130 mmHg and a history of hypertension or on antihypertensive medications prior to the stroke or TIA. Exclusion criteria are: (1) younger than 40 years old; (2) unable to communicate understanding of the study during the informed consent process, or (3) not fluent in English, Spanish, Korean, Mandarin or Cantonese. Individuals younger than 40 years of age are excluded because the mechanisms for their strokes are often not due to atherosclerosis (e.g. arterial dissections, inherited coagulation defects, cardiac conditions); therefore, the interventions in this trial may not target their risk factors. The included languages reflect the languages spoken by the majority of the LAC-DHS safety net population.

Intervention structure and activities

Individuals randomized to the intervention arm receive usual care plus care from a team consisting of an APC, supported by the site principal investigator (who is a Vascular Neurologist or Cardiologist), and a CHW. Over the course of the year, the intervention consists of: (1) a minimum of three clinic visits with the APC (CHW attends when possible); (2) a minimum of three home visits by the CHW; (3) the option to participate in Chronic Disease Self-Management Program (CDSMP) workshops, and (4) telephone coordination of care (Fig. 2). Beyond the minimum set of interactions, the care team has the ability to deliver additional interactions based on participants' needs; therefore, individuals with more complex needs are tagged as "high needs" and receive more 'touches' than those who are more stable. Criteria that flag an intervention arm participant as "high needs" are: (1) SBP > 180 mmHg; (2) HbA1c > 10% or fingerstick glucose >200 mg/dL in the last 2 weeks; (3) depression (Patient Health Questionnaire [PHQ]-9 score > 10) or suicidal ideation, (4) morbid obesity (body mass index [BMI] > 35 kg/m^2; (5) cognitive deficits impairing capability for self-management, and (6) alcohol or drug abuse. This is a fluid designation, and all participants are evaluated by the care team each week for their "needs status". Participants have the choice to opt out of any aspect of the intervention. Intervention teams and the two study PIs have weekly conference calls to monitor and troubleshoot intervention implementation.

Care ManagementTechnology (CMT)

To increase effectiveness and efficiency, we contracted with Dimagi, whose platform, CommCare, is an open-source, mobile device-based tool for CHWs. The platform consists of two components - a mobile application, CommCare Mobile, and a cloud-based application management and reporting tool, CommCareHQ.

The goal of CommCare Mobile was to enhance the CHWs' capabilities during home visits. We programmed all protocols into CommCare Mobile, which was accessible via Android tablets (Fig. 3). CommCare Mobile was intended to enable the CHWs to: have immediate access to patient-specific care management information, including problem lists, care plans, risk factor goals, and health status; follow protocols, with decision support; administer depression, self-management, and lifestyle habit assessments; review participants' goals; track tasks, complete and record assessments, and communicate with the APCs, and select culturally-tailored educational materials, including handouts, self-management tools, and videos. Data entered into CommCare Mobile is

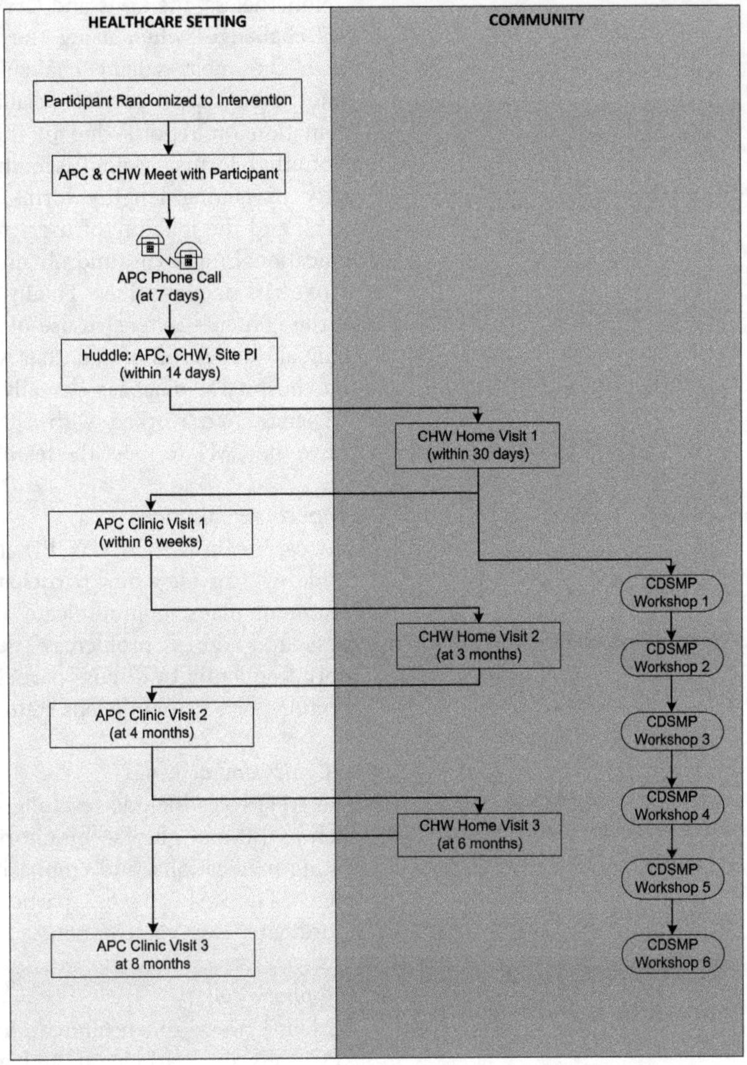

Fig. 2 Participant flow in intervention

stored on the mobile device until a cellular connection is established to perform a two-way synchronization to CommCareHQ. CommCare HQ has reporting tools to provide real-time updates and can export data into other common software programs. Prior to this RCT, the platform had not been adapted to the specific topic of vascular risk factor management.

The APCs have the choice of using CommCareHQ on a desktop or CommCare Mobile on a tablet or smart phone. Updated data on any patient or task is passed back and forth between the CHWs' and APCs' tools. We pilot-tested the CMT with the CHWs and APCs using simulation data. Tracking tools installed on the CommCare platform enable the study team and the intervention teams to track forms submitted on a weekly basis.

CommCare formative evaluation

During the first 12 months of rollout of the CMT, we conducted a formal formative evaluation, to enable APCs and CHWs to provide feedback to revise the tools and protocols for more effective and efficient operation [31]. Overall, the APCs and CHWs expressed that the CMT assisted them in care management. The CMT helped APCs and CHWs track their interactions with participants and plan their work accordingly to ensure that participants received at least the minimum interactions per the SUCCEED protocol. For CHWs, the CMT facilitated efficient data collection, provided decision support during home visits, tracked participants' stroke risk factor values, guided them in developing care plans, and provided remote access to care plans and important patient health information while in the community.

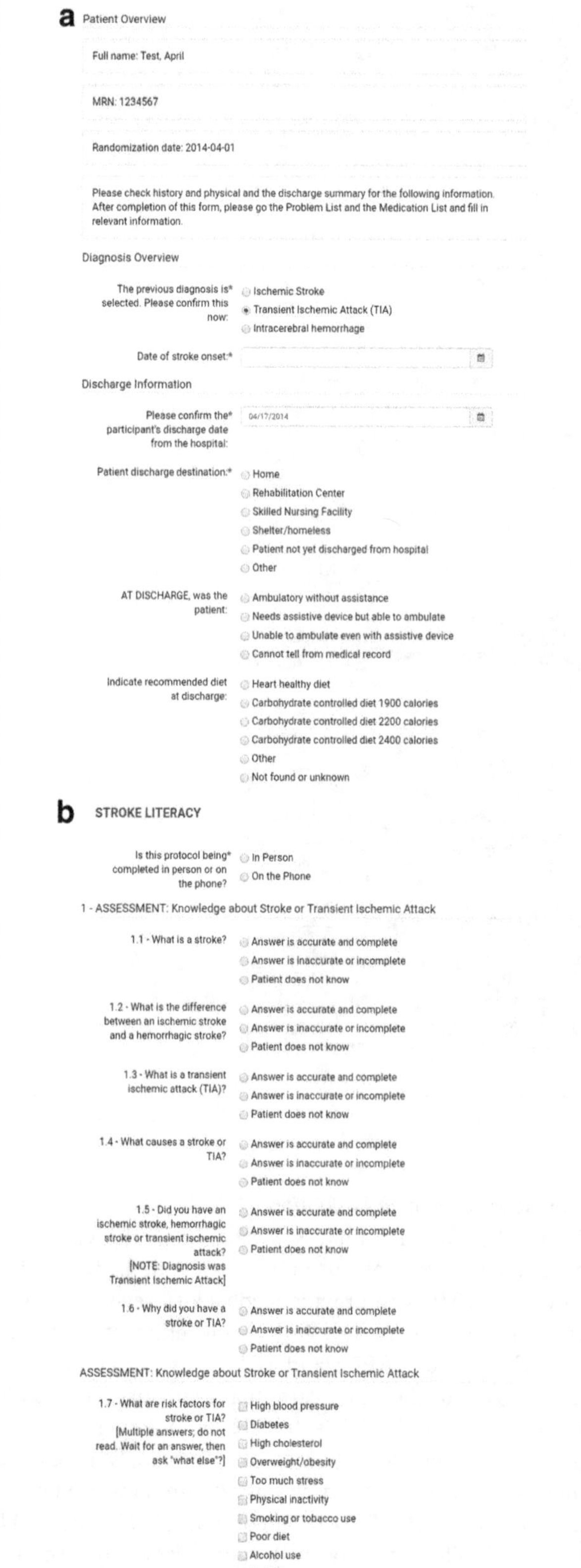

Fig. 3 **a** Screenshot of CommCare application for APC. **b** Screenshot of CommCare application for CHW

Nonetheless, the CMs and CHWs experienced numerous challenges when using the CMT. At the platform level, the most salient challenges were long loading times, inconsistent service reliability, and inaccurate information on reports due to the CMT not registering submitted forms. Major usability issues included difficulty navigating lengthy forms, the effort to manage tasks, and the inability of users to tailor reports, display educational materials, and obtain useful visualizations of stroke risk factor values. Finally, issues with the design of the content—extensive use of free-text responses and manual duplication of data that was already contained in the hospital's database—greatly hindered care team efficiency. We worked with DiMagi to iteratively improve the CMT to meet the team's needs.

Team communication

The care team (APC/CHW/PI) at each site holds weekly "huddles" to review new participants and jointly develop treatment plans, communicate about participants' progress, and address problems. The CHW and APC meet more frequently to discuss participants in detail and determine participants' "needs status".

APC roles and activities

The APC roles include teaching self-management skills, such as BP and glucose monitoring, prescribing and titrating medications, and emphasizing medication adherence. The APC sees participants in clinic and coordinates care via telephone.

APC phone call

Within 1 week of enrollment in the intervention, the APC calls the participant and assesses current health status (any changes in stroke symptoms since enrollment), blood pressure, medication adherence and side effects, smoking, transportation, and reminds him/her of the next clinic appointment.

APC clinic visits

At clinic visits, the APC is guided by evidence-based care protocols developed by the research team, covering: stroke literacy, blood pressure, cholesterol, diabetes, antithrombotic medications, smoking cessation, depression, diet, and physical activity. Each protocol is organized into six sections: (1) assessment; (2) information provision; (3) self-management and adherence; (4) adjustment of medications (if applicable); (5) clinical support (e.g. from the site PI), and (6) resource provision for the participant. Clinic visits are conducted using patient-centered principles of care that include the patient's chosen support network (caregivers, family, and friends). The APCs have smart cellular telephones that enable the participants to reach the APC during business hours by phone call or text message, as well as send photos of BP and glucose logs or new medications. The APCs also assist the participants with goal setting.

CHW roles

The CHWs key roles are to: (1) reinforce and enhance self-management skills; (2) serve as a liaison between the patient and the health care system; (3) mobilize resources, system support, and friend and family networks to reduce social isolation; and (4) educate participants about vascular risk factors, signs and symptoms of stroke, and activation of emergency medical services for stroke symptoms. These functions are performed through two mechanisms: CDSMP workshops held in the community, and home visits. The CHWs also have cellular telephones enabling participants to call the CHWs during business hours with questions and concerns. The CHWs assist the participants with transportation arrangements.

CHW home visits

The CHWs follow protocols to assess and address: (1) stroke literacy; (2) BP; (3) antithrombotic use; (4) cholesterol; (5) diabetes; (6) psychosocial issues, including depression and social isolation; (7) diet; (8) physical activity; (9) smoking; (10) alcohol and illicit drug use; (11) transportation, (12) communication preferences, and (13) access to care. The CHWs provide the participants with appropriate literacy-level, culturally-adapted educational materials (for Hispanic, African American, Chinese and Korean racial/ethnic groups) that were developed in conjunction with community-academic teams.

Chronic disease self-management program (CDSMP) workshops

Each workshop series is facilitated by two lead CHWs. Each series is comprised of 6 weekly workshops addressing key themes: use of symptom management techniques to deal with chronic disease symptoms, including fear, depression, anger, frustration, fatigue, pain and isolation; appropriate exercise for maintaining and improving strength and endurance; appropriate use of medications; communicating effectively with family, friends and health care professionals; and nutrition. Each session is framed by action planning, disease-related problem solving, and decision making. Trained CDSMP facilitators follow a scripted Leaders' Manual each time they lead the program. Since the workshops are highly participatory, they work best when attended by at least seven participants. In order to increase the likelihood of meeting the seven minimum participants, intervention subjects are encouraged to invite caregivers, friends, family members, and community members with chronic conditions ranging from hypertension to obesity to participate. If the attendance is below seven, our community-based partners assist us in identifying participants for the workshop and we invite individuals not enrolled in the RCT to participate by advertising the workshops in outpatient clinics. Each intervention subject in the workshop receives a personal copy of the companion book, *Living a Healthy Life with Chronic Conditions, 3rd Edition* and an audio relaxation CD, *Time for Healing*. Participants are provided with small incentives for participation in the CDSMP workshops, such as $25 gift cards for grocery stores and an alarm/CD player to play the CDSMP meditation CD. Attendance at CDSMP workshops is recorded in CommCare.

The CHWs received 9 days of training to lead CDSMP workshops. In order to address cultural differences, the trainings for English and Spanish were separate. Two CHWs facilitate CDSMP workshops; separate workshops are conducted for English and Spanish-speaking intervention participants.

Education and support materials

In addition to the materials described above, other materials are provided to support the decision-making and behavioral choices of participants.

Goal cards and tools

At the first clinic visit with the APC, participants receive a customized goal card delineating current versus optimal control of key factors: BP, low density lipoprotein (LDL) cholesterol, diabetes, smoking, diet, physical activity, BMI, emotional health, and antithrombotic medications (Fig. 4). Factors are classified as "at goal" (green), "near goal" (yellow), and "not at goal" (red). Participants have the option of choosing media with this information; choices include refrigerator magnets, whiteboards, accordion pocket cards, coffee mugs, water bottles, and spiral bound index cards. Some of the goal tools, such as the white board, include a space labeled "where I am" and space to write action plans. Goal tools were developed using input and feedback from approximately 10 individuals attending a Stroke Community Engagement Symposium, a local event dedicated to raising awareness and arming participants with information on stroke warning signs, risk factors, treatment, and disparities. Attendees included stroke survivors, community advocates, and members of community-based organizations. Further input on the design, content, language, practicality, cultural sensitivity, and usefulness of the goal cards was obtained from 15 stroke survivors recruited from Rancho Los Amigos.

Blood pressure self-management and glucose monitoring

Once participants are randomized to the intervention, they receive Omron HEM-711 DLX BP monitors for

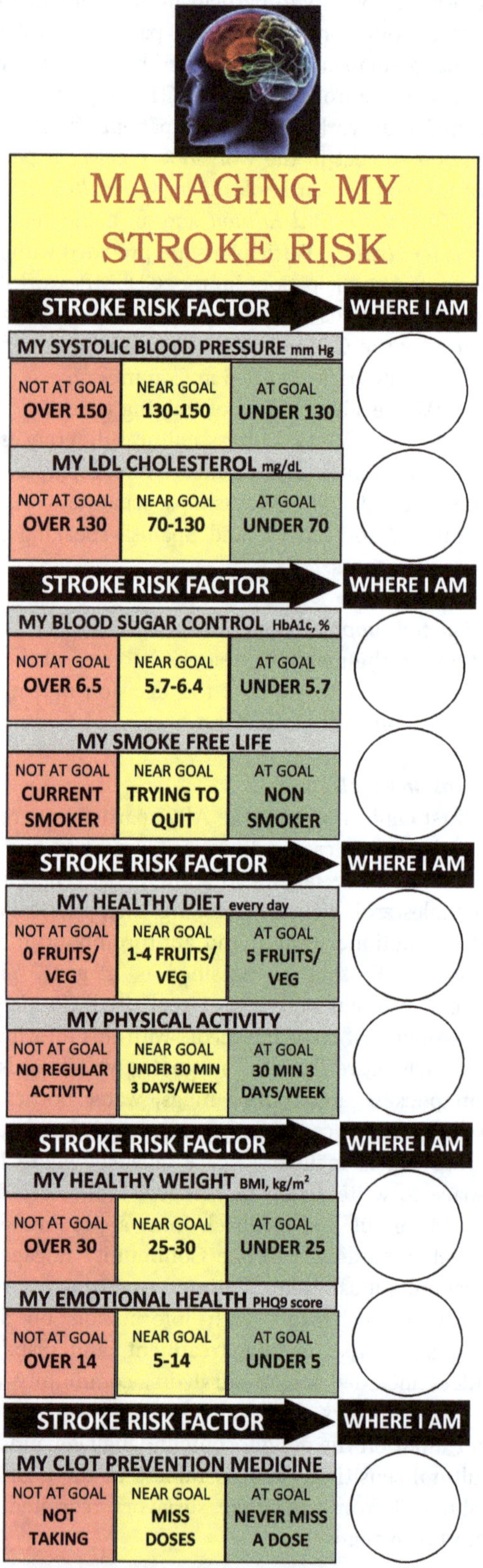

Fig. 4 Risk factor goal card: trifold wallet card

home monitoring and are instructed on how to use the BP monitor and log and track the results. Participants also receive instructions on how to check and monitor blood glucose levels, if clinically indicated. These skills are assessed and re-enforced at subsequent clinic visits and home visits.

Intervention team recruitment and training

The PIs and site PIs trained the APCs to follow evidence-based protocols, teach self-management skills, and educate participants. Dimagi conducted remote and on-site training to use CommCare Mobile and CommCare HQ. The APCs also received training on motivational interviewing.

We partnered with three community-based organizations to recruit CHWs: (1) the Los Angeles Healthcare Workforce Development Program (HCWDP)/Worker Education and Resource Center (WERC), (2) Esperanza Community Housing Corporation (Esperanza), and (3) Watts Labor Community Action Committee (WLCAC). HCWDP is a labor/management partnership between LAC-DHS and the Service Employees International Union, that provides workforce development courses for healthcare workers, and specifically for CHWs who work in the Los Angeles healthcare safety-net system of hospitals and clinics. Esperanza and WLCAC are nonprofit organizations empowering residents of South Central Los Angeles through programs focused on affordable housing, health, arts and sciences, education, and economic development. To date, Esperanza's Community Health Promoters Training Program has trained over 400 bi- and trilingual low-income residents to become community health leaders, patient advocates, health educators, and community organizers.

We conducted CHW training and selection in two phases. First, Esperanza, WLCAC, and WERC advertised the opportunity to obtain training in CDSMP and stroke to their community members and CHWs. We selected bilingual (English and Spanish) individuals to complete a 36-h training workshop for CDSMP. Second, we invited graduates of the CDSMP training to participate in an 80-h training on SUCCEED-specific topics, including stroke and vascular risk factors. We selected CHWs from the second phase of training.

We developed the 80-h curriculum for CHWs in collaboration with WERC. Topics included basic CHW skills, stroke etiology, signs and symptoms of stroke, hypertension, obesity, diabetes, dyslipidemia, diet, physical activity, smoking cessation, communication, speech, and swallowing, mental health and cognition, self-management skills, motivational interviewing, assessing therapy needs, potential stroke complications, common medications for stroke, tools for medication adherence, healthcare system navigation, goal cards and tools, panel management, and staff safety. The courses were taught by study staff, subject matter experts, and WERC curriculum developers and instructors. We trained two cohorts of CHWs—one in 2013 and another in 2015 (due to attrition of one CHW during the trial and expansion of the trial to the private medical center).

Control structure and activities

Participants randomized to the control arm receive usual care, which varies by study site, but typically includes primary care visits, a post-hospital follow up visit with a vascular neurologist, and AHA educational handouts regarding stroke, physical activity and diet, and antithrombotics.

Clinical outcomes

The primary outcome is the proportion of participants who achieve BP control (SBP <130 mmHg) at 1 year and the average change in SBP (Table 1. Secondary outcomes include: (1) mean change in systolic BP; (2) control of other vascular risk factors including lipids and hemoglobin A1c, (3) inflammation (C reactive protein [CRP]), (4) medication adherence, (5) lifestyle factors (smoking, diet, and physical activity), (6) estimated relative reduction in risk for recurrent stroke or MI, and (7) cost-effectiveness of the intervention versus usual care (Table 1). In addition, we will estimate the combined impact of changes in multiple risk factors on the relative risk of cardiovascular disease (CVD) or recurrent stroke in intervention and control groups. This secondary outcome of "global CVD risk reduction" will be modeled using observed changes in risk factor values for each participant and the relative risk reductions reported in randomized controlled trials of respective interventions (ie: statin therapy, anti-hypertensive medications). Detailed methods used to calculate the global risk reduction will be published in a forthcoming manuscript.

Participant timeline

At baseline, 3 and 12 months, research assistants (RAs) interview participants and measure BP, anthropometrics (including height, weight and waist circumference), and laboratory studies (by fingerstick, using a CardioChek® handheld device and dried blood spot collection; Table 2, Fig. 5). After the participant sits still for five minutes, three BP measurements are obtained five minutes apart; the mean BP is used. Participants complete a telephone-administered interview at 8 months. Subsequently, after the 12-month study period, participants receive surveillance telephone calls every 6 months to assess for vascular events or death up to 36 months. Weekly reports of screening, enrollment, and data collection by time point and by site are generated from Research Electronic Data Capture (REDCap™) and circulated and discussed on weekly investigator/evaluation RA conference calls.

Sample size calculation and power analysis

Our sample size calculation and power analyses were based on the primary outcome of SBP. Meta-analyses have revealed a 25 to 40% reduction in recurrent stroke risk with BP-lowering therapies [32–34]. We initially defined BP control as SBP < 120 mmHg, consistent with the Seventh Report of the Joint National Committee on Prevention, Detection, Evaluation, and Treatment of High Blood Pressure (JNC-7). During the course of the trial, evidence of a potential J-shaped curve emerged among individuals with existing cardiovascular disease or diabetes, with higher cardiovascular events and mortality associated with tight BP control [35–38]. Retrospective analyses of RCTs and observational studies suggested a potential J-shaped curve among individuals with stroke as well, particularly in the first 6 months post-stroke [39–42]. Sixteen months after initiating the trial (after enrolling 150 participants), we increased our SBP goal to <130 mmHg at 1 year. We simultaneously revised our inclusion criteria from SBP ≥120 mmHg, to either SBP ≥130 mmHg, or SBP between 120 and 130 mmHg and a history of hypertension or on antihypertensive medications prior to the stroke or TIA event.

Power analyses were conducted with comparison of the primary outcome (SBP) between the intervention and the control arm. Based on availability of our patients and our capacity, we plan to enroll 516 participants. Using intra-class correlation of the five sites at 0.0085 level, standard deviation of 20 mmHg, three repeated measurements (at baseline, 3 and 12 months), type I error of 0.05, type II error of 0.2 (or equivalent to power of 80%), 2.4 average data points for each subject (corresponding to 30% attrition), and an auto-correlation of 0.2, the effective sample size for the entire study will be 261 (after adjusting for clustering effect of the five recruitment sites). The effect size for SBP as small as 0.25 in standard deviation units or 5.06 mmHg can be considered clinically meaningful in the presence of both moderators and mediators.

With a planned enrollment of 516 and conservative attrition estimates, SUCCEED is powered to detect a clinically meaningful difference in BP between intervention and usual care arms in the presence of moderator and mediator effects. For potential moderators (e.g., age, sex, stroke type and severity, education, country of birth/primary language), we will test power of moderation using f^2, the most common measure of effect size [43]. To analyze power of potential mediators (e.g., self-efficacy, self-management, social isolation, depression, perceived risk of stroke), we will use indirect effect.

Recruitment

We recruit participants from both the inpatient and outpatient settings. The research team presents information

Table 1 Primary and secondary outcomes, moderators, and mediators

Outcome	Measure
Primary Outcome	
Systolic blood pressure control (<130 mmHg)	Physical exam
Secondary Outcomes	
Change in systolic blood pressure	Physical exam
Dyslipidemia: non-HDL cholesterol	CardioChek®
Glucose control: hemoglobin A1c	Dried blood spot
Inflammation: C-reactive protein	Dried blood spot
Adiposity: BMI, WC, WHR	Physical exam
Physical activity	Adapted from International Physical Activity Questionnaire [59]
Diet	California Health Interview Survey (CHIS) 2011–2012 [60]
Smoking	CHIS 2011–2012, Behavioral Risk Factor Surveillance System (BRFSS) 2013 [61]
Recurrent stroke or TIA	Questionnaire for Verifying Stroke-Free Status (QVSFS) [62]
Myocardial infarction	Medical history Common Data Element [45]
Cost	
Moderators	
Sociodemographics: age, sex, race/ethnicity	NINDS Demographics Common Data Element [45]
Acculturation and Education: country of birth, primary language, education level	Adapted from NINDS Demographics CDE, subscale of Bidimensional Acculturation Scale for Hispanics [63]
Health-care system	Study site
Type of cerebrovascular event (TIA, ischemic stroke, intracerebral hemorrhage)	Medical record
Stroke severity	NIH Stroke Scale
Functional status	Modified Rankin Scale
Mediators	
Stroke Literacy	Stroke warning signs and risk factors for stroke [64]
Health Literacy	4-Item Brief Health Literacy Screening Tool (BRIEF) [65]
Medication adherence	Adapted from Simoni et al. [66] and Chesney et al. [67]
Self-management skills	Adapted from Self-Efficacy for Managing Chronic Disease 6-item scale [68]
Self-efficacy	General Self-Efficacy Scale [69]
Perceived risk of stroke	Adapted from Stroke Risk and Worry Survey [70]
Social isolation	8-Item Social Support Scale [71]
Depression	Center for Epidemiologic Studies Depression Scale (CES-D) [72]
Health related quality of life	SF-6D [73]
Perceptions of quality of care	Adapted from Patient Assessment of Chronic Illness Care (PACIC) [74] and Consumer Assessment of Healthcare Providers and Systems (CAHPS®) [75]
Intervention Mediators	
Coordination and communication with care team: number CHW home visits, CDSMP workshops attended, APC clinic visits, telephone visits; communication between APC and CHW	CommCare tracking technology

Abbreviations: *BMI* body mass index, *WC* waist circumference, *WHR* waist-to-hip ratio, *CDE* common data element

about SUCCEED to clinicians in the Neurology, Internal Medicine, Family Medicine, Emergency Medicine, and Physical Medicine and Rehabilitation and Therapy departments. We post study flyers in the wards, outpatient clinics, and housestaff offices of these departments. In the inpatient setting, we discuss the study with the inpatient and consult teams taking care of patients with stroke or TIA. In the outpatient setting, we discuss the

Table 2 Evaluation timeline

		"On" intervention or usual care			"Off" or post-intervention or usual care follow up		
Time, months	Baseline	3	8	12	18	24	30
Informed consent	X						
Physical exam • Blood pressure • Body mass index • Waist circumference • Waist-to-hip ratio • NIH SS • mRS	X	X		X			
Fingerstick labs • Total cholesterol • HDL • Triglycerides • Calculated LDL • Total cholesterol/HDL • Hemoglobin A1c • C-reactive protein	X	X		X			
Full in-person[a] questionnaire	X	X		X			
Brief telephone questionnaire			X				
Telephone surveillance (vascular events, death)					X	X	X

Abbreviations: NIH SS National Institutes of Health Stroke Scale, *mRS* modified Rankin Score, *HDL* high density lipoprotein cholesterol, *LDL* low density lipoprotein cholesterol

[a]Sometimes obtained by phone if an in-person visit was infeasible

study with the physicians, clinic coordinators, nurses, and medical assistants.

A potential participant's clinician obtains verbal permission from the patient before passing his/her name to a member of the research team. In the inpatient setting, the RA either attends inpatient rounds (fostering awareness about the study and prompting the study team during rounds to ask patients for permission for the RA to meet the patient later) or confers with the team after morning rounds to review eligible participants. In the outpatient setting, we use several methods to identify participants: (1) review clinic patient lists for potentially eligible participants; (2) attend clinic and reviewing the list with the clinician, and (3) remind the clinicians to call the RA for potentially eligible patients. Since outpatients may need to leave the clinic immediately after the visit with the clinician, the RA may not be able to speak to an outpatient before he or she leaves, but can call the patient later. Alternatively, potential subjects can also directly call the RA to learn more about the RCT, using the number listed on flyers.

Methods: assignment of interventions

Allocation: sequence generation, allocation concealment mechanism, implementation

Before the RCT began, we used computer-assisted stratified randomization of block size of four to develop randomization schedules. The three stratification variables are site, spoken language (English, Spanish, or other [Mandarin/Cantonese and Korean]), and type of stroke (ischemic vs. hemorrhagic). The schedules have an allocation ratio of 1:1 of control and intervention. We use permuted block randomization that stratifies by site to promote periodic balance through the trial and group balance at the end of the trial. The study programmer/analyst generated 28 lists, one for each stratum; we subsequently programmed these lists into the electronic database, Research Electronic Data Capture (REDCap™), for automated randomization. Each row of the list includes a unique subject ID and arm assignment of the study.

The randomization program in REDCap™ is only accessible by the Project Manager, Principal Investigators and Data Manager, and only the Project Manager enters new data to obtain a randomization assignment. For individuals who consent to the study and meet inclusion criteria, the RA assigns a unique study ID and collects baseline data before randomization. After an eligible participant has consented and completed the baseline survey, the RA informs the Project Manager, who enters the appropriate variables to obtain a randomization assignment. The Project Manager notifies the intervention team of participants randomized to the intervention. If possible, the intervention team meets participants upon enrollment; otherwise, the team calls participants to introduce themselves and the study.

Screening and consent procedure

When a clinician notifies the RA of a potential participant, the RA arranges a face-to-face meeting to

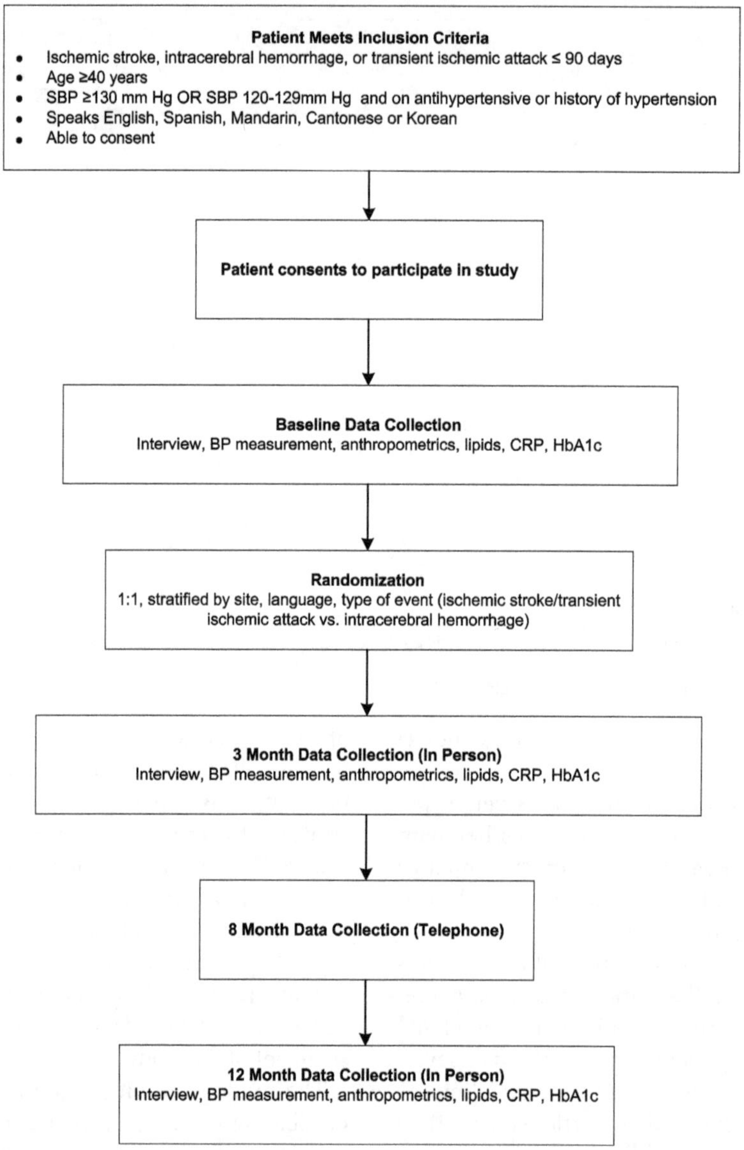

Fig. 5 Enrollment of subjects and schedule for collecting evaluation data

determine whether the patient meets eligibility criteria for enrollment. The RA reads to the patient an institutional review board (IRB)-approved script that further describes the SUCCEED trial. If a potential participant directly contacts the RA, the RA reads the IRB-approved script and if the potential participant is interested, a face-to-face meeting will be scheduled. The RAs are bilingual in English and Spanish, and in the case that a subject speaks a language other than English or Spanish, the research team uses volunteers fluent in the appropriate language to translate for the RA. All consent materials were translated into Spanish by an American Translators Association-certified translator. Consent forms were translated into Korean and Chinese with a three-step process using Transperfect® [44]. If the potential participant is interested in participating in the study, the RA (1) asks questions about age and time of stroke onset or TIA occurrence to confirm eligibility; (2) asks the participant questions to determine comprehension of study participation; and (3) measures BP. For those found to be ineligible, the reasons for ineligibility are recorded. If eligible participants choose not to consent to the study, the RA records the reason. Further, the RA asks permission to use the demographic information of those who decline study participation (without obtaining any personally identifiable information) to generate enrollment propensity weights. Enrollment propensity weights will be used to analyze whether characteristics of those eligible for the trial but who declined to participate may impact generalizability of study outcomes.

Blinding

The RA collects the baseline survey and examination data prior to randomization. Only the Project Manager randomizes participants, and all data related to participants' activities with the intervention are managed in a separate database that cannot be accessed by the RAs. RAs remain blinded to group assignment throughout the follow-up. The RAs work in offices that are geographically separate from the intervention team to avoid unblinding. If a participant informs the RA at a subsequent evaluation that they are in either arm, a different RA is assigned to perform the evaluation, without discussion regarding the reason.

Methods: data collection, management, and analysis

Data collection methods

All RAs are trained using a manual developed by study staff to promote fidelity across sites. The manual instructs in use of REDCap™, recruitment and telephone scripts, eligibility criteria, surveys, study instruments, measurement procedures, and general study office organization. A co-investigator with expertise in biomarker collection developed the sections regarding the collection of BP, anthropometric measurements, and fingerstick blood sample collection with the CardioChek® device and the DBS. Each RA was certified in two phases: (1) after completion of a 2-day training course which included observation; and (2) after successful observation of a collection at the study site. Anthropometric measurements, BP measurements and blood sample collections are periodically reviewed by this co-investigator with biomarker collection expertise to ensure consistency and fidelity, via reports of collected data and in-person observations.

For each measure, we assessed the appropriateness for our patient population, including considerations such as literacy and cultural appropriateness. We used the National Institutes of Neurological Disorders and Stroke (NINDS) Common Data Elements (CDE) if they were available and appropriate [45]. If survey instruments were not CDEs, we tested them with a pilot group of 24 volunteer participants who fit the study's eligibility criteria. This group provided feedback on the clarity of the questions, evaluation duration, fingerstick DBS and CardioChek®, anthropometric measurements, and survey questions. We performed cognitive testing of the survey measures. We made revisions to the overall instrument for clarity, order, and length. An additional 10 participants provided feedback for the Korean and Chinese surveys.

Participant retention

We use multiple strategies to promote participant retention and follow-up for the 3-, 8-, and 12-month evaluations. First, we arrange appointments according to the participants' availability, and include the possibility of evening and weekend visits. Additionally, we attempt to schedule evaluations around participants' usual care appointments at the healthcare facility. Participants are given the option to have data collected at other study sites, if more convenient. We offer to pay for transportation for those without access to transportation. For individuals unable to return to the healthcare facilities, we offer telephone interviews and data collection at a home visit. Participants receive cash payment at completion of each of the evaluation time points ranging from \$10 to \$40.

Data management

Each of the five sites maintains a linking file that includes identifying information (name, address, phone number) and the subject ID. These files are for the purpose of subject tracking, and subject payment tracking. These files are password-protected on a designated computer in a locked office and only the site's Principal Investigator and research staff have access to the tracking file. Electronic files are kept until the completion of all data collection and the successful creation of the final analytic dataset.

Once data are entered into REDCap™, these data are only retrievable by the Data Management team at UCLA. The Data Management team analyzes these data, which are stored on a UCLA server. No direct identifiers (only study IDs) are kept with these data.

Statistical methods

We will compare baseline characteristics between the SUCCEED intervention and usual care groups. We will compare continuous variable means using the *t*-test and ordinal or non-Gaussian continuous variables using the Wilcoxon rank sum test. We will compare unordered categorical variables using Chi-square test or Fisher's exact test.

Enrollment weights based on a logistic regression model will be calculated using demographic data collected from eligible non-participants. If needed, attrition weights will be determined from logistic regression models using demographic data on participants who drop out of the study. We will combine these two weights to form an overall weight (using the inverse of the product of the probabilities of participation). Both raw and adjusted rates using the overall weight will be compared between SUCCEED and usual care arms.

We will conduct intention-to-treat analyses on all directly measured primary and secondary clinical outcomes using ordinal logistic or multiple linear regression models, incorporating the overall weights. Intervention status will be an independent variable in all models. We will compare study outcomes between the control and intervention groups before and after adjusting for potential covariates associated with the outcome measure.

We will use modified Monte Carlo simulation methods to model outcomes related to cost, cost effectiveness, and global risk reduction

There may be underlying intra-site correlations of outcome measures in the collected data, which will potentially impact statistical significance tests of parameter estimates in the analyses. To account for this in our analyses and modeling, robust standard errors will be calculated using Huber-White Sandwich method. Although we will assess for the impact of clustering data structure, we do not expect a large intra-site correlation because four of the five sites are part of the same county healthcare system and we are not aware of differences of outcomes by site. Furthermore, we will include independent dummy variables for each study site to evaluate possible site-level variation in treatment effects.

We will use statistical tests (such as the Shapiro-Wilk test) and graphical analyses (e.g., histograms and box plots) to assess normality of the measures. Based on the nature of distributions, either parametric (e.g., *t*-test and ANOVA for means) or nonparametric tests (Kruskal-Wallis test for medians) will be used. The approaches will include univariate, bivariate, and multivariate modeling.

We will test moderator and mediator effects separately. To assess the moderating effects, we will compare regression models including interaction terms between the independent variables and each possible moderator, and the models that do not include the corresponding interaction terms, using the likelihood ratio test.

We will use the Sobel test [46] and bootstrapping to test mediating effects. We will use the Sobel test to generate a t statistic, which compares the magnitude of the indirect effect to the standard error of measurement. We will compare the t statistic to the normal distribution to determine its significance. Bootstrapping [47] methods will be used to generate a sampling distribution to assess indirect effects of mediators. Baron and Kenny [48] methods will be used to assess the mediating effects through a series of manual regressions. We will use macros from SPSS and SAS that provide output simultaneously for the 3 methods [47, 49, 50]. We will use structural equation modeling to accommodate mediating or moderating effects at the same time.

To check the fidelity (uptake) of the SUCCEED intervention, we will also analyze attendance at SUCCEED clinics, home visits, and the number of telephone coordination of care calls made during enrollment. To evaluate the implementation of the SUCCEED intervention, observations and interviews will be conducted with the intervention staff. Observations of the first APC clinic visit and CHW home visits will clarify the procedures that occur at each clinical study site. Interviews with APC, CHW, and site PIs will further elucidate the intervention processes; barriers and challenges to implementing the intervention; and key intervention components. The observations and interviews will be compared across study sites and between staff to determine the optimal processes for implementation of the intervention.

SUCCEED is a multi-component intervention. It is infeasible to randomize all permutations of these components; thus, our approach to acquiring knowledge of contributions of these different components is to assess, using both qualitative and quantitative methods: (1) extent of implementation of different intervention components, (2) associations of intensity of use or uptake of different intervention components with mediators and with risk factor control outcomes among intervention participants, and (3) perceptions of staff (via interviews with SUCCEED care managers and CHWs) to identify themes about intervention components judged key to effectiveness. Variables will include, for example, number and type of interactions between patients and different care team providers, interactions among care team members, distributions of patient participation in self-management groups, and so forth.

Cost analysis

To estimate intervention costs, we will take into account equipment costs (e.g. tablets, home BP monitors) and staff time (ACP, CHW, physician, mobile health programmers), including time for intervention development and time spent in training the various providers. We will collect data on intervention costs through interviews and reviews of expense reports for the project. In our analysis of intervention costs, we will distinguish between start-up costs of implementing the new care model, the fixed annual maintenance costs of sustaining the model, and the marginal cost of adding another patient to the model.

We will calculate health care utilization costs from the perspective of LAC-DHS and from a more general perspective applicable nationwide. For the LAC-DHS analysis, we will query the county administrative database to determine the total number of hospitalization days (bed-days), Intensive Care Unit days, Emergency Department visits, outpatient primary care visits, outpatient subspecialty visits related to stroke prevention, stroke prevention-related prescription medications, and laboratory and imaging tests related to stroke prevention. We will obtain the cost equivalents of each of these services from LAC-DHS. For the national analysis, we will obtain unit costs for each health care service from reimbursement rates provided in Medicare fee schedules.

There are several limitations to administrative database utilization data in LAC-DHS. First, Los Angeles County is geographically large; therefore, participants may seek care from non-LAC-DHS facilities. Second, participants without insurance may not qualify for non-emergency insurance coverage; therefore, they may not receive care within LAC-DHS. Third, prior to 2014, LAC-DHS did not have a single medical record number for each individual and the utilization data was incomplete. Since 2014, however, LAC-DHS has developed robust electronic databases to track utilization, and as of March 2015, all facilities are on a single electronic medical record (Cerner) and each individual has a single patient identifier across the system. To address these limitations, we will use survey methods to obtain participants' healthcare utilization at baseline, 3, 8, 12 months. We have successfully used surveys for tracking healthcare utilization in previous projects [51, 52]. Although surveys are subject to recall bias, randomization will balance this bias across intervention and control groups.

Another important reason for collecting survey data is to obtain information regarding time spent by family members and friends providing informal assistance to the participant. This is particularly important for individuals with stroke, where much of the long-term cost associated with stroke may be related to informal caregiving [53]. The time of informal caregivers will be valued using national average wage rates in the appropriate age-sex cells as recommended by the Panel on Cost-Effectiveness in Health and Medicine [54].

Once we obtain cost data from administrative and survey sources, we will compare total costs for the intervention group (intervention costs plus health services utilization costs) with costs for the control group. If the intervention improves health and saves costs when compared to the control group, the cost analysis will terminate at this point. If the SUCCEED intervention improves health but the costs of the intervention are higher than in the control group, we will conduct a cost-effectiveness analysis. Our primary estimate of within-trial intervention effectiveness, the reduction in SBP, will be derived directly from SUCCEED. This will allow us to compute the cost of the intervention per mm Hg reduction in SBP, an approach used previously [55], which can also be calculated as the cost per clinically meaningful reduction in BP. This method requires minimal assumptions or modeling, since it uses data collected from participants in the trial. Estimating cost-effectiveness based on within-trial data on BP lowering is limited by two factors – 1) inability to compare the cost-effectiveness of this intervention with other interventions not focused on BP and 2) not accounting for long-term costs and benefits beyond the trial. To improve comparability of SUCCEED with other interventions, we will measure effectiveness using quality adjusted life years (QALYs), [54] combining information on health related quality of life (HRQOL) and mortality. To calculate the HRQOL of the intervention and control patients, we will survey participants using the SF-6D [56]. We will obtain vital status of individuals throughout the study for mortality calculations.

In order to demonstrate the clinical relevance of the reduction of multiple stroke risk factors we will estimate the combined impact of SUCCEED on cardiovascular risk at 3 years. As noted above, the "global risk reduction" outcome estimates the relative reduction in risk for recurrent stroke, and for fatal and nonfatal cardiovascular disease (stroke or myocardial infarction) at 12 months. We will modify the relative global risk reduction calculation to estimate risk for stroke and CVD at 36 months, using an alternative ratio of stroke: CVD in order to account for the rapid decline in risk of recurrent stroke relative to risk of myocardial infarction following a stroke event [57]. Two sources of uncertainty affect the precision of our estimate of the reduction in risk of fatal and nonfatal stroke and CVD. We will use bootstrapping techniques to account for uncertainty in our data (observed changed in risk factors); and we will use Monte Carlo simulation methods to account for uncertainty in the effectiveness of each component intervention. Additional details on the bootstrapping-simulation methods will be available in a subsequent global risk reduction manuscript.

Methods: monitoring

Data monitoring

For Care Management studies such as SUCCEED, a Data Safety Monitoring Board is not usually required. The APCs and CHWs monitor vascular risk factor control and resource utilization of subjects randomized to the intervention. Through telephone calls, clinic visits, home visits, and CDSMP workshops, they ask subjects about the steps they are taking to lower the risk of stroke.

Harms

Adverse experiences are reported as required by the IRB at each site. There are no additional US Food and Drug Administration regulations because we are not studying a biological agent. The Manual of Operations includes detailed definitions of adverse experiences, a table for grading their severity, and details of how clinical sites are to report them.

Auditing

A co-investigator with expertise in biomarker collection periodically conducts site visits for quality assurance regarding biomarker collection by the RAs and reviews data on protocol fidelity periodically downloaded by the study programmer from REDcap™. Additionally, the Project Manager reviews the data entered by the RAs and locks the forms monthly.

Sensitivity analyses

Moderator analyses described above provide estimates of possible effect modification among pre-specified subgroups in Table 1. Exploring possible variation in outcomes among sociodemographic subgroups facilitates equity analyses to determine whether the intervention preferentially benefits socially disadvantaged individuals. Additional sensitivity analyses will be performed to examine how various assumptions related to the efficacy and cost of individual components impact simulated estimates of the overall impact of the intervention on clinical global risk reduction and cost-effectiveness.

Discussion

The optimal BP goal after stroke remains unclear in the absence of RCTs designed to answer the question. The goal, therefore, may change as new RCT findings become available. Nevertheless, the SUCCEED intervention is designed to address all major cardiovascular risk factors, in addition to BP. Although a composite cardiovascular risk score would have been a reasonable alternative to BP as a primary outcome, existing composite scores were derived from populations free of stroke. We have developed and will use this trial to test a composite tool for assessing relative risk of recurrent stroke [58]. Second, since this is a pragmatic trial, the clinical settings vary between sites and we have allowed for heterogeneity; however, we have strategies in place to heighten fidelity in the core aspects of the intervention. In addition, there may be site-specific differences in usual care and temporal changes in usual care. By testing this intervention in real world settings, we will maximize external validity. Third, it will be difficult to assess which components of the intervention explain the effectiveness (or lack thereof); however, we will employ post-hoc subgroup analyses and assess the effects of mediators and moderators. Fourth, contamination of the usual care arm is possible. However, the only providers who potentially care for participants in both arms of the trial are the site PIs; they do not share intervention tools or educational materials with participants. The APCs and CHWs do not interact with usual care participants.

Individuals with stroke or TIA are often high-cost, high-needs patients; therefore, if this coordinated care management intervention is effective, it can have far-reaching consequences. By using an interdisciplinary team, we have drawn upon various skillsets in a cost-effective manner, and anticipate improving the quality and effectiveness of care. In addition, we anticipate improving efficiency and care quality by using evidence-based protocols embedded into a mobile electronic platform that offers real-time decision support, an avenue for communication, and a tool for panel management. By including community representatives and stroke survivors in the development of the intervention, and employing CHWs from the communities that are served, we have culturally tailored the intervention and are better equipped to address potential barriers, understand participants' needs, and provide patient-centered care.

Although this intervention is designed to address disparities in care and outcomes in vulnerable, socioeconomically disadvantaged populations, it may be applicable to a variety of healthcare settings. Furthermore, since individuals with stroke and TIA have multiple cardiovascular comorbidities, many of the tools we developed may be applicable to a large proportion of high-cost, high-needs patients at high risk for CVD. Finally, the care management model developed in this trial is applicable to most chronic conditions.

Once the RCT is completed, the materials and products will be available to the research, clinical and public health communities. Dimagi's software is open source.

Progress to date

We have enrolled 357 of the 516 participants (Table 3). The mean age is 57.2 years (SD 8.7). The majority are men (64.5%). With respect to race, 66.2% are White, 17.7% Black, 7.3% Asian, 2.5% Native American or Alaskan Native, and 3.7% >1 race. The majority (70.9%) are Hispanic. Most participants are born outside of the United States (72.7%) and 61.9% have less than a high school education. Approximately half (52.5%) were working prior to the stroke. The majority of events were ischemic strokes or TIAs (83.2%) and the remainder were intracerebral hemorrhages. The mean systolic BP at baseline was 145.5 mmHg. Three quarters of the population was either overweight or obese. Most had mild to moderate strokes (NIH SS <15). Nearly half of the participants had moderately severe or severe disability at enrollment. Nearly half the participants had a history of smoking; 24.1% smoked in the year prior to the stroke. With respect to medical comorbidities, 23% had a prior history of stroke, 51.7% had dyslipidemia and 48.3% had diabetes by self report.

Table 3 Sociodemographic and clinical characteristics of participants enrolled to date

	Eligible enrolled ($N = 357$)
Sociodemographic Characteristics	
Age, years, mean (SD)	57.2 (8.7)
Male, *n* (%)	229 (64.5)
Race, *n* (%)	
White	235 (66.2)
Black	63 (17.7)
Asian	26 (7.3)
American Indian/Alaskan Native	9 (2.5)
Native Hawaiian/Other Pacific Islander	3 (0.8)
More than one race	13 (3.7)
Unknown	6 (1.7)
Ethnicity: Hispanic, *n* (%)	251 (70.9)
Born in the United States, *n* (%)	97 (27.3)
Living with at least one other adult, *n* (%)	314 (88.5)
Education, *n* (%)	
Some college	107 (30.4)
Associate degree: academic, occupational, technical or vocational program	1 (0.3)
At least high school graduate or equivalent	26 (7.4)
Some high school	81 (23.0)
8th grade or less	137 (38.9)
Working for pay, part- or full-time, prior to stroke, *n* (%)	189 (53.5)
Clinical Characteristics	
Stroke Type, *n* (%)	
Ischemic / TIA	297 (83.2)
Intracerebal hemorrhage	60 (16.8)
Systolic blood pressure, mm Hg, mean (SD)	145.4 (18.4)
BMI category, *n* (%)	
Underweight (<18 kg/m^2)	1 (0.7)
Normal (18–24.9 kg/m^2)	37 (24.7)
Overweight (25–29.9 kg/m^2)	61 (40.7)
Obese (≥30 kg/m^2)	51 (34.0)
NIH stroke score, *n* (%)	
Mild (1–5)	225 (63.4)
Moderate (6–14)	121 (34.1)
Severe (15–24)	9 (2.5)
Very severe (≥25)	0
Modified Rankin Scale, *n* (%)	
No disability	25 (7.0)
No significant disability	60 (16.9)
Slight disability	60 (16.9)
Moderate disability	53 (14.9)
Moderately severe disability	112 (31.5)
Severe disability	45 (12.7)
History of smoking, *n* (%)	160 (45.3)
Smoked in the year prior to the stroke, *n* (%)	85 (24.1)
Medical History, *n* (%)	
Prior stroke	80 (23.0)
Heart attack	32 (9.0)
Atrial fibrillation	25 (7.1)
Congestive heart failure	26 (7.4)
Dyslipidemia	182 (51.7)
Cancer	14 (4.0)
Diabetes	171 (48.3)

Abbreviations

APC: Advanced Practice Clinician; BMI: Body mass index; BP: Blood pressure; CCM: Chronic care model; CDE: Common data elements; CDMP: Chronic Disease Self-Management Program; CHW: Community Health Worker; CRP: C reactive protein; DBS: Dried blood spot; HbA1c: Hemoglobin A1c; HCWDP: Healthcare Workforce Development Program; HDL: High density lipoprotein; HIPAA: Health Insurance Portability and Accountability Act; ICC: Intraclass correlation; IRB: Institutional Review Board; LAC-DHS: Los Angeles County Department of Health Services; LDL: Low density lipoprotein; LRT: Likelihood ratio test; NINDS: National Institute of Neurological Disorders and Stroke; NP: Nurse Practitioner; PA: Physician Assistant; PHQ: Patient health questionnaire; RA: Research Assistant; RCT: Randomized controlled trial; REDCap™: Research electronic data capture; SAS: Statistical analysis system; SBP: Systolic blood pressure; SPSS: Statistical Package for the Social Sciences; SUCCEED: Secondary stroke prevention by Uniting Community and Chronic care model teams Early to End Disparities; SUSTAIN: Systemic Use of STroke Averting INterventions; TIA: Transient ischemic attack; WERC: Worker Education and Resource Center; WLCAC: Watts Labor Community Action Committee

Acknowledgments

Dorothy Harris, MD, PhD for assistance with development of the goal cards. Lilian Moreno, Diamond Garcia, BA, Maura Fernandez, MD, Bianca Alcatar, MBA, Cynthia Munoz Ayala, BA, and Marlene Keymolen-Ramirez, BS for recruitment and data collection. Tom Bailey, MA, Michael Chachere, BS, and Tim Wager, PhD for CHW curriculum development and training. Regine Goh and Joanne Lee for translation of selected outcome measures. Betty Shaby, DNP, MSN, ANP-c and Samantha Theaker, RN, MSN, CNRN for care management activities. Marissa Castro and Paty Gomez for CHW activities. Sarah Song, MD, Catherine Sarkisian, MD, Joseph Kim, MD, Hui Gong, MD, Peggy Nguyen, MD, and Pei Liu, MD for assistance with culturally tailoring intervention for Korean, Mandarin, and Cantonese speakers.

Funding

This study was supported by the National Institute of Neurological Disorders and Stroke U54NS081764 and the California Community Foundation BAPP-15-118096.

Authors' contributions

AT co-led development of the study design and implementation, drafted the manuscript, has full access to the data, and takes responsibility for the integrity and accuracy of the analysis. EMC participated in the design of the study and development of the analysis plan. MAR oversees RA training, project implementation, and project coordination. HM designed the protocol for obtaining, storing and analyzing all indicated biomarkers and trained the RAs to collect measures. NS is the site principal investigator at LAC-USC Medical Center and approved final advanced practice clinician protocols. TD is the site principal investigator at Rancho Los Amigos and approved final advanced practice clinician protocols. RB is the site principal investigator at Olive View Medical Center and approved final advanced practice clinician protocols. NR assisted with recruitment at Olive View Medical Center. BMehta is the site principal investigator at Harbor-UCLA Medical Center and approved final advanced practice clinician protocols. SS is the site principal investigator at Cedars Sinai Medical Center. AR was the site principal investigator at Rancho Los Amigos and approved final advanced practice clinician protocols. MR contributed to designing the mobile application and completed a formative evaluation of technology implementation. TST, the lead APC, contributed to developing care management protocols for the mobile care management application, CHW curriculum development and training, and development of a tool to assess "needs" status. JT is an APC and contributed to developing the protocols. EMH is a CHW and assisted in culturally tailoring the intervention. AM is a CHW and assisted in culturally tailoring the intervention. MC is a CHW and assisted in culturally tailoring the intervention. BMartinez participated in reviewing outcome measures and participated in participant recruitment and data collection. PW helped recruit CHWs and trained them to lead Chronic Disease Self-Management workshops. MM assisted in developing the CHW curriculum. NI helped recruit CHWs. SW contributed to designing the mobile application. JW contributed to designing and programming the mobile application and training the staff to use the CommCare software. AR developed a composite tool for risk stratification after stroke. FB creates data reports for study monitoring. VH conducted a formative evaluation of SUCCEED implementation. HH contributed to designing and programming the mobile application and training the staff to use the CommCare software. BMittman assisted in developing the formative evaluation of trial implementation. WC contributed to identifying outcome measures. HL provided statistical expertise. DG contributed to the design of the cost-effectiveness analysis of the intervention. DF assisted in developing the CHW curriculum. BGV co-led development of the study design and implementation, made key edits to the manuscript, has full access to the data, and takes responsibility for the integrity and accuracy of the analysis. All authors read and contributed to the preparation of the manuscript. All authors read and approved the final manuscript.

Competing interests
The authors declare that they have no competing interests.

Ethics approval and consent to participate
Research Ethics Approval: IRB approval was obtained from all study sites as well as UCLA.
Protocol Amendments: All protocol amendments undergo IRB review and approval at UCLA, Rancho Los Amigos, USC, and Olive View Medical Center. The UCLA IRB has reliance mechanisms with Mount Sinai, LA Biomed and Cedars-Sinai.
Consent: Informed consent is obtained from all participants in the primary language.
Dissemination Policy: The scientific integrity of the project requires that the data from all SUCCEED sites be analyzed study-wide and reported as such. Thus, the individual centers are not expected to report data collected from their sites alone. All presentations and publications will be expected to protect the integrity of the major objectives of the study. Every attempt will be made to reduce to an absolute minimum the interval between the completion of data collection and release of study results. The study results will be released to study participants and the general medical community.
Authorship: Topics suggested for presentation or publication will be circulated to the PIs. The PIs will suggest and justify names for authorship. Individuals who fulfill authorship criteria will not remain hidden and will have final authority over manuscript content.

Confidentiality
All study staff received training on Human Subjects Research and Information Privacy and Security through the Collaborative Institutional Training Institute and maintain certification per institutional guidelines. CommCare Mobile and CommCare HQ are Health Insurance Portability and Accountability Act (HIPAA) compliant.

Author details
[1]Los Angeles County Department of Health Services, Los Angeles, California, USA. [2]University of Southern California, Los Angeles, California, USA. [3]Rancho Los Amigos National Rehabilitation Center, Downey, California, USA. [4]University of California, Los Angeles (UCLA), Los Angeles, California, USA. [5]Los Angeles County-University of Southern California (USC) Medical Center, Los Angeles, California, USA. [6]Kaiser Permanente, Sacramento, California, USA. [7]Harbor-UCLA Medical Center, Torrance, California, USA. [8]Olive View-UCLA Medical Center, Sylmar, California, USA. [9]Cedars Sinai Medical Center, Los Angeles, California, USA. [10]Kaiser Permanente, Irvine, California, USA. [11]Fielding School of Public Health, Department of Health Policy and Management, University of California, Los Angeles, Los Angeles, California, USA. [12]Watts Labor Community Action Committee, Watts, California, USA. [13]Worker Education and Resource Center, Los Angeles, California, USA. [14]Esperanza Community Housing, Los Angeles, California, USA. [15]School of Social Work, Edward R. Roybal Institute on Aging, and Daniel J. Epstein Department of Industrial and Systems Engineering, University of Southern California, Los Angeles, California, USA. [16]RAND Corporation, Santa Monica, California, USA. [17]Dimagi, Inc., Cambridge, Massachusetts, USA. [18]Department of Veterans Affairs Greater Los Angeles Healthcare System, Los Angeles, California, USA. [19]Icahn School of Medicine at Mount Sinai, New York, New York, USA.

References
1. Bodenheimer T, Berry-Millett R. Follow the money—controlling expenditures by improving care for patients needing costly services. N Engl J Med. 2009;361(16):1521–3.
2. Bodenheimer TS, Smith MD. Primary care: proposed solutions to the physician shortage without training more physicians. Health Aff (Millwood). 2013;32(11):1881–6.
3. Reuben DB. Physicians in supporting roles in chronic disease care: the CareMore model. J Am Geriatr Soc. 2011;59(1):158–60.
4. Milstein A, Gilbertson E. American medical home runs. Health Aff (Millwood). 2009;28(5):1317–26.
5. Bell JF, Krupski A, Joesch JM, West II, Atkins DC, Court B, Mancuso D, Roy-Byrne P. A randomized controlled trial of intensive care management for disabled Medicaid beneficiaries with high health care costs. Health Serv Res. 2015;50(3):663–89.
6. Mozaffarian D, Benjamin EJ, Go AS, Arnett DK, Blaha MJ, Cushman M, Das SR, de Ferranti S, Despres JP, Fullerton HJ, et al. Heart disease and stroke statistics-2016 update: a report from the American heart association. Circulation. 2016;133(4):e38–e360.
7. Egan BM, Zhao Y, Axon RN. US trends in prevalence, awareness, treatment, and control of hypertension, 1988–2008. JAMA. 2010;303(20):2043–50.
8. Furie KL, Kasner SE, Adams RJ, Albers GW, Bush RL, Fagan SC, Halperin JL, Johnston SC, Katzan I, Kernan WN, et al. Guidelines for the prevention of stroke in patients with stroke or transient ischemic attack: a guideline for healthcare professionals from the American heart association/American stroke association. Stroke. 2011;42(1):227–76.
9. O'Donnell MJ, Xavier D, Liu L, Zhang H, Chin SL, Rao-Melacini P, Rangarajan S, Islam S, Pais P, Mcqueen MJ, et al. Risk factors for ischaemic and intracerebral haemorrhagic stroke in 22 countries (the INTERSTROKE study): a case-control study. Lancet. 2010;376(9735):112–23.
10. Whitworth JA. 2003 World Health Organization (WHO)/International Society of Hypertension (ISH) statement on management of hypertension. J Hypertens. 2003;21(11):1983–92.
11. Cheng EM, Jolly D, Jones LA, Cohen SN. Modest improvement in risk factor control after admission for a stroke or transient ischemic attack. J Stroke Cerebrovasc Dis. 2005;14(4):174–8.
12. Razmara A, Ovbiagele B, Markovic D, Towfighi A. Patterns and predictors of blood pressure treatment, control, and outcomes among stroke survivors in the United States. J Stroke Cerebrovasc Dis. 2016;25(4):857–65.
13. Lin MP, Ovbiagele B, Markovic D, Towfighi A: "Life's simple 7" and long-term mortality after stroke. *J Am Heart Assoc* 2015, 4 (11).

14. McManus M, Ovbiagele B, Markovic D, Towfighi A. Association of Insurance Status with Stroke-Related Mortality and Long-term Survival after Stroke. J Stroke Cerebrovasc Dis. 2015;24(8):1924–30.
15. Cruz-Flores S, Rabinstein A, Biller J, Elkind MS, Griffith P, Gorelick PB, Howard G, Leira EC, Morgenstern LB, Ovbiagele B, et al. Racial-ethnic disparities in stroke care: the American experience: a statement for healthcare professionals from the American Heart Association/American Stroke Association. Stroke. 2011;42(7):2091–116.
16. Bodenheimer T, Wagner EH, Grumbach K. Improving primary care for patients with chronic illness. JAMA. 2002;288(14):1775–9.
17. Bodenheimer T, Wagner EH, Grumbach K. Improving primary care for patients with chronic illness: the chronic care model, Part 2. JAMA. 2002;288(15):1909–14.
18. Cheng EM, Cunningham WE, Towfighi A, Sanossian N, Bryg RJ, Anderson TL, Guterman JJ, Gross-Schulman SG, Beanes S, Jones AS, et al. Randomized, controlled trial of an intervention to enable stroke survivors throughout the Los Angeles County safety net to "stay with the guidelines". Circ Cardiovasc Qual Outcomes. 2011;4(2):229–34.
19. Brownstein JN, Chowdhury FM, Norris SL, Horsley T, Jack Jr L, Zhang X, Satterfield D. Effectiveness of community health workers in the care of people with hypertension. Am J Prev Med. 2007;32(5):435–47.
20. Gary TL, Batts-Turner M, Yeh HC, Hill-Briggs F, Bone LR, Wang NY, Levine DM, Powe NR, Saudek CD, Hill MN, et al. The effects of a nurse case manager and a community health worker team on diabetic control, emergency department visits, and hospitalizations among urban African Americans with type 2 diabetes mellitus: a randomized controlled trial. Arch Intern Med. 2009;169(19):1788–94.
21. Allen JK, Dennison-Himmelfarb CR, Szanton SL, Bone L, Hill MN, Levine DM, West M, Barlow A, Lewis-Boyer L, Donnelly-Strozzo M, et al. Community Outreach and Cardiovascular Health (COACH) Trial: a randomized, controlled trial of nurse practitioner/community health worker cardiovascular disease risk reduction in urban community health centers. Circ Cardiovasc Qual Outcomes. 2011;4(6):595–602.
22. Hill MN, Han HR, Dennison CR, Kim MT, Roary MC, Blumenthal RS, Bone LR, Levine DM, Post WS. Hypertension care and control in underserved urban African American men: behavioral and physiologic outcomes at 36 months. Am J Hypertens. 2003;16(11 Pt 1):906–13.
23. Fedder DO, Chang RJ, Curry S, Nichols G. The effectiveness of a community health worker outreach program on healthcare utilization of west Baltimore City Medicaid patients with diabetes, with or without hypertension. Ethn Dis. 2003;13(1):22–7.
24. Babamoto KS, Sey KA, Camilleri AJ, Karlan VJ, Catalasan J, Morisky DE. Improving diabetes care and health measures among hispanics using community health workers: results from a randomized controlled trial. Health Educ Behav. 2009;36(1):113–26.
25. Dennison CR, Post WS, Kim MT, Bone LR, Cohen D, Blumenthal RS, Rame JE, Roary MC, Levine DM, Hill MN. Underserved urban african american men: hypertension trial outcomes and mortality during 5 years. Am J Hypertens. 2007;20(2):164–71.
26. Philis-Tsimikas A, Fortmann A, Lleva-Ocana L, Walker C, Gallo LC. Peer-led diabetes education programs in high-risk Mexican Americans improve glycemic control compared with standard approaches: a Project Dulce promotora randomized trial. Diabetes Care. 2011;34(9):1926–31.
27. Norris SL, Chowdhury FM, Van Le K, Horsley T, Brownstein JN, Zhang X, Jack Jr L, Satterfield DW. Effectiveness of community health workers in the care of persons with diabetes. Diabet Med. 2006;23(5):544–56.
28. Dromerick AW, Gibbons MC, Edwards DF, Farr DE, Giannetti ML, Sanchez B, Shara NM, Fokar A, Jayam-Trouth A, Ovbiagele B, et al. Preventing recurrence of thromboembolic events through coordinated treatment in the district of Columbia. Int J Stroke. 2011;6(5):454–60.
29. Egan M, Anderson S, Mctaggart J. Community navigation for stroke survivors and their care partners: description and evaluation. Top Stroke Rehabil. 2010;17(3):183–90.
30. Towfighi A, Gallup M, Tai W, Guevara E, Ovbiagele B. Differences in index ischemic stroke characteristics in a multiethnic medically underserved population. International Stroke Conference, San Antonio; 2010.
31. Ramirez M, Wu S, Towfighi A, Wacksman J, Sivers-Teixeira T, Haber H, Vickrey BG. International Symposium on Human Factors and Ergonomics in Health Care. Using mobile health tools to support team-based approaches for chronic disease care. San Diego; 2016.
32. Rashid P, Leonardi-Bee J, Bath P. Blood pressure reduction and secondary prevention of stroke and other vascular events: a systematic review. Stroke. 2003;34(11):2741–8.
33. Turnbull F, Blood Pressure Lowering Treatment Trialists C. Effects of different blood-pressure-lowering regimens on major cardiovascular events: results of prospectively-designed overviews of randomised trials. Lancet. 2003;362(9395):1527–35.
34. Lawes CM, Bennett DA, Feigin VL, Rodgers A. Blood pressure and stroke: an overview of published reviews. Stroke. 2004;35(4):1024.
35. Dorresteijn JA, van der Graaf Y, Spiering W, Grobbee DE, Bots ML, Visseren FL, Secondary Manifestations of Arterial Disease Study G. Relation between blood pressure and vascular events and mortality in patients with manifest vascular disease: J-curve revisited. Hypertension. 2012;59(1):14–21.
36. Cooper-Dehoff RM, Gong Y, Handberg EM, Bavry AA, Denardo SJ, Bakris GL, Pepine CJ. Tight blood pressure control and cardiovascular outcomes among hypertensive patients with diabetes and coronary artery disease. JAMA. 2010;304(1):61–8.
37. Accord Study Group, Cushman WC, Evans GW, Byington RP, Goff Jr DC, Grimm Jr RH, Cutler JA, Simons-Morton DG, Basile JN, Corson MA, et al. Effects of intensive blood-pressure control in type 2 diabetes mellitus. N Engl J Med. 2010;362(17):1575–85.
38. Vamos EP, Harris M, Millett C, Pape UJ, Khunti K, Curcin V, Molokhia M, Majeed A. Association of systolic and diastolic blood pressure and all cause mortality in people with newly diagnosed type 2 diabetes: retrospective cohort study. BMJ. 2012;345:e5567.
39. Boan AD, Lackland DT, Ovbiagele B. Lowering of blood pressure for recurrent stroke prevention. Stroke. 2014;45(8):2506–13.
40. Ovbiagele B. Low-normal systolic blood pressure and secondary stroke risk. J Stroke Cerebrovasc Dis. 2013;22(5):633–8.
41. Ovbiagele B, Diener HC, Yusuf S, Martin RH, Cotton D, Vinisko R, Donnan GA, Bath PM, Investigators P. Level of systolic blood pressure within the normal range and risk of recurrent stroke. JAMA. 2011; 306(19):2137–44.
42. Lin MP, Ovbiagele B, Markovic D, Towfighi A. Systolic blood pressure and mortality after stroke: too low, no go? Stroke. 2015;46(5):1307–13.
43. Aiken LS, West SG. Multiple regression: testing and interpreting interactions. Newbury Park: Sage Publications; 1991.
44. TransPerfect Translations International. 3 Park Avenue, 39th Floor New York, New York 10016.
45. Grinnon ST, Miller K, Marler JR, Lu Y, Stout A, Odenkirchen J, Kunitz S. National Institute of Neurological Disorders and Stroke Common Data Element Project—approach and methods. Clin Trials. 2012;9(3): 322–9.
46. Sobel Mel S. Asymptotic confidence intervals for indirect effects in structural equation models. Sociol Methodol. 1982;13:290–312.
47. Shrout PE, Bolger N. Mediation in experimental and nonexperimental studies: new procedures and recommendations. Psychol Methods. 2002;7(4):422–45.
48. Baron RM, Kenny DA. The moderator-mediator variable distinction in social psychological research: conceptual, strategic, and statistical considerations. J Pers Soc Psychol. 1986;51(6):1173–82.
49. Paffenbarger Jr RS, Wing AL, Hyde RT. Physical activity as an index of heart attack risk in college alumni. 1978. Am J Epidemiol. 1995;142(9):889–903. discussion 887–888.
50. Preacher KJ, Hayes AF. Asymptotic and resampling strategies for assessing and comparing indirect effects in multiple mediator models. Behav Res Methods. 2008;40(3):879–91.
51. Mangione CM, Brown A, Sarkisian C, Brusuelas RJ, Norris K, Steers N, Davison M, Ettner S, Ganz D, Funnell MM, et al. Randomized community-based intervention to improve self-management of diabetes among older African Americans and Latinos. J Gen Intern Med. 2007;22:158.
52. Duru OK, Ettner SL, Vassar SD, Chodosh J, Vickrey BG. Cost evaluation of a coordinated care management intervention for dementia. Am J Manag Care. 2009;15(8):521–8.

53. Hickenbottom SL, Fendrick AM, Kutcher JS, Kabeto MU, Katz SJ, Langa KM. A national study of the quantity and cost of informal caregiving for the elderly with stroke. Neurology. 2002;58(12):1754–9.
54. Gold MR. Cost-effectiveness in health and medicine. New York: Oxford University Press; 1996.
55. Logan AG, Milne BJ, Achber C, Campbell WP, Haynes RB. Cost-effectiveness of a worksite hypertension treatment program. Hypertension. 1981;3(2):211–8.
56. Brazier J, Roberts J, Deverill M. The estimation of a preference-based measure of health from the SF-36. J Health Econ. 2002;21(2):271–92.
57. Hankey GJ. Secondary stroke prevention. Lancet Neurol. 2014;13(2):178–94.
58. Richards A, Jackson N, Cheng E, Towfighi A, Bryg R, Brown A, Sanossian N, Barry F, Li N, Vickrey BG. Global risk reduction: a novel method to estimate the impact of multiple intervention trials to reduce stroke disparities. International Stroke Conference, Los Angeles; 2016.
59. Craig CL, Marshall AL, Sjostrom M, Bauman AE, Booth ML, Ainsworth BE, Pratt M, Ekelund U, Yngve A, Sallis JF, et al. International physical activity questionnaire: 12-country reliability and validity. Med Sci Sports Exerc. 2003;35(8):1381–95.
60. UCLA Center for Health Policy Research. California Health Interview Survey 2011-2012 (CHIS 2011-2012).
61. Centers for Disease Control and Prevention. Behavioral risk factor surveillance system survey questionnaire. Atlanta: US Department of Health and Human Services, Centers for Disease Control and Prevention; 2013.
62. Meschia JF, Brott TG, Chukwudelunzu FE, Hardy J, Brown Jr RD, Meissner I, Hall LJ, Atkinson EJ, O'Brien PC. Verifying the stroke-free phenotype by structured telephone interview. Stroke. 2000;31(5):1076–80.
63. Marin G, Gamba RJ. A New measurement of acculturation for hispanics: the bidimensional acculturation scale for Hispanics (BAS). Hisp J Behav Sci. 1996;18(3):297–316.
64. Schneider AT, Pancioli AM, Khoury JC, Rademacher E, Tuchfarber A, Miller R, Woo D, Kissela B, Broderick JP. Trends in community knowledge of the warning signs and risk factors for stroke. JAMA. 2003;289(3):343–6.
65. Haun J, Luther S, Dodd V, Donaldson P. Measurement variation across health literacy assessments: implications for assessment selection in research and practice. J Health Commun. 2012;17 Suppl 3:141–59.
66. Simoni JM, Kurth AE, Pearson CR, Pantalone DW, Merrill JO, Frick PA. Self-report measures of antiretroviral therapy adherence: a review with recommendations for HIV research and clinical management. AIDS Behav. 2006;10(3):227–45.
67. Chesney MA, Ickovics JR, Chambers DB, Gifford AL, Neidig J, Zwickl B, Wu AW. Self-reported adherence to antiretroviral medications among participants in HIV clinical trials: the AACTG adherence instruments. Patient Care Committee & Adherence Working Group of the Outcomes Committee of the Adult AIDS Clinical Trials Group (AACTG). AIDS Care. 2000;12(3):255–66.
68. Lorig KR, Sobel DS, Ritter PL, Laurent D, Hobbs M. Effect of a self-management program on patients with chronic disease. Eff Clin Pract. 2001;4(6):256–62.
69. Luszczynska A, Scholz U, Schwarzer R. The general self-efficacy scale: multicultural validation studies. J Psychol. 2005;139(5):439–57.
70. Powers BJ, Oddone EZ, Grubber JM, Olsen MK, Bosworth HB. Perceived and actual stroke risk among men with hypertension. J Clin Hypertens (Greenwich). 2008;10(4):287–94.
71. Wong ST, Nordstokke D, Gregorich S, Perez-Stable EJ. Measurement of social support across women from four ethnic groups: evidence of factorial invariance. J Cross Cult Gerontol. 2010;25(1):45–58.
72. Radloff L. The CES-D scale: A self report depression scale for research in the general population. Applied Psychological Measurement. 1977;1(3):385–401.
73. Kharroubi SA, Brazier JE, Roberts J, O'Hagan A. Modelling SF-6D health state preference data using a nonparametric Bayesian method. J Health Econ. 2007;26(3):597–612.
74. Glasgow RE, Wagner EH, Schaefer J, Mahoney LD, Reid RJ, Greene SM. Development and validation of the Patient Assessment of Chronic Illness Care (PACIC). Med Care. 2005;43(5):436–44.
75. Harris-Kojetin LD, Fowler Jr FJ, Brown JA, Schnaier JA, Sweeny SF. The use of cognitive testing to develop and evaluate CAHPS 1.0 core survey items. Consumer Assessment of Health Plans Study. Med Care. 1999;37(3 Suppl):MS10–21.

Chronic kidney disease and poor outcomes in ischemic stroke: is impaired cerebral autoregulation the missing link?

Pedro Castro[1*], Elsa Azevedo[1], Isabel Rocha[2], Farzaneh Sorond[3] and Jorge M. Serrador[4,5,6]

Abstract

Background: Chronic kidney disease increases stroke incidence and severity but the mechanisms behind this cerebro-renal interaction are mostly unexplored. Since both vascular beds share similar features, microvascular dysfunction could be the possible missing link. Therefore, we examined the relationship between renal function and cerebral autoregulation in the early hours post ischemia and its impact on outcome.

Methods: We enrolled 46 ischemic strokes (middle cerebral artery). Dynamic cerebral autoregulation was assessed by transfer function (coherence, phase and gain) of spontaneous blood pressure oscillations to blood flow velocity within 6 h from symptom-onset. Estimated glomerular filtration rate (eGFR) was calculated. Hemorrhagic transformation (HT) and white matter lesions (WML) were collected from computed tomography performed at presentation and 24 h. Outcome was evaluated with modified Rankin Scale at 3 months.

Results: High gain (less effective autoregulation) was correlated with lower eGFR irrespective of infarct side ($p < 0.05$). Both lower eGFR and higher gain correlated with WML grade ($p < 0.05$). Lower eGFR and increased gain, alone and in combination, progressively reduced the odds of a good functional outcome [ipsilateral OR = 4.39 (CI95% 3.15–25.6), $p = 0.019$; contralateral OR = 8.15 (CI95% 4.15–15.6), $p = 0.002$] and increased risk of HT [ipsilateral OR = 3.48 (CI95% 0.60–24.0), $p = 0.132$; contralateral OR = 6.43 (CI95% 1.40–32.1), $p = 0.034$].

Conclusions: Lower renal function correlates with less effective dynamic cerebral autoregulation in acute ischemic stroke, both predicting a bad outcome. The evaluation of serum biomarkers of renal dysfunction could have interest in the future for assessing cerebral microvascular risk and relationship with stroke complications.

Keywords: Cardiovascular disease, Chronic kidney disease, Glomerular filtration rate, Stroke; transcranial Doppler

Background

Chronic kidney disease (CKD) increases the risk of ischemic stroke [1, 2], its severity and the chance of poor outcome [3, 4]. The exact mechanisms that govern this cerebro-renal interaction are poorly understood [5]. A possible explanation may involve the similar features of kidney and brain microvascular beds. Both vascular beds are low resistance arterial beds that rely on continuous blood flow that ismaintained at relatively constant levels by a fine-tuned myogenic regulatory system. This confers protection to both the brain and kidney from arterial blood pressure (ABP) fluctuations that could cause large swings in blood flow [6–8]. This property, called autoregulation, has been long known to exist in renal [9] and cerebral [10, 11] vasculatures. Despite differences between organ systems, autoregulation is viewed as a generalized vascular protective mechanism [8] witch failure results in microvessel damage (e.g. from uncontrolled hypertension and diabetes [12–15]). In fact, glomerular sclerosis of chronic kidney failure [16], as well as lacunar infarcts and white matter lesions (WML) in the brain [12, 17], are all characterized by similar pathological conditions: endothelial dysfunction; ischaemic arteriosclerosis; low perfusion and small vessel leakage [12, 17]. Recent evidence shows that kidney impairment is associated with a greater severity of cerebral WML [18].

* Correspondence: pedromacc@gmail.com
[1]Department Neurology, São João Hospital Center, Faculty of Medicine of University of Porto, Alameda Professor Hernani Monteiro, 4200-319 Porto, Portugal
Full list of author information is available at the end of the article

Because microvascular dysfunction impairs myogenic autoregulation, this could be the missing link between renal dysfunction and stroke morbidity and worthwhile of being explored. Dynamic cerebral autoregulation (CA) is rapidly and noninvasively assessed at the patient bedside by transfer function analysis (TFA) using spontaneous oscillations in ABP and cerebral blood flow velocity (CBFV) [14, 19–22] which is known to be impaired in acute ischemic stroke [23].

In this study, we examined the relationship between renal function and CA, assessed from TFA measured within 6 h of symptom-onset and its impact on long-term outcome.

Methods

Population studied

The study was conducted in Hospital Center São João, Porto, and its local ethical committee approved the study and all participants or proxy signed written informed consent. We included consecutive patients with acute ischemic stroke admitted to our stroke unit and with time from symptom onset, or from last seen well, within 6 h. Most patients admitted after 8:00 p.m. or weekends were not enrolled because transcranial Doppler (TCD) monitoring was not available. Exclusion criteria included hemodynamic instability requiring vasoactive agents, other central neurological co-morbidities, acute renal injury [24] or insufficient temporal window. We recruited 46 patients with ischemic stroke in middle cerebral artery (MCA) territory. All participants underwent cervical and transcranial ultrasound studies (Vivid e; GE) before evaluation to exclude hemodynamically significant extra- (> 50% in carotid artery calculated by NASCET method) or intracranial stenosis (≥ 50% by angle-corrected velocimetric criteria). Blood samples were collected at admission. We calculated Estimated glomerular filtration rate (eGFR) using the Chronic Kidney Disease Epidemiology Collaboration formula [25–27]. In the first fasting sample, we obtained total, low-density lipoprotein (LDL) and high-density lipoprotein (HDL) cholesterol, glucose and glycated hemoglobin (HgA1C).

Clinical assessment

All patients underwent a neurological examination at presentation and National Institute of Health Stroke Scale (NIHSS) scores were calculated at baseline. The outcome, assessed by clinical interview, corresponded to mortality and functional independence [modified Rankin Scale (mRS) 0–2] at 90 days.

Monitoring protocol

Evaluations were carried out in the stroke unit with the head of the bed at 0°. ABP was continuously monitored with a finger cuff in the unaffected side using Finometer MIDI (FMS, Amsterdam, Netherlands). Additionally, ABP was assessed with oscillometric cuff (Dash 2500, GE, UK). Heart rate was assessed from lead II of a standard 3-lead electrocardiogram. CBFV was recorded bilaterally from M1 segment of MCA (depth of 50–55 mm) with 2-MHz monitoring probes secured with a headband (Doppler BoxX, DWL, Singen, Germany). End-tidal carbon dioxide was evaluated by nasal cannula attached to Respsense capnograph (Nonin, Amsterdam, The Netherlands). All data was synchronized at 400 Hz with Powerlab (AD Instruments, Oxford, UK) and stored for offline analysis. Data collection occurred for 10 min within 6 h from symptoms-onset.

Cerebral autoregulation data analysis

All signals were inspected using a custom based Matlab® program and artifacts removed by linear interpolation [28]. Systolic, mean and diastolic values of ABP and CBFV were calculated. For each heart-beat estimated cerebrovascular resistance (CVRi) was calculated by mean ABP/CBFV, reflecting vasomotor function [29]. TFA was used to assess dynamic CA by calculating coherence, gain and phase parameters from 10 min of beat-to-beat spontaneous oscillations of CBFV and ABP as previously reported [26, 27, 30, 31]. Coherence, gain and phase are reported for the low-frequency range (LF: 0.03–0.15 Hz), which is the autoregulatory frequency [6, 20, 21, 30], and also at high-frequency (HF: 0.15–0.5 Hz) band. In short, coherence is the coefficient of correlation between the signals; higher coherence between the oscillations is reflective of less effective CA. Gain quantifies the damping effect of CA on the magnitude of ABP oscillations. Phase shift represents the time delay between ABP and CBFV oscillations. Lower gain and higher phase represent tighter, more effective autoregulatory response [20].

Neuroimaging assessment

Computed Tomography brain scan (Siemens Somaton Emotion Duo, Erlangen, Germany), with 3 to 6 mm slices, was performed at presentation and repeated at 24 h. Hemorrhagic transformation was defined as any hemorrhage ranging from petechial hyperdensities to parenchymal hematoma [32]. WML, a correlate of cerebral microvascular disease, [17] were graded by the van Swieten [33] scale based on the first scan, a method validated against MRI in ischemic stroke [34].

Statistical analysis

Normality was determined by Shapiro-Wilk test. Baseline data are presented for all subjects. The relationship between baseline characteristics, including eGFR, and CA parameters were determined by multivariate and univariate linear regression analysis adjusting for age, gender and other significantly related variables at previous univariate analysis. To better depict the relationship between CA and eGFR, we divided the first by median and the latter into subgroups of low and high (< 60 and ≥60 mL/min/1.73 m^2, respectively) subgroups. Any subgroups were compared with Kruskal-Wallis and Mann-Whitney tests. The impact of eGFR on the outcome (mRS 0–6) and association with WML grades (0–4) were characterized by ordinal regression analysis. The risk of hemorrhagic transformation was assessed by logistic regression analysis. To avoid spurious associations, we considered statistically significant at $P < 0.01$ level for univariate regression analysis. Otherwise, $P < 0.05$ cut-off was used. All statistics were performed using IBM Statistical Package for Social Sciences (SPSS) Statistics v21™.

Results

Renal function and cerebral autoregulation

Baseline characteristics and hemodynamic data are reported in Tables 1 and 2, respectively. In a multivariate linear regression analysis, greater LF and HF gain values (indicating less effective CA) within 6 h of symptoms were significantly associated with lower eGFR irrespective of infarct side ($p < 0.05$, Table 3). Phase and coherence were not related to any baseline variable. Additional file 1: Table S4 shows the results of univariate linear regression. Figure 1 shows the distribution of CA parameters throughout all spectrum of frequencies. We found significantly higher gain values in low eGFR subgroup compared to the high one ($p < 0.05$).

Previous use of Calcium Channel Blockers (CCB) was associated with higher gain values bilaterally ($p < 0.05$, Table 3). To explore further the influence of chronic medication with CCB we compared gain values in those using CCB ($n = 10$) compared to patients who were not on CCB (Fig. 2a and b) as well as renal function (Fig. 2c). CCB use was associated with higher gain values ($p < 0.05$) and also lower eGFR (57 and 75 ml/min, $p = 0.022$) but this was not statistically significant if we only compared chronically hypertensive patients ($N = 37$, 57 and 70 ml/min, $p = 0.082$). ABP at presentation was not different between those on CCB compared to those not on CCB (systolic 137 ± 21 vs 138 ± 20 mmHg, $p = 0.901$; diastolic 47 ± 12 vs 55 ± 14 mmHg, $p = 0.125$).

Relationship with cerebral microvascular disease (WML)

WML severity was correlated in an inverse manner with lower levels of eGFR (rho Spearman = – 0.52, $p < 0.0001$) and proportionally to higher levels of LF gain (ipsilateral $r = 0.368$, $p = 0.040$; contralateral $r = 0.402$, $p = 0.006$). This can be depicted clearly in figs. 3c and 4c+F, where we explored the distribution of WML grades accordingly to subgroups of low and high eGFR and LF gain, respectively. In Fig. 5c and f, we demonstrate the interaction between renal function and dynamic CA, by studying subgroups of eGFR versus subgroups of LF gain. Lower eGFR and higher LF gain (worse CA) were associated with more

Table 1 Demographics and baseline characteristics of patients ($N = 46$)

Demographics	
Male, n (%)	19 (41)
Age, years (mean ± SD)	73 ± 12
BMI, Kg.m^{-2} (mean ± SD)	27 ± 5
Previous stroke/TIA, n (%)	6 (13)
Hypertension, n (%)	28 (61)
Diabetes Mellitus, n (%)	14 (30)
Dyslipidemia, n (%)	27 (59)
Tobacco, n (%)	4 (9)
Previous MI, n (%)	2 (4)
Atrial Fibrillation, n (%)	20 (43)
Chronic Medication, n (%)	
Antiplatelet	18 (39)
Statin	17 (37)
Beta-Blocker	10 (22)
ACEI/ARB	15 (33)
CCB	9 (20)
Stroke characteristics	
Etiology (TOAST), n (%)	
Large Vessel	6 (13)
Cardioembolic	18 (39)
Small vessel	2 (4)
Other	1 (2)
Undetermined	12 (26)
Occlusion of affected MCA	16 (35)
Baseline NIHSS score *[median(IQR)]*	14 (9–22)
Neuroimaging [median(IQR)]	
Infarct Volume, mL	19 (2–139)
Leucoencephalopathy grade (VanSwieten scale [33])	2 (1–3)
Laboratorial (mean ± SD)	
Total cholesterol, mg/dL	174 ± 72
LDL cholesterol, mg/dL	105 ± 42
HDL cholesterol, mg/dL	46 ± 11
Triglycerides, mg/dL	111 ± 68
Glucose, mg/dL	140 ± 81
HbA1C, %	6.4 ± 1.4
Creatinine, mg/dL	1.0 ± 1.0
Renal Function	
eGFR, ml/min/1.73 m^2	80 ± 39
CDK-EPI Stage 0–1, n (%)	10 (22)
CDK-EPI Stage 2, n (%)	23 (50)
CDK-EPI Stage 3, n (%)	13 (28)
CDK-EPI Stage 4, n (%)	1 (2)
CDK-EPI Stage 5, n (%)	1 (2)

Body-Mass Index (*BMI*), Transitory Ischemic Attack (*TIA*), angiotensin-conversion-enzyme inhibitor (*ACEI*), angiotensin receptor blocker (*ARB*), calcium channel blocker (*CCB*), Trial of ORG10172 in Acute Stroke Treatment (*TOAST*), middle cerebral artery (*MCA*), National Institutes of Health Stroke Scale (*NIHSS*), Low-density lipoprotein (*LDL*), High-density lipoprotein (*LDL*), glycated hemoglobin (*HbA1C*), eGFR (estimated glomerular filtration rate) by Chronic Kidney Disease Epidemiology Collaboration (*CKD-EPI*) formula [25]

Table 2 Systemic and cerebral hemodynamic characteristics of patients ($N = 46$)

Systemic hemodynamics (mean ± SD)	
Systolic ABP, mmHg	144 ± 19
Mean ABP, mmHg	98 ± 11
Diastolic ABP, mmHg	75 ± 11
Heart rate, bpm	67 ± 11
LF mean ABP variability, $mmHg^2$	85 ± 111
HF mean ABP variability, $mmHg^2$	13 ± 20
$EtCO_2$, mmHg	36 ± 7
Cerebral hemodynamics (mean ± SD)	
Ipsilateral	
MFV, cm/s	40 ± 20
CVRi, mmHg/(cm/s)	2.3 ± 0.9
LF MFV variability, $(cm/s)^2$	128 ± 142
HF MFV variability, $(cm/s)^2$	35 ± 49
Contralateral	
MFV, cm/s	48 ± 17
CVRi, mm Hg/(cm/s)	1.7 ± 0.7
LF MFV variability, $(cm/s)^2$	200 ± 250
HF MFV variability, $(cm/s)^2$	47 ± 68
Dynamic cerebral autoregulation	
Ipsilateral	
LF coherence, a.u.	0.5 ± 0.2
LF gain, $\%^2/mmHg^2$	1.0 ± 0.3
LF phase, degrees	32 ± 23
HF coherence, a.u.	0.6 ± 0.2
HF gain, $\%^2/mmHg^2$	1.5 ± 0.6
HF phase, degrees	− 0.1 ± 13
Contralateral	
LF coherence, a.u.	0.5 ± 0.2
LF gain, $\%^2/mmHg^2$	1.2 ± 0.5
LF phase, degrees	44 ± 26
HF coherence, a.u.	0.7 ± 0.2
HF gain, $\%^2/mmHg^2$	1.5 ± 0.6
HF phase, degrees	− 0.7 ± 13

Arterial blood pressure (*ABP*), mean flow velocity (*MFV*), estimated cerebrovascular resistance (*CVRi*), end-tidal carbon dioxide (*EtCO2*), Low (LF: 0.3–0.15 Hz) and high (HF: 0.15–0.5 Hz) frequency spectral bands; a.u., arbitrary units

severe white matter lesion grades (ordinal shift analysis of infarct side $p = 0.045$ and non-infarct side $p = 0.009$).

Renal function, cerebral autoregulation and outcome

As presented in Fig. 4a, lower GFR reduces significantly the odds of a good outcome (grade of 0–2) measured by mRS at 3 months [Fig. 3a, lower eGFR as reference, ordinal regression odds ratio, OR = 0.32 (confidence interval, CI, 95% 0.10–0.56), $p = 0.005$] and higher risk of hemorrhagic transformation [Fig. 3b, logistic regression OR 0.97 (CI95% 0.95–0.99), $p = 0.026$].

Figure 4 depicts outcome accordingly to CA status. Higher LF gain (worse CA) also increased the odds of a poor outcome (mRS > 2) [Fig. 4a, ipsilateral OR = 2.18 (CI95% 1.01–5.28), $p = 0.048$; fig. 4d, contralateral OR = 2.17 (CI95% 1.12–4.17), $p = 0.022$], and the risk of developing hemorrhagic transformation [Fig. 4b, ipsilateral OR = 1.98 (CI95% 1.002–8.12), Fig. 4e, p=0.042; contralateral OR = 2.79 (CI95% 1.03–7.56), $p = 0.043$].

An ordinal regression model with interaction between decreasing eGFR and increasing LF gain (Fig. 5a and d) found that both factors combine to progressively reducing the odds of a good functional outcome [ipsilateral OR = 4.39 (CI95% 3.15–25.6), $p = 0.019$; contralateral OR = 8.15 (CI95% 4.15–15.6), $p = 0.002$]. Multinomial logistic regression also found an interaction between lower eGFR and higher LF gain with an increased risk of hemorrhagic transformation that was only statistically significant on the contralateral side [Fig. 5b and e, ipsilateral OR = 3.48 (CI95% 0.60–24.0), $p = 0.132$; contralateral OR = 6.43 (CI95% 1.40–32.1), $p = 0.034$].

Discussion

Our data shows significant association between impaired cerebral autoregulation (higher dynamic CA gain values) assessed during acute ischemic stroke (< 6 h) and impaired renal function (lower glomerular filtration rate) independent of age, vascular risk factors and relevant laboratory metabolic control parameters. Moreover, both impaired renal function and impaired cerebral autoregulation (i.e. high gain values) were associated with greater white matter abnormalities and with reduced likelihood of a good functional outcome (scale of 0–2) as assessed by mRS at 3 months.

To understand why impaired renal function might be linked to impaired cerebral autoregulation, we need to consider the physiology of autoregulation. Renal autoregulation adjusts vascular resistance to stabilize renal blood flow and filtration rate during changes in renal perfusion pressure [7]. Basically, as pressure changes stretch the smooth muscles of the afferent and cortical arterioles, a myogenic response occurs to adjust the vascular resistance to maintain flow. Since blood flow in a vascular bed is determined by perfusion pressure and resistance (Blood flow = perfusion pressure/vascular resistance), if perfusion pressure increases, stretching the smooth muscle surrounding the arterioles, the arterioles will then constrict to increase resistance and maintain the ratio of pressure to resistance and thus maintain blood flow [7]. In fact, renal autoregulation status has been well documented by the same method of TFA we used to assess dynamic CA. This method quantifies the transfer of blood pressure

Table 3 Association between estimated glomerular filtration rate and cerebral autoregulation parameters in acute stroke (< 6 h)

	Multiple Linear Regression – Beta coefficients and estimated 95% confidence interval					
	Coherence (a.u.)		Gain (%^{2}/ mmHg^2)		Phase (degrees)	
	LF band	HF band	LF band	HF band	LF band	HF band
Ipsilateral (N = 37)						
eGFR, ml/min	– 0.01 (– 0.01, 0.01)	– 0.08 (– 0.23, 0,15)	*– 0.01 (– 0.01,–0.004)	*– 0.02 (– 0.18,–0.003)	0.10 (– 0.24, 0.43)	– 0.08 (– 0.26, 0.14)
CCB Use	– 0.32 (– 10.6, 0.75)	– 0.12 (– 10.6, 0.75)	* 0.52 (0.22, 0.71)	* 0.35 (0.06, 1.12)	0.17 (– 0.09, 0.26)	0.17 (– 0.05, 0.12)
Mean ABP, mmHg	0.01 (– 0.01, 0.01)	0.06 (– 0.27, 0.37)	– 0.39 (– 0.02, 0.001)	– 0.01 (– 0.03, 0.01)	0.28 (– 1.21, 0.60)	0.28 (– 1.21, 0.60)
Heart Rate, bpm	– 0.11 (– 0.01, 0.00)	– 0.02 (– 0.43, 0.37)	– 0.30 (– 0.03, 0.03)	– 0.32 (– 0.01, 0.02)	0.13 (– 0.33, 1.26)	0.24 (– 1.23, 0.23)
$EtCO_2$, mmHg	– 0.13 (– 0.01, 0.01)	– 0.03 (– 0.78, 0.67)	– 0.34 (– 0.08, 0.05)	– 0.23 (– 0.10, 0.02)	0.31 (– 0.10, .34)	0.13 (– 0.13, 2.31)
Contralateral (N = 46)						
eGFR, ml/min	– 0.19 (–0.01, 0.01)	0.09 (– 0.13, 0.25)	*– 0.01 (– 0.01,–0.004)	*– 0.02 (– 0.02,–0.004)	0.06 (– 0.23, 0.35)	0.09 (– 0.13, 0.25)
CCB Use	– 0.15 (– 34.5, 10.2)	– 0.32 (– 45.6, 7.5)	* 0.40 (0.16, 0.81)	0.25 (– 0.04, 0.76)	0.14 (– 0.06, 0.24)	0.17 (– 0.05, 0.12)
Mean ABP, mmHg	– 0.20 (– 0.01, 0.001)	0.10 (– 0.22, 0.45)	*– 0.02 (– 0.03,–0.01)	*– 0.02 (– 0.03, – 0.01)	0.17 (– 0.26, 0.84)	0.21 (– 1.23, 1.01)
Heart Rate, bpm	– 0.08 (– 0.01, 0.003)	– 0.02 (– 0.45, 0.38)	– 0.15 (– 0.02, 0.01)	– 0.32 (– 0.01, 0.13)	– 0.04 (– 0.58, 1.03)	– 0.10 (– 2.33, 0.12)
$EtCO_2$, mmHg	– 0.03 (– 0.01, 0.01)	– 0.17 (– 1.12, 0.28)	– 0.29 (– 0.04, 0.00)	– 0.24 (– 0.01, 0.12)	0.13 (0.14, 2.56)	– 0.25 (– 0.23, 3.12)

Estimated glomerular filtration rate (eGFR), arterial blood pressure (MBP), end-tidal carbon dioxide ($EtCO_2$), low (LF: 0.03–0.15 Hz) and high (HF: 0.15–0.5 Hz) frequency spectral bands, a.u., arbitrary units
*$P < 0.01$ for multivariate linear regression analysis adjusting for age, gender and all significantly related variables in univariate analysis (Additional file 1: Table S4)

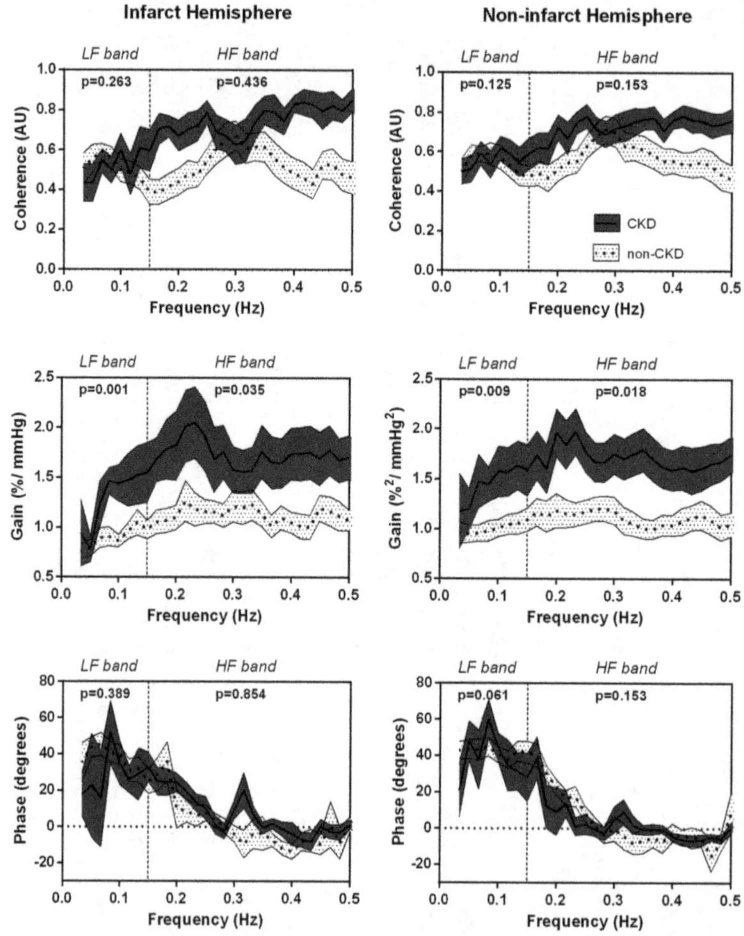

Fig. 1 Frequency spectra from 0.03 to 0.5 Hz of Coherence and Transfer Function Gain and Phase measured in acute stroke patients (< 6 h) accordingly to their estimated glomerular filtration rate (eGFR). Continuous and spotted lines within dark grey and spotted white strips corresponds to means±SE of groups of low (< 60 mL/min/1.73 m^2) and high (≥60 mL/min/1.73 m^2) subgroups of eGFR, respectively. Groups were compared with Mann-Whitney and *P* values presented at right superior corner of each plot. Lower GFR shows higher gain values bilaterally which indicate less effective dynamic cerebral autoregulation

changes into flow change, thus high gain means that pressure changes are causing flow changes, and thus autoregulation is impaired. In the kidney, previous work in hypertensive rats with adenine-induced chronic renal failure has shown that gain is increased in the < 0.1 Hz band, suggesting higher gain is an indicator of impaired renal autoregulation [35].

The same characteristics are found in the cerebrovasculature with increased gain in the low-frequency range associated with impaired cerebral autoregulation [10, 20]. In fact, myogenic autoregulation is widely distributed over various vascular beds including the brain, coronary, pulmonary, mesenteric, and skeletal muscle [8].

Considering the similarities in the characteristics of autoregulation in the kidney and brain, one could propose that microvascular damage (e.g. caused by hypertension, diabetes) that causes impairment of kidney function [7, 16] could also affect the brain in a similar fashion. Support for this idea is found in stroke-prone spontaneously-hypertensive rats that have a genetic predisposition to rapid glomerulosclerosis and stroke [36]. In fact, in these rats, both renal autoregulation (assessed by TFA) and cerebral autoregulation are impaired prior to the development of stroke and death [37, 38]. Examination of the histopathology of cerebral arteries in the spontaneously hypertensive rats have also shown medial hypertrophy and remodeling, [39] that are hallmarks of small vessel disease, as in humans [17]. Thus it would appear that the stroke-prone spontaneously hypertensive rats show impairments of autoregulation in both the kidney and brain, prior to stroke. These data would suggest, in this animal model, that impairment of autoregulation is occurring in multiple vascular beds.

Taken together, this would suggest that if patients demonstrate less effective autoregulation in the cerebral vasculature (high gain) they would likely also have impaired renal

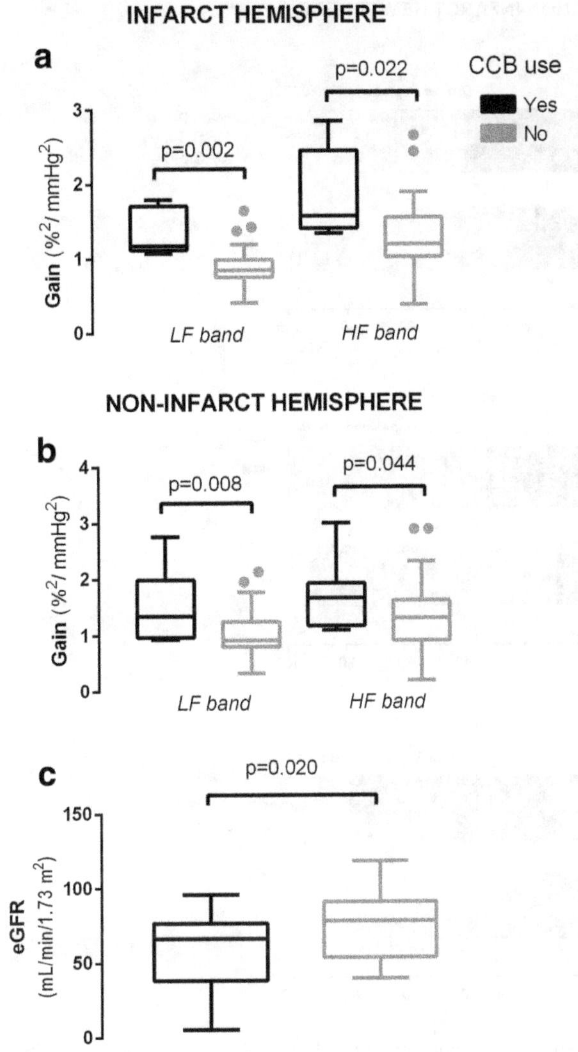

Fig. 2 Box plots comparing median and quartiles distribution of cerebral autoregulation. Gain, at low (LF: 0.03–0.15 Hz) and high (HF: 0.15–0.5 Hz) frequency bands (subpanels A and B), and estimated glomerular filtration rate (GFR, subpanel C) by groups with and without chronic use of calcium channel blockers (CCB). Statistical *P* value of Mann-whitey test (**a**, **b**) and T-test (**c**) is presented

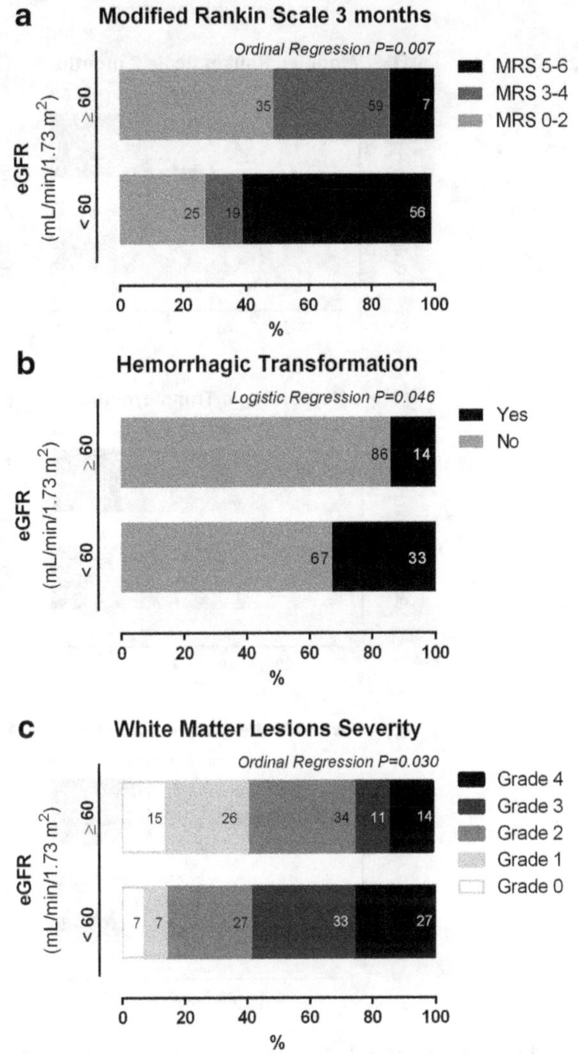

Fig. 3 Relationship between renal function subgroups of low (< 60 mL/min/1.73 m^2) and high (≥60 mL/min/1.73 m^2) subgroups of estimated glomerular filtration rate (eGFR) and outcome accordingly to modified Rankin scale (**a**), risk of hemorrhage (**b**) and the severity of white matter lesions assessed at 24-h head Computed Tomography, accordingly to vanSwieten scale [33]. Subgroups were compared with ordinal regression or logistic regression as appropriate

myogenic autoregulation, which would cause glomerular dysfunction.

One interesting finding was that previous CCB use was correlated to increased LF gain values in both cerebral hemispheres as well as reduced eGFR. A possible explanation for this finding lies in the effect of CCB on autoregulation. In fact, previous work has demonstrated that CCB impairs the myogenic response in the kidney in animal models [7, 40] and perhaps in humans [41, 42]. CCB block the L-type voltage-gated calcium channels that are activated by the stretch of the arterial vessel wall [7]. Thus changes in pressure that result in changes in stretch of the walls will no longer activate the release of calcium and contraction of smooth muscle to modulate vascular resistance to maintain flow, which we would expect to result in an increased gain (i.e. worse autoregulation). The finding that CCB are associated with increased gain and poor eGFR may be due to CCB impairing autoregulation in both organs (brain and kidney), consistent with our hypothesis. However, the effect of CCB on cerebral autoregulation in humans is not as clear with studies, using measures other than TFA, showing impaired autoregulation, [41–43] while another study found no change in TFA derived gain in 8 healthy individuals [44].

Our finding that both low eGFR and high gain were significantly associated with severe WML grade does suggest that impaired autoregulation in the brain and kidney

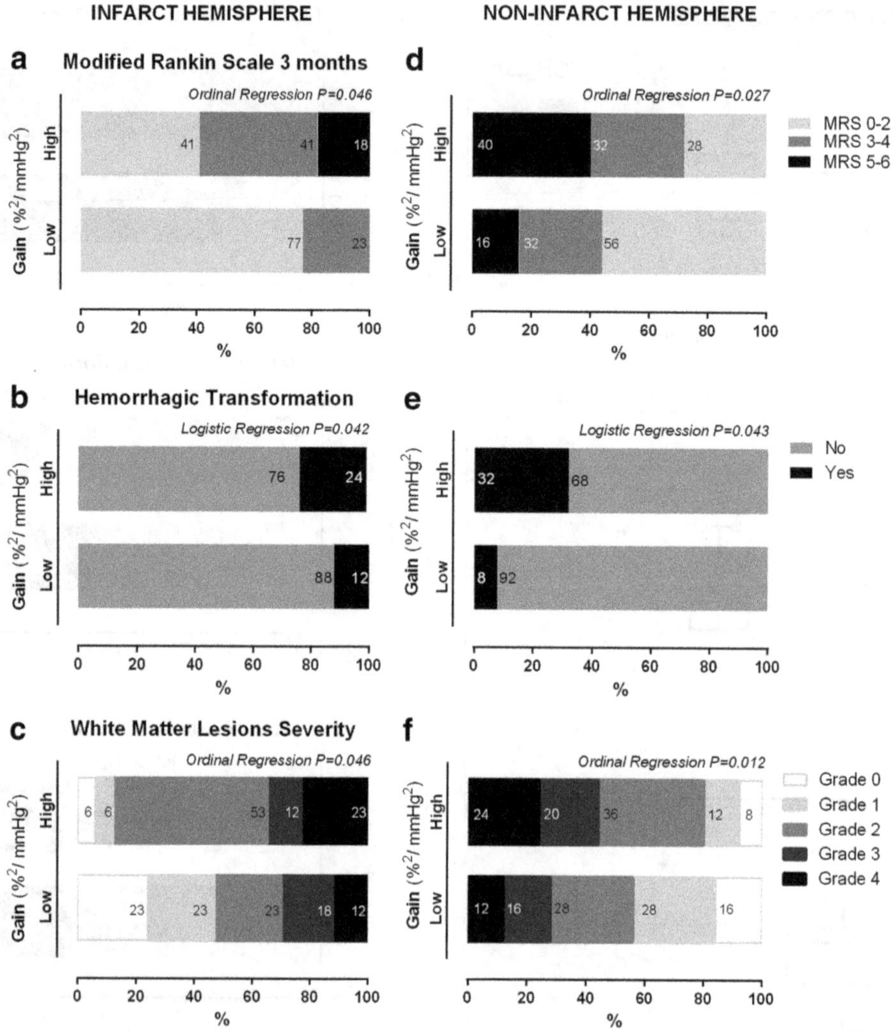

Fig. 4 Relationship between cerebral autoregulation within 6 h of symptoms by subgroups of low and high LF gain subgroups for infarct (≤0.90, > 0.9%^{2}/mmHg^2, respectively) and non-infarct hemisphere (≤1.10, > 1.10%^{2}/mmHg^2, respectively) and outcome accordingly to modified Rankin scale (**a**), risk of hemorrhage (**b**) and the severity of white matter lesions assessed at 24-h head Computed Tomography, accordingly to vanSwieten scale [33]. Subgroups were compared with ordinal regression or logistic regression as appropriate

may be associated. A suggested mechanism for this is that microvascular damage is the basis of this autoregulatory dysfunction. Our work is the first to demonstrate that low eGFR is significantly associated with high gain and severe WML. From our data, we cannot rule out if WML cause cerebral autoregulation impairment or the opposite. Previous work has demonstrated that WML are correlated with cerebral autoregulation efficiency [14]. However, we hypothesize that both WML, as well as worse cerebral autoregulation, are expressions of a systemic microvascular dysfunction that can also impair renal function. Further prospective studies could untangle what's cause or consequence.

Another finding in our study was the relationship between high gain, low eGFR and hemorrhagic transformation. Higher gain values reflect less effectiveness in the dampening capability of cerebral resistance vessels in the insonated vascular territory to ABP oscillations [6]. These dysfunctional vessels disrupt Starling's principle by increasing the hydrostatic pressure across the capillary bed and contribute to the existing blood-brain barrier leakage [45]. Therefore, this might explain the association of higher gain and the risk of hemorrhagic transformation and cerebral edema [27]. Also, high gain values have been implicated in acute intracerebral hemorrhage [21, 46] and hematoma expansion [46].

In the infarcted hemisphere, gain had more non-significant relationships with outcome measurements. This can be observed by inspecting figs. 4 and 5. One obvious explanation is that some patients had occluded MCA at infarct side and CA cannot be assessed at infarct side in the severe cases. Therefore, gain apparently

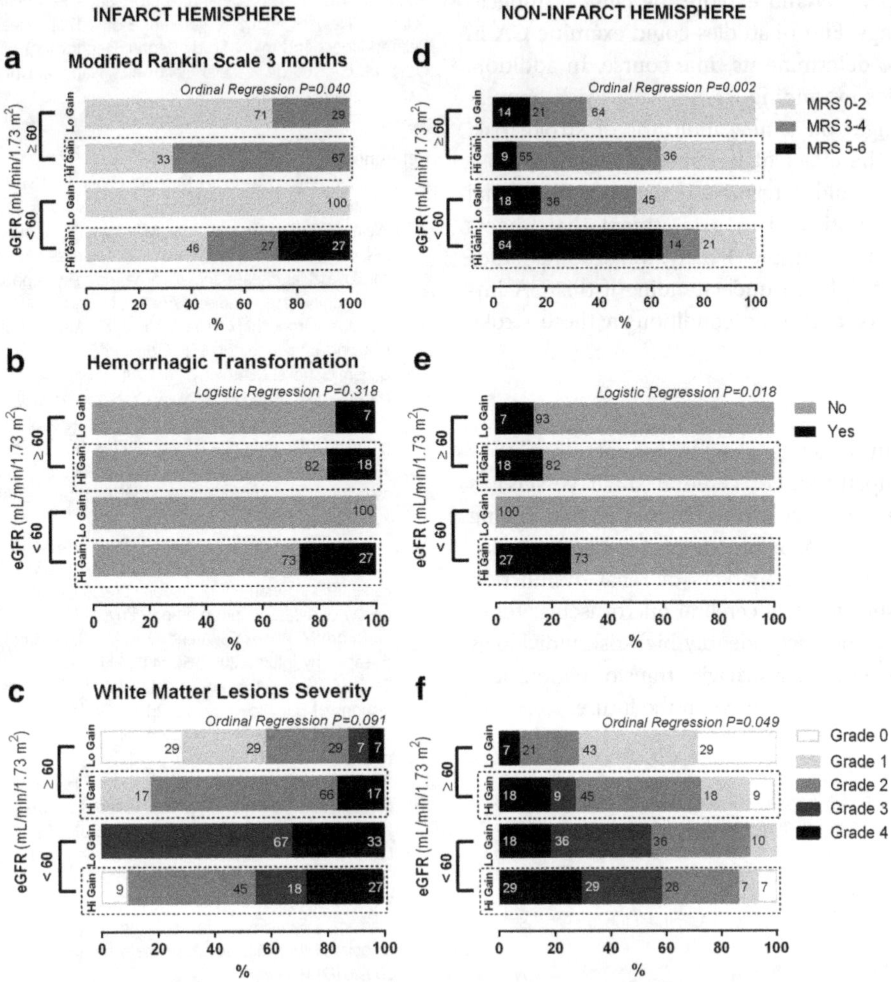

Fig. 5 Interaction between cerebral autoregulation and renal function on outcome accordingly to modified Rankin scale (**a**), risk of hemorrhage (**b**) and on severity of white matter lesions assessed at 24-h head Computed Tomography, accordingly to vanSwieten scale [33]. Subgroups were created by splitting renal function into low (< 60 mL/min/1.73 m^2) and high (≥60 mL/min/1.73 m^2) estimated glomerular filtration rate (eGFR); cerebral autoregulation into low (Lo gain) and high (Hi gain) subgroups of LF gain in infarct (≤ 0.90 and > 0.90%^{2}/mmHg^2) and non-infarct hemisphere (≤ 1.10 and > 1.10%^{2}/mmHg^2). Notice that higher gain values represents worse levels of cerebral autoregulation. The interaction effect in outcome and white matter lesions was tested in multinomial logistic or ordinal regression models as appropriate

had weaker associations with outcome measures. A second possibility may be that the gain in the ischemic hemisphere is artificially lowered and cerebral autoregulation falsely normalized due to the increased vascular resistance caused by microthrombosis [47] and/or cytotoxic edema [48] in the infarcted area [49]. Clearly, much more work on the physiological determinants influencing each TFA parameter is needed.

One possible confounder on ABP variability and transfer function estimates of CA is the effect of atrial fibrillation. To address this we compared values between patients with and without atrial fibrillation and found no statistical difference between groups, suggesting atrial fibrillation did not have a significant effect on our estimates of ABP variability or CA.

The small sample is a limitation of this study. Also, we cannot rule out that this brain-kidney interaction is specific of a stroke population, rather than present in all individuals including healthy subjects since we don't have a control group. Other angiographic imaging modalities (CT or MRI) are more accurate in excluding significant stenosis and since we relied mainly on ultrasound exams this may be a possible limitation. ABP was assessed using non-invasive oscillometric as well as finger photoplethysmography which are known to have limitations but generally provide a relatively accurate estimate of ABP [10].

Our results show that CA assessment may be an important factor to consider in advancing treatment of acute cerebrovascular disease. Given our finding that impaired CA is associated with worse functional outcome, further work is needed to verify and explore the clinical implications of our findings. Future studies could examine CA in ischemic stroke to determine its time course. In addition, longitudinal studies examining CA in a high-risk population could shed light on a new indicator of stroke risk. Studies assessing the effect of treatments targeting those with impaired CA could determine if the poor functional outcome could be mitigated by a treatment that targets cerebral perfusion for example. Finally, longitudinal studies would also be helpful in understanding if this CA impairment is acute or a chronic condition in these stroke patients.

Conclusions

In conclusion, our findings provide support that early autoregulatory impairment of cerebral small vessels, as well as renal vessels, may be a possible mechanism linking low renal function with poor outcome of ischemic stroke. Rapid assessment of serum markers of renal dysfunction could be used as surrogates of cerebral microvascular function integrity which may help identify high-risk individuals for complications like hemorrhagic transformation and possibly provide a therapeutic target in the future.

Abbreviations

ABP: Arterial blood pressure; CA: Cerebral autoregulation; CBFV: Cerebral blood flow velocity; CKD: Chronic kidney disease; CVRi: Cerebrovascular resistance; eGFR: Estimated glomerular filtration rate; HDL: High-density lipoprotein cholesterol; HgA1C: Glycated hemoglobin; LDL: Low-density lipoprotein cholesterol; MCA: Middle cerebral artery; mRS: modified Rankin Scale; NIHSS: National Institute of Health Stroke Scale; TFA: Transfer function analysis

Funding

This study received public national grant from Fundação para a Ciência e a Tecnologia (FCT), Portugal, PTDC/SAU-ORG/113329/2009.The funding body had no role or interference in the design of the study and collection, analysis, and interpretation of data and in writing the manuscript.

Authors' contributions

PC Reviewed the literature, designed the study, extracted the data, analyzed the results and wrote the paper. IR Designed the study, analyzed the results, reviewed the paper. EA Designed the study, analyzed the results, and co-wrote the paper. FS Reviewed the literature, designed the study, analyzed the results. JS Designed the study, analyzed the results, and co-wrote the paper and reviewed the paper. All authors read and approved the final manuscript.

Competing interests

Jorge Serrador is a member of the editorial board (Associate Editor) of this journal.

Author details

[1]Department Neurology, São João Hospital Center, Faculty of Medicine of University of Porto, Alameda Professor Hernani Monteiro, 4200-319 Porto, Portugal. [2]Cardiovascular Autonomic Function Lab, Institute of Physiology, Faculty of Medicine of University of Lisbon, Lisbon, Portugal. [3]Department of Neurology, Division of Stroke and Neurocritical, Northwestern University Feinberg School of Medicine, Chicago, IL, USA. [4]Department of Pharmacology, Physiology and Neuroscience, Rutgers Biomedical Health Sciences, Newark, NJ, USA. [5]Veterans Biomedical Research Institute and War Related Illness and Injury Study Center, Department of Veterans Affairs, East Orange, USA. [6]Cardiovascular Electronics, National University of Ireland Galway, Galway, Ireland.

References

1. Lee M, Saver JL, Chang KH, Liao HW, Chang SC, Ovbiagele B. Low glomerular filtration rate and risk of stroke: meta-analysis. BMJ. 2010;341:c4249.
2. Weiner DE, Tighiouart H, Amin MG, Stark PC, MacLeod B, Griffith JL, Salem DN, Levey AS, Sarnak MJ. Chronic kidney disease as a risk factor for cardiovascular disease and all-cause mortality: a pooled analysis of community-based studies. J Am Soc Nephrol. 2004;15(5):1307–15.
3. Kumai Y, Kamouchi M, Hata J, Ago T, Kitayama J, Nakane H, Sugimori H, Kitazono T, Investigators FSR. Proteinuria and clinical outcomes after ischemic stroke. Neurology. 2012;78(24):1909–15.
4. Naganuma M, Koga M, Shiokawa Y, Nakagawara J, Furui E, Kimura K, Yamagami H, Okada Y, Hasegawa Y, Kario K, et al. Reduced estimated glomerular filtration rate is associated with stroke outcome after intravenous rt-PA: the stroke acute management with urgent risk-factor assessment and improvement (SAMURAI) rt-PA registry. Cerebrovasc Dis. 2011;31(2):123–9.
5. Toyoda K, Ninomiya T. Stroke and cerebrovascular diseases in patients with chronic kidney disease. Lancet Neurol. 2014;13(8):823–33.
6. Panerai RB. Assessment of cerebral pressure autoregulation in humans–a review of measurement methods. Physiol Meas. 1998;19(3):305–38.
7. Carlstrom M, Wilcox CS, Arendshorst WJ. Renal autoregulation in health and disease. Physiol Rev. 2015;95(2):405–511.
8. Davis MJ. Perspective: physiological role(s) of the vascular myogenic response. Microcirculation. 2012;19(2):99–114.
9. Bayliss WM. On the local reactions of the arterial wall to changes of internal pressure. J Physiol. 1902;28(3):220–31.
10. Panerai RB, Rennie JM, Kelsall AW, Evans DH. Frequency-domain analysis of cerebral autoregulation from spontaneous fluctuations in arterial blood pressure. Med Biol Eng Comput. 1998;36(3):315–22.
11. Lassen NA. Cerebral blood flow and oxygen consumption in man. Physiol Rev. 1959;39(2):183–238.
12. Wardlaw JM, Doubal F, Armitage P, Chappell F, Carpenter T, Munoz Maniega S, Farrall A, Sudlow C, Dennis M, Dhillon B. Lacunar stroke is associated with diffuse blood-brain barrier dysfunction. Ann Neurol. 2009;65(2):194–202.
13. O'Rourke MF, Safar ME. Relationship between aortic stiffening and microvascular disease in brain and kidney: cause and logic of therapy. Hypertension. 2005;46(1):200–4.
14. Purkayastha S, Fadar O, Mehregan A, Salat DH, Moscufo N, Meier DS, Guttmann CR, Fisher ND, Lipsitz LA, Sorond FA. Impaired cerebrovascular hemodynamics are associated with cerebral white matter damage. J Cereb Blood Flow Metab. 2014;34(2):228–34.
15. Sorond FA, Galica A, Serrador JM, Kiely DK, Iloputaife I, Cupples LA, Lipsitz LA. Cerebrovascular hemodynamics, gait, and falls in an elderly population: MOBILIZE Boston study. Neurology. 2010;74(20):1627–33.
16. Bidani AK, Griffin KA. Pathophysiology of hypertensive renal damage: implications for therapy. Hypertension. 2004;44(5):595–601.
17. Fazekas F, Kleinert R, Offenbacher H, Schmidt R, Kleinert G, Payer F, Radner H, Lechner H. Pathologic correlates of incidental MRI white matter signal hyperintensities. Neurology. 1993;43(9):1683–9.
18. Khatri M, Wright CB, Nickolas TL, Yoshita M, Paik MC, Kranwinkel G, Sacco RL, DeCarli C. Chronic kidney disease is associated with white matter hyperintensity volume: the northern Manhattan study (NOMAS). Stroke. 2007;38(12):3121–6.
19. Meel-van den Abeelen AS, van Beek AH, Slump CH, Panerai RB, Claassen JA. Transfer function analysis for the assessment of cerebral autoregulation using spontaneous oscillations in blood pressure and cerebral blood flow. Med Eng Phys. 2014;36(5):563–75.
20. Zhang R, Zuckerman JH, Giller CA, Levine BD. Transfer function analysis of dynamic cerebral autoregulation in humans. Am J Phys. 1998;274(1 Pt 2): H233–41.
21. Nakagawa K, Serrador JM, LaRose SL, Sorond FA. Dynamic cerebral autoregulation after intracerebral hemorrhage: a case-control study. BMC Neurol. 2011;11:108.

22. Castro P, Santos R, Freitas J, Rosengarten B, Panerai R, Azevedo E: Adaptation of cerebral pressure-velocity hemodynamic changes of neurovascular coupling to orthostatic challenge. Perspectives in Medicine 2012: https://doi.org/10.1016/j.permed.2012.1002.1052 [Available online 1028 March 2012].
23. Aries MJ, Elting JW, De Keyser J, Kremer BP, Vroomen PC. Cerebral autoregulation in stroke: a review of transcranial Doppler studies. Stroke. 2010;41(11):2697–704.
24. Group KDIGOKAKIW. KDIGO clinical practice guideline for acute kidney injury. Kidney International Supplements. 2012;2(1):1.
25. Levey AS, Stevens LA, Schmid CH, Zhang YL, Castro AF 3rd, Feldman HI, Kusek JW, Eggers P, Van Lente F, Greene T, et al. A new equation to estimate glomerular filtration rate. Ann Intern Med. 2009;150(9):604–12.
26. Castro P, Serrador J, Rocha I, Sorond F, Azevedo E. Efficacy of cerebral autoregulation in early ischemic stroke predicts smaller infarcts and better outcomes. Front Neurol. 2017;8(113)
27. Castro P, Azevedo E, Serrador J, Rocha I, Sorond F. Hemorrhagic transformation and cerebral edema in acute ischemic stroke: link to cerebral autoregulation. J Neurol Sci. 2017;372:256–61.
28. Deegan BM, Serrador JM, Nakagawa K, Jones E, Sorond FA, Olaighin G. The effect of blood pressure calibrations and transcranial Doppler signal loss on transfer function estimates of cerebral autoregulation. Med Eng Phys. 2011;33(5):553–62.
29. Panerai RB. The critical closing pressure of the cerebral circulation. Med Eng Phys. 2003;25(8):621–32.
30. Aaslid R, Lindegaard KF, Sorteberg W, Nornes H. Cerebral autoregulation dynamics in humans. Stroke. 1989;20(1):45–52.
31. Serrador JM, Sorond FA, Vyas M, Gagnon M, Iloputaife ID, Lipsitz LA. Cerebral pressure-flow relations in hypertensive elderly humans: transfer gain in different frequency domains. J Appl Physiol. 2005;98(1):151–9.
32. Fiorelli M, Bastianello S, von Kummer R, del Zoppo GJ, Larrue V, Lesaffre E, Ringleb AP, Lorenzano S, Manelfe C, Bozzao L. Hemorrhagic transformation within 36 hours of a cerebral infarct: relationships with early clinical deterioration and 3-month outcome in the European cooperative acute stroke study I (ECASS I) cohort. Stroke. 1999;30(11):2280–4.
33. van Swieten JC, Hijdra A, Koudstaal PJ, van Gijn J. Grading white matter lesions on CT and MRI: a simple scale. J Neurol Neurosurg Psychiatry. 1990;53(12):1080–3.
34. Curtze S, Melkas S, Sibolt G, Haapaniemi E, Mustanoja S, Putaala J, Sairanen T, Tiainen M, Tatlisumak T, Strbian D. Cerebral computed tomography-graded white matter lesions are associated with worse outcome after thrombolysis in patients with stroke. Stroke. 2015;46(6):1554–60.
35. Saeed A, DiBona GF, Grimberg E, Nguy L, Mikkelsen ML, Marcussen N, Guron G. High-NaCl diet impairs dynamic renal blood flow autoregulation in rats with adenine-induced chronic renal failure. Am J Physiol Regul Integr Comp Physiol. 2014;306(6):R411–9.
36. Churchill PC, Churchill MC, Griffin KA, Picken M, Webb RC, Kurtz TW, Bidani AK. Increased genetic susceptibility to renal damage in the stroke-prone spontaneously hypertensive rat. Kidney Int. 2002;61(5):1794–800.
37. Abu-Amarah I, Bidani AK, Hacioglu R, Williamson GA, Griffin KA. Differential effects of salt on renal hemodynamics and potential pressure transmission in stroke-prone and stroke-resistant spontaneously hypertensive rats. Am J Physiol Renal Physiol. 289(2):F305–13.
38. Smeda JS, VanVliet BN, King SR. Stroke-prone spontaneously hypertensive rats lose their ability to auto-regulate cerebral blood flow prior to stroke. J Hypertens. 1999;17(12 Pt 1):1697–705.
39. Izzard AS, Graham D, Burnham MP, Heerkens EH, Dominiczak AF, Heagerty AM. Myogenic and structural properties of cerebral arteries from the stroke-prone spontaneously hypertensive rat. Am J Physiol Heart Circ Physiol. 2003;285(4):H1489–94.
40. Nakamura Y, Ono H, Frohlich ED. Differential effects of T- and L-type calcium antagonists on glomerular dynamics in spontaneously hypertensive rats. Hypertension. 1999;34(2):273–8.
41. Endoh H, Honda T, Komura N, Shibue C, Watanabe I, Shimoji K. The effects of nicardipine on dynamic cerebral autoregulation in patients anesthetized with propofol and fentanyl. Anesth Analg. 2000;91(3):642–6.
42. Hamner JW, Tan CO. Relative contributions of sympathetic, cholinergic, and myogenic mechanisms to cerebral autoregulation. Stroke. 2014;45(6):1771–7.
43. Tan CO, Hamner JW, Taylor JA. The role of myogenic mechanisms in human cerebrovascular regulation. J Physiol. 2013;591(20):5095–105.
44. Tzeng YC, Chan GS, Willie CK, Ainslie PN. Determinants of human cerebral pressure-flow velocity relationships: new insights from vascular modelling and ca(2)(+) channel blockade. J Physiol. 2011;589(Pt 13):3263–74.
45. Simard JM, Kent TA, Chen M, Tarasov KV, Gerzanich V. Brain oedema in focal ischaemia: molecular pathophysiology and theoretical implications. Lancet Neurol. 2007;6(3):258–68.
46. Reinhard M, Neunhoeffer F, Gerds TA, Niesen WD, Buttler KJ, Timmer J, Schmidt B, Czosnyka M, Weiller C, Hetzel A. Secondary decline of cerebral autoregulation is associated with worse outcome after intracerebral hemorrhage. Intensive Care Med. 2010;36(2):264–71.
47. Wang X, Lo EH. Triggers and mediators of hemorrhagic transformation in cerebral ischemia. Mol Neurobiol. 2003;28(3):229–44.
48. Balami JS, Chen RL, Grunwald IQ, Buchan AM. Neurological complications of acute ischaemic stroke. Lancet Neurol. 2011;10(4):357–71.
49. Panerai RB. Cerebral autoregulation: from models to clinical applications. Cardiovasc Eng. 2008;8(1):42–59.

3

Neurogranin and tau in cerebrospinal fluid and plasma of patients with acute ischemic stroke

Ann De Vos[1], Maria Bjerke[2], Raf Brouns[3], Naomi De Roeck[2], Dirk Jacobs[1], Lien Van den Abbeele[1], Kaat Guldolf[2,4], Henrik Zetterberg[5,6,7], Kaj Blennow[5,6], Sebastiaan Engelborghs[2,4] and Eugeen Vanmechelen[1*]

Abstract

Background: While neurogranin has no value as plasma biomarker for Alzheimer's disease, it may be a potential blood biomarker for traumatic brain injury. This evokes the question whether there are changes in neurogranin levels in blood in other conditions of brain injury, such as acute ischemic stroke (AIS).

Methods: We therefore explored neurogranin in paired cerebrospinal fluid (CSF)/plasma samples of AIS patients (n = 50) from a well-described prospective study. In parallel, we investigated another neuronal protein, i.e. tau, which has already been suggested as potential AIS biomarker in CSF and blood. ELISA as well as Single Molecule Array (Simoa) technology were used for the biochemical analyses. Statistical analyses included Shapiro-Wilk testing, Mann-Whitney analyses and Pearson's correlation analysis.

Results: In contrast to tau, of which high levels in both CSF and plasma were related to stroke characteristics like severity and long-term outcome, plasma neurogranin levels were only correlated with infarct volume. Likewise, CSF neurogranin levels were significantly higher in patients with an infarct volume > 5 mL than in patients with smaller infarct volumes. Finally, neurogranin and tau were significantly correlated in CSF, whereas a weaker relationship was observed in plasma.

Conclusions: These findings indicate that although plasma and CSF neurogranin may reflect the volume of acute cerebral ischemia, this synaptic protein is less likely to be a potential AIS biomarker. Levels of tau correlated with severity and outcome of stroke in both plasma and CSF, in the present study as well as previous reports, confirming the potential of tau as an AIS biomarker.

Keywords: AIS, Neurogranin, Tau, Plasma, CSF, Elisa, Simoa, NIHSS, mRS, Biomarker

Background

Several studies illustrate the potential of neurogranin as biomarker for Alzheimer's disease (AD), the most common cause of dementia. Concentrations of this post-synaptic protein are higher in CSF of AD patients compared with cognitively healthy individuals [1–7] and such increased levels probably reflect degeneration of synapses, which has been linked to the cognitive decline [8, 9]. Contrary to CSF, neurogranin in plasma does not differ between AD patients and controls, indicating that the protein may not be an AD blood biomarker [3, 10]. Yet, in conditions where sudden severe neurological damage occurs, such as in the event of traumatic brain injury (TBI), increased blood neurogranin concentrations have been found. As recently reported, serum neurogranin levels were elevated in TBI patients compared to controls [11]. This urges the need for additional studies examining the potential value of CSF and plasma neurogranin in conditions associated with brain injury, like acute ischemic stroke (AIS). So far, neurogranin has not been investigated in AIS although this condition is also characterized by sudden brain damage [12].

We therefore studied neurogranin in paired CSF/plasma samples of individuals who have suffered from AIS (n = 50). We analyzed CSF and plasma levels on

* Correspondence: Eugeen.vanmechelen@adxneurosciences.com
[1]ADx NeuroSciences NV, Technologiepark 4, 9052 Ghent, Belgium
Full list of author information is available at the end of the article

admission to the hospital, as well as plasma concentrations of neurogranin at different time points after stroke onset. For each of these time points, the relationship was explored between neurogranin levels and stroke severity (as defined by the National Institutes of Health Stroke Scale (NIHSS) [13]), as well as long-term stroke outcome (represented by the modified Rankin Scale (mRS) [14]) and infarct volume. To enable a further assessment of neurogranin as biomarker reflecting stroke characteristics, we performed analysis on protein tau as well. Although, to the best of our knowledge, there have been no studies up to date in paired CSF/plasma samples from AIS patients, the brain injury coherent with stroke is seemingly reflected by elevated levels of tau, in both CSF and plasma [15–20]. In the current study, we verified the correlation between tau levels and stroke characteristics.

Methods

Study population

The study population is part of the Middelheim's Interdisciplinary Stroke Study, a project on the clinical, biochemical, neuroimaging, electrophysiological, and neuropsychological evaluation of AIS patients. These individuals were admitted to the stroke unit of Ziekenhuis Netwerk Antwerpen (ZNA)-Middelheim hospital between October 2005 and February 2008. All patients with suspicion of a cerebrovascular accident or transient ischemic attack were assessed for eligibility: patients were included if clinical evaluation and neuroimaging of the brain (within 24 h after admission) were consistent with AIS. A transient ischemic attack was defined as a clinical presentation believed to be secondary to focal cerebral ischemia, but with symptoms lasting less than 1 h and without proof of acute infarction on structural neuroimaging [21, 22]. Biochemical analyses from the Middelheim's Interdisciplinary Stroke Study project have been reported elsewhere [23–26].

At admission, CSF sampling was performed 8.7 h (6.2 h) (mean (standard deviation)) after onset of stroke symptoms as well as blood collection (5.2 h (5.8 h) after stroke onset). Plasma samples were available at admission and at minimal 3 consecutive time points after stroke onset: at 24 h, 72 h, 7 days, 1 month and/or 3 months post-stroke. CSF samples were obtained by lumbar puncture at the L3/L4 or L4/L5 interspaces, using a 20 Gauge, 3.5 in. Quincke point spinal needle (BD, Belgium), collected in polypropylene cryovials (Nalgene, cat.no.5000–1020 and 5000–0050), immediately frozen in liquid nitrogen and stored at −80 °C until analysis. Venous blood samples were collected in 4.9 mL tubes containing EDTA (Sarstedt Monovette, Germany) and immediately centrifuged at 4000 g during 10 min. Plasma was frozen in liquid nitrogen before storing at −80 °C at the biobank facilities.

The NIHSS was used to assess the neurological deficit by qualified stroke physicians at admission. A NIHSS cut-off score of ≤7 and >8 was used to dichotomize the study population based on stroke severity. To estimate the infarct volume, all patients underwent magnetic resonance imaging (MRI) of the brain at admission or during the first week after stroke onset. The infarct volume was assessed on diffusion weighted MRI by two independent raters as described before [27], using the public domain software Image J (NIH, Bethesda, Md, http://rsb.info.nih.gov/ij). All lesion areas were manually outlined on a slice-by-slice basis and volumes were automatically produced by the multiplication of the total lesion area times the sum of slice thickness and interslice gap. The final infarct volume was calculated as the mean of the infarct volumes obtained by the two raters. The distance between brain infarct and the lateral ventricles was assessed as well. Long-term functional outcome of the AIS was evaluated using the mRS. A favorable outcome was defined by mRS 0 to 3 and a poor outcome as mRS 4 to 6, which is a commonly used and accepted method for dichotomization of the mRS score [28]. From all but one patient, data were available on the CSF/serum albumin ratio, calculated as previously described [29].

Neurogranin in CSF and plasma

To measure neurogranin in both CSF and plasma, we used a research ELISA described in our previous study [30]. This assay, based on two mouse monoclonal antibodies (mAbs), i.e. ADx403 (clone ADxNGCI2) and ADx451 (clone ADxNGCT1), quantifies specifically neurogranin fragments that are C-terminally truncated at P75. This type of neurogranin is the most abundant form circulating in CSF and plasma based on mass spectrometry data [10]. CSF samples, in duplicate, were analyzed undiluted, whereas plasma samples, also in duplicate, were diluted 1:20 in sample diluent preceding analysis (15 μL). The serial plasma samples were analyzed anonymously, i.e. samples were randomized. Final concentrations of neurogranin in both CSF and plasma were intrapolated (log(X); 5PL) based on a synthetic peptide calibrator. For the analysis of CSF, both the intra-assay (n = 2) and inter-plate (n = 2) variability of the ELISA was 5% coefficient of variation (CV), based on three run validation (RV) samples with different neurogranin concentrations. For plasma, RV samples with low, mid and high concentrations were quantified, resulting in an intra-assay (n = 2) variability of 3%, 2% and 5%CV, and an inter-plate (n = 9) precision of 8%, 10% and 14%.

Total-tau in CSF and plasma

To measure total protein levels of tau in CSF, we used the total-tau ELISA by Euroimmun (Lübeck, Germany).

The kit includes lyophilized, ready-to-use calibrators, a standardized protocol, and was performed according to the kit-insert. All CSF samples were run in duplicate. Intra-assay (n = 2) variability was 4%CV for RV samples with a low or a high tau concentration. Inter-plate (n = 2) precision was 3% and 4%CV respectively.

For quantification of total-tau levels in plasma samples, an in-house research prototype ELISA was used [3]. Undiluted plasma samples were analyzed in duplicate. Tau levels were calculated via intrapolation (log(X); 5PL) based on the calibrator, i.e. *E.coli* recombinant tau 441 (rPeptide, USA), but the quantifications were expressed as arbitrary units (AU) since this concerns a not yet fully developed research assay. The research ELISA enabled detection of tau in 92% of the plasma samples. Two RV samples with different tau levels were run in parallel with the patient samples, resulting in an intra-plate (n = 2) variability of 5% and 3%CV, and inter-plate (n = 9) precision of 8% and 5%.

Tau plasma levels were also measured using the Simoa assay by Quanterix (Boston, USA), as described elsewhere [31, 32], for which samples, in duplicate, were diluted 4-fold. Based on two samples with different tau concentrations, intra-assay (n = 2) variability was 11% and 3%CV, whereas inter-mediate (n = 4) precision was 11% and 5%CV. Tau could be quantified in all plasma samples.

As in case of the analysis of neurogranin, tau levels were quantified in randomized plasma samples, blinded from the test performer.

Statistical analysis

GraphPad Prism 6 was used for statistical analyses and figures. To test normality of data, a Shapiro-Wilk test was performed. In case of a non-normal distribution, all subsequent analyses were based on log-transformed data. To compare quantitative data between two groups, a Mann-Whitney test was applied, whereas correlations were determined using Pearson's correlation analysis. Results were considered significant for P-values <0.05.

Results

Study population

Demographic and stroke-related characteristics, as well as stroke syndrome and TOAST (Trial of Org 10,172 in Acute Stroke Treatment) classification are summarized in Table 1. The study population included 23 female and 27 male patients, with mean age at stroke onset 71 ± 14 years. At month 3, 39 patients had a favorable outcome (mRS 0–3) and 11 patients had a poor outcome (mRS 4–6). Of these 11 patients with a poor outcome, 8 died within 3 months after stroke (mRS at month 3 = 6). At month 12, there were 33 patients with a favorable outcome, whereas 10 patients had a poor outcome. Eight of these patients with a poor outcome died within 3 months after stroke, one patient died between month 3 and 12. For the 9 patients who died during follow-up, the cause of death was documented: related to stroke (5 patients), hepatocellular carcinoma (1 patient), post-operative complications of a coronary artery bypass (1 patient) or unknown (2 patients). For 7 patients, the mRS scale was not available at month 12.

Table 1 Summary of the demographic, clinical and biomarker data of the AIS patients

Patient characteristics	
Age (years)	71 (±14)
Gender (female/male)	23/27
Time to CSF sampling, at admission (h)	8.7 (± 6.2)
Time to plasma sampling, at admission (h)	5.2 (± 5.8)
Stroke characteristics	
Ischemic stroke/ transient ischemic attack	40/10
NIHSS at admission	6.8 (±7.8)
mRS at 3 months	2.4 (±1.9)
mRS at 12 months	2.1 (±2.3)[a]
Infarct volume (mL)	26.0 (±50.1)[b]
Shortest distance between infarct and ventricles (mm)	5.5 (±8.6)[b]
Stroke syndrome:	
- Lacunar stroke syndrome	8 (±16.0)
- Partial anterior circulation syndrome	20 (±40.0)
- Total anterior circulation stroke	8 (±16.0)
- Posterior circulation syndrome	12 (±24.0)
TOAST classification:	
- Lacunar	8 (±16.0)
- Atherothrombotic	6 (±12.0)
- Cardioemboligenic	17 (±34.0)
- Specific	4 (±8.0)
- Undetermined	13 (±26.0)
- Mimic	2 (±4.0)
Biochemical analysis at admission	
CSF neurogranin (pg/mL)	380 (279–482)
CSF tau (pg/mL)	434 (322–535)

Data are represented as mean (±standard deviation) or median values (interquartiles) as appropriate

[a] n = 43 since for seven patients mRS at 12 m was not available

[b] MRI data was available for a subset of patients: n = 33

CSF neurogranin and tau in relation to stroke severity and outcome

In Table 1, the median CSF concentrations of neurogranin and tau are represented. There was a strong correlation between CSF levels of these two analytes (Pearson's correlation coefficient r = 0.608; P < 0.0001).

Furthermore, CSF levels from tau were correlated to stroke severity, represented by the NIHSS values at admission (Table 2). CSF tau was also significantly correlated with mRS score at 12 months after stroke ($r = 0.403$; $P < 0.01$). Notably, there was no correlation between CSF levels of tau and the distance of the infarct to the lateral ventricles, whereas for neurogranin, an inverse relationship was noted ($r = -0.545$; $P < 0.05$). No significant association was seen between the CSF analytes and infarct volume. Yet, in case the infarct volume was dichotomized at 5 mL, CSF neurogranin, but not CSF tau, was significantly increased in the subset of patients with an infarct volume greater than 5 mL ($P < 0.05$) (Fig. 1). Receiver Operating Curve (ROC) analysis demonstrated an Area Under the ROC Curve (AUC)-value of 0.704 ($P < 0.05$).

Neurogranin and tau in plasma of stroke patients

In this study, all consecutive plasma samples were analyzed in duplicate by ELISA (for neurogranin) or by ELISA and Simoa technology (for tau). A few number of samples were re-analyzed since the %CV between duplicates was above 20%, i.e. $n = 5$ for neurogranin, $n = 7$ for tau by ELISA and $n = 5$ for tau by Simoa. As consecutive plasma samples from patients were always run on the same plate, the entire patient's series was re-analyzed in that case. Since plasma tau levels obtained by ELISA correlated significantly with levels quantified by the Simoa assay ($r = 0.678$; $P < 0.0001$) (see Additional file 1), only tau levels resulting from ELISA are discussed in the following paragraphs, unless stated otherwise.

Plasma levels of neurogranin and tau are depicted as median values with interquartile range in Fig. 2. There was no strong relationship between neurogranin and tau in plasma. Levels of both analytes only correlated weakly ($r = 0.313$; $P < 0.05$) 7 days after stroke onset.

At none of the time points, CSF and plasma levels of neurogranin were correlated. CSF tau levels were related to plasma tau levels at admission ($r = 0.353$; $P < 0.05$) and 1 m after stroke onset ($r = 0.357$; $P < 0.05$).

Plasma neurogranin did not correlate with stroke severity, as represented by NIHSS, nor with long-term outcome, i.e. with mRS at 3 months or 12 months after stroke, at any of the time points (Table 3). A relationship was observed between infarct volume, measured at admission, and concentrations of plasma neurogranin at 24 h ($r = 0.510$; $P < 0.01$) and 72 h ($r = 0.478$; $P < 0.01$) after stroke onset. Notably, plasma levels of neurogranin 72 h after stroke were weakly inversely related to the CSF/serum ratio of albumin ($r = -0.330$; $P < 0.05$) and, at 3 months after stroke onset, to the distance between the infarction and the ventricles ($r = -0.688$; $P < 0.05$). Stronger correlations with stroke characteristics were seen for tau. Plasma levels of tau were significantly related to stroke severity, stroke outcome as well as infarct volume at several time points after stroke (Table 3).

To further explore the value of plasma tau in reflecting stroke characteristics, we calculated the AUC-values for the analyte at each time point, wherefore stroke severity or outcome were dichotomized. As illustrated in Table 4, strong predictive power was demonstrated at time points between 24 h and 1 m after stroke onset. When assessing the AUC-values based on tau quantified by the Simoa assay, which allowed quantification of tau-levels in an additional 22 samples, statistical significance increased at time points (see Additional file 2).

Discussion

Although progressive brain damage, as in case of AD, is clearly not reflected in plasma levels of neurogranin, it remains to be investigated how acute brain injury affects the blood levels. In the current study, we focused on acute ischemic stroke and observed a relationship between increased plasma neurogranin and infarct volume. Yet, neither stroke severity nor long-term outcome were reflected by neurogranin in plasma, or CSF. Levels of axonal protein tau, on the other hand, were significantly associated with stroke severity and long-term outcome, indicating that different neuronal proteins may entail different kinds of information, at least in AIS.

Due to the high plasma concentrations of neurogranin in normal individuals, i.e. more than 1000 pg/mL, small increases are possibly not detected in plasma in case of slow progressive neurodegeneration like AD [3, 10]. Only in conditions of acute severe brain trauma, such as TBI, neurogranin may serve as potential plasma biomarker. Serum neurogranin concentrations in TBI cases were recently reported as significantly higher than in controls [11]. In our study on AIS, we monitored plasma neurogranin from admission to the hospital until 3 months post-stroke. This aspect was suggested in the recent study [11] on neurogranin in TBI since this could offer insights in the temporal profile of the protein in blood, following acute brain damage. We observed a trend in increasing plasma levels of the protein, with the highest concentration at 3 m. Blood brain barrier

Table 2 Pearson's correlation analysis of the relationship between CSF neurogranin or CSF tau, and stroke characteristics

Analyte	NIHSS admission	mRS 3 months	mRS 12 months	Infarct volume	Distance to ventricles
CSF neurogranin	−0.075	−0.140	−0.061	0.274	**−0.545***
CSF tau	**0.356***	0.219	**0.403****	0.235	−0.216

The correlation coefficient is presented with the corresponding statistical significance (*$P < 0.05$; **$P < 0.01$). Values with statistical significance are in bold and underlined

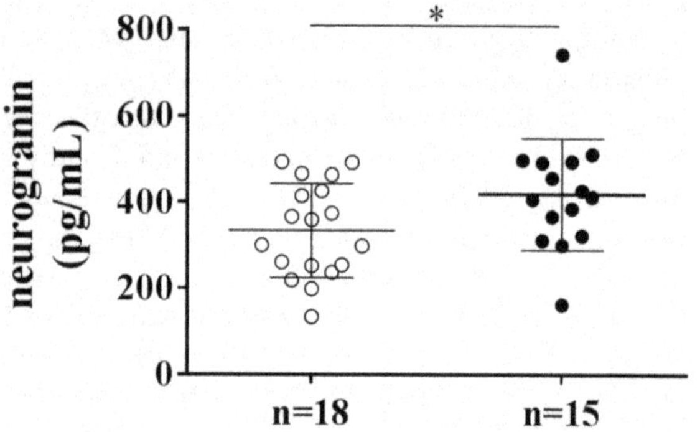

Fig. 1 Scatter dot plot of neurogranin in CSF in case infarct volume was dichotomized at 5 mL. The median levels are represented as a line in each dot plot, whereas the bars represent the interquartile range. The open circles represent patient neurogranin levels in case of an infarct volume of 5 mL or smaller (n = 18), while the black circles depict a volume greater than 5 mL (n = 15). The statistically significant difference between the two groups of stroke patients is represented by * = $P < 0.05$

dysfunction has been reported in stroke [33], which could allow progressive leakage of brain-derived neurogranin into the plasma. However, this contradicts the observation of the lowest plasma neurogranin levels at 72 h being inversely related to a high CSF/serum albumin ratio, suggesting that lower neurogranin levels may be linked to a dysfunctional blood brain barrier. To the best of our knowledge, this is the first report on neurogranin in AIS and further studies are needed, preferentially in moderate or even severe conditions of brain damage. Based on the relatively low NIHSS scores, the patients suffered from a mild stroke in the current study, which is corroborated by the rather low CSF tau values at admission. CSF tau has been reported to substantially increase in case of stroke, i.e. about a 4-fold increase in case of higher NIHSS values [15]. Hence, more severe stroke may result in higher neurogranin levels. Nonetheless, our current dataset suggests that neurogranin may not have great value as plasma biomarker, or as CSF biomarker, for acute brain injury in case of stroke. Besides only observing a trend in increasing levels in function of time, plasma levels were inversely related to the distance between the infarct and the ventricles, which represents a confounding factor. In case the infarct occurs at a larger distance from the ventricles, this could lead to a possible underestimate of the infarct volume. Moreover, even though levels in plasma and CSF of neurogranin were significantly associated with infarct volume, levels were not related to stroke severity, neither to long-term outcome, which are clinical relevant characteristics. Perhaps neurogranin could still have value as biomarker, reflecting infarct volume, when combined with other proteins, such as GFAP, and UCH-L1, which show potential in case of TBI [34, 35]. Or, it could even be combined with tau since our findings are strongly indicative for a high performance of tau, even as single analyte, as measure for stroke severity and outcome in AIS.

Plasma tau significantly peaked 7 days after stroke, where levels were linked to stroke severity, i.e. NIHSS, long-term outcome, represented by the mRS, as well as infarct volume, which confirms prior reports [19, 20]. No relationship with the distance between the infarct and the ventricles, nor with the CSF/serum albumin ratio was seen at that time point. Similarly, CSF levels of tau, which correlated to the plasma levels of the protein, were related to NIHSS assessment at admission and mRS rating 12 months after stroke. This result was in line with previously published studies on tau in CSF from AIS patients [15, 17, 36]. Interestingly, CSF tau at admission was not associated with infarct volume unlike plasma tau. Since plasma tau only peaked 7 days after stroke, it is plausible that CSF tau does not adequately reflects infarct volume at admission, but rather 72 h to 1 week after stroke onset. This was actually suggested by Hesse and colleagues, who demonstrated increasing CSF tau levels over time that peaked one or 3 weeks after stroke onset. Only at maximum CSF tau concentrations, there was a correlation with infarct volume [16, 17]. This corroborates earlier findings on higher CSF tau levels in patients with large infarcts in the subacute stage, i.e. less

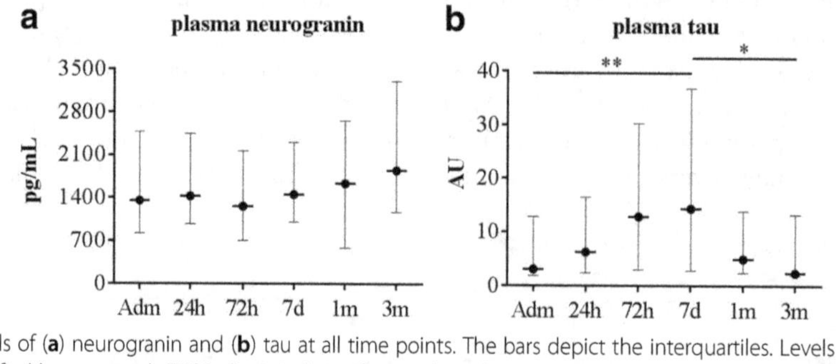

Fig. 2 Median plasma levels of (**a**) neurogranin and (**b**) tau at all time points. The bars depict the interquartiles. Levels of tau are represented as arbitrary units, since quantified by a research ELISA. Statistical significance, based on Tukey's multiple comparison analyses on log-transformed data, is represented by * = $P < 0.05$, ** = $P < 0.01$

Table 3 Pearson's correlation analysis of the relationship between plasma neurogranin or tau and stroke characteristics

Plasma neurogranin	NIHSS admission	mRS 3 m	mRS 12 m	Infarct volume	Distance to ventricles	CSF/serum albumin ratio
Admission	−0.073	−0.214	−0.214	0.288	−0.212	−0.186
24 h	−0.037	0.067	0.024	**0.510****	−0.132	−0.163
72 h	0.135	0.114	−0.038	**0.478****	−0.115	**−0.330***
7d	−0.110	−0.144	−0.192	0.330	−0.249	−0.266
1 m	−0.003	−0.207	−0.149	0.353	−0.154	−0.218
3 m	0.201	0.078	0.203	0.231	**−0.688***	−0.007
Admission	0.230	0.201	0.143	**0.380***	**−0.503***	0.236
24 h	**0.379***	0.286	0.233	**0.528****	**−0.492***	0.197
72 h	**0.451****	**0.434****	**0.411****	**0.614*****	−0.302	0.202
7d	**0.484*****	**0.459****	**0.465****	**0.753******	−0.408	0.063
1 m	0.120	0.314	0.295	0.392	−0.138	0.202
3 m	−0.239	0.203	−0.050	0.243	−0.474	0.021

The correlation coefficient is presented with the corresponding statistical significance (*$P < 0.05$; **$P < 0.01$; ***$P < 0.001$; ****$P < 0.0001$). The values with statistical significance are in bold and underlined

than 1 month after stroke onset, compared to patients in the acute stage, i.e. less than 1 week [37]. Importantly, the latter report mentioned that even small infarct volumes resulted in elevated CSF tau levels several days after stroke.

Although plasma tau was the best candidate biomarker in the current study, compared to neurogranin, the search continues for non-invasive AIS biomarkers providing an early evaluation of the stroke. Ideally, physicians can gauge the severity and long-term outcome of the acute brain damage on admission to the hospital. Most likely this will be enabled by analysis of a panel of proteins, possibly including plasma tau.

Table 4 Value of tau as plasma AIS biomarker reflecting stroke severity and long-term outcome

		AUC value	*P*-value
NIHSS	At admission	0.581	0.355
	24 h	**0.701**	**0.022**
	72 h	**0.751**	**0.004**
	7d	**0.730**	**0.009**
	1 m	0.672	0.113
	3 m	0.518	0.890
mRS 12 m	At admission	0.638	0.198
	24 h	0.645	0.180
	72 h	**0.750**	**0.019**
	7d	**0.804**	**0.005**
	1 m	**0.850**	**0.027**
	3 m	0.783	0.348

Severity (NIHSS) or outcome at 12 months (mRS 12 m) were first dichotomized: patients with NIHSS scores ≤7 were pooled versus NIHSS >7, or with mRS scores 0–3 versus scores 4–6. ROC analysis was performed at all time points on both groups for tau, quantified by ELISA. Statistically significant AUC-values are in bold font and underlined

Conclusion

Based on the present findings, we conclude that neuronal proteins like neurogranin and tau do not entail the same information in brain injury concurring with acute ischemic stroke. Neurogranin may be a plasma biomarker for acute ischemic stroke, unlike for AD, by reflecting infarct volume. However, plasma tau has added clinical relevant value compared to neurogranin, since plasma levels of this analyte reflect stroke severity and long-term outcome. Also in CSF, tau is the most promising candidate biomarker for stroke.

Additional files

Additional file 1: Correlation.tiff. Correlation analysis of plasma tau levels measured with the ELISA ($n = 241$) or Simoa ($n = 263$) assay. The Pearson's correlation coefficient, on log-transformed data, was 0.678 ($P < 0.0001$).

Additional file 2: Plasma AIS biomarker tau.xls. Value of tau as plasma AIS biomarker reflecting stroke severity and long-term outcome. Severity (NIHSS) or outcome at 12 months (mRS 12 m) were first dichotomized: patients with NIHSS scores ≤7 were pooled versus NIHSS >7, or with mRS scores 0–3 versus scores 4–6. ROC analysis was performed at all time points on both groups for tau, quantified by Simoa. Statistical significant AUC-values are depicted in bold font and underlined.

Abbreviations

AD: Alzheimer's disease; AIS: Acute ischemic stroke; AU: Arbitrary units; AUC: Area under the curve; CSF: Cerebrospinal fluid; CV: Coefficient of variation; ELISA: Enzyme linked immunoSorbent assay; MRI: Magnetic resonance imaging; mRS: Modified rankin scale; NFL: Neurofilament light; NIHSS: National institutes of health stroke scale; ROC: Receiver operating characteristic; RV: Run validation; Simoa: Single molecule array; TBI: Traumatic brain injury; TOAST: Trial of Org 10,172 in acute stroke treatment; ZNA: Ziekenhuis Netwerk Antwerpen

Acknowledgements

The authors would like to acknowledge Kimberley Mauroo, Cindy François and Erik Stoops for their technical work on the development of the neurogranin ELISA.

Funding

This work was funded in part by the Agency for Innovation by Science and Technology (VLAIO, www.vlaio.be, grant nr 140,105); University of Antwerp Research Fund; the Alzheimer Research Foundation (SAO-FRA, http://alzh.org); the Institute Born-Bunge (IBB, www.bornbunge.be); the Belgian Science Policy Office Interuniversity Attraction Poles (IAP) program (BELSPO, www.belspo.be); the Flemish Government initiated Methusalem excellence grant (EWI, www.ewi-vlaanderen.be); the Flanders Impulse Program on Networks for Dementia Research (VIND); the Research Foundation Flanders (FWO, www.fwo.be); VINNOVA; the Swedish Research Council (www.vr.se/inenglish); the Swedish Brain Foundation (www.hjarnfonden.se) and Torsten Söderberg Foundation at the Royal Swedish Academy of Sciences. The funding sources had no role in the design of the study and collection, analysis, and interpretation of data and in writing the manuscript.

Authors' contributions

ADV: conception and design of the study, analysis and interpretation of the data, first drafting and revising the manuscript. MB: analysis and interpretation of the data, revising the manuscript. RB: conception and design of the study, analysis and interpretation of the data, revising the manuscript. NDR: conception and design of the study, acquisition of the data. DJ and LVdA: acquisition and analysis of the data, revising the manuscript. KG: interpretation of the data, revising the manuscript. HZ: design of the study, interpretation of the data, revising the manuscript. KB: design of the study, interpretation of the data, revising the manuscript. SE: conception and design of the study, analysis and interpretation of the data, revising the manuscript. EV: conception and design of the study, analysis and interpretation of the data, revising the manuscript. All authors read and approved the final manuscript.

Competing interests

ADV and DJ are both employee and shareholder of ADx NeuroSciences. RB was/is consultant for Pfizer, Medtronic, Shire Human Genetics Therapies, Sanofi-Aventis, Boehringer Ingelheim, Daiichi Sankyo, Amen, Bayer, and is co-founder of Zebra Academy cvba. HZ and KB are co-founders of Brain Biomarker Solutions in Gothenburg AB, a GU Venture-based platform company at the University of Gothenburg. KB has served as consultant and at advisory boards for Fujirebio Europe, IBL International and Roche Diagnostics. SE was/is consultant for and/or received research funding from Janssen, ADx NeuroSciences, Innogenetics/Fujirebio Europe, Nutricia/Danone and Lilly. EV is co-founder of ADx NeuroSciences. MB, NDR, LVdA and KG have nothing to disclose.

Author details

[1]ADx NeuroSciences NV, Technologiepark 4, 9052 Ghent, Belgium. [2]Reference Center for Biological Markers of Dementia (BIODEM), Institute Born-Bunge, University of Antwerp, Antwerp, Belgium. [3]Department of Neurology, Hospital ZorSaam, Terneuzen, The Netherlands. [4]Department of Neurology and Memory Clinic, Hospital Network Antwerp (ZNA) Middelheim and Hoge Beuken, Antwerp, Belgium. [5]Clinical Neurochemistry Laboratory, Sahlgrenska University Hospital, Mölndal, Sweden. [6]Institute of Neuroscience and Physiology, Department of Psychiatry and Neurochemistry, the Sahlgrenska Academy at the University of Gothenburg, Mölndal, Sweden. [7]Department of Molecular Neuroscience, UCL Institute of Neurology, London, UK.

References

1. Thorsell A, Bjerke M, Gobom J, Brunhage E, Vanmechelen E, Andreasen N, et al. Neurogranin in cerebrospinal fluid as a marker of synaptic degeneration in Alzheimer's disease. Brain Res. 2010;1362:13–22.
2. Kvartsberg H, Duits FH, Ingelsson M, Andreasen N, Öhrfelt A, Andersson K, et al. Cerebrospinal fluid levels of the synaptic protein neurogranin correlates with cognitive decline in prodromal Alzheimer's disease. Alzheimers Dement. 2015a;11:1180–90.
3. De Vos A, Jacobs D, Struyfs H, Fransen E, Andersson K, Portelius E, Andreasson U, et al. C-terminal neurogranin is increased in cerebrospinal fluid but unchanged in plasma in Alzheimer's disease. Alzheimers Dement. 2015;11:1461–9.
4. Kester MI, Teunissen CE, Crimmins DL, Herries EM, Ladenson JH, Scheltens P, et al. Neurogranin as a cerebrospinal fluid biomarker for synaptic loss in symptomatic Alzheimer disease. JAMA Neurol. 2015;72:1275–80.
5. Portelius E, Zetterberg H, Skillbäck T, Törnqvist U, Andreasson U, Trojanowski JQ, et al. Cerebrospinal fluid neurogranin: relation to cognition and neurodegeneration in Alzheimer's disease. Brain. 2015;138:3373–85.
6. Janelidze S, Hertze J, Zetterberg H, Landqvist Waldö M, Santillo A, Blennow K, Hansson O. Cerebrospinal fluid neurogranin and YKL-40 as biomarkers of Alzheimer's disease. Ann Clin Transl Neurol. 2015;3:12–20.
7. Tarawneh R, D'Angelo G, Crimmins D, Herries E, Griest T, Fagan AM, et al. Diagnostic and prognostic utility of the synaptic marker neurogranin in Alzheimer disease. JAMA Neurol. 2016;73:561–71.
8. Terry RD, Masliah E, Salmon DP, Butters N, DeTeresa R, Hill R, et al. Physical basis of cognitive alterations in Alzheimer's disease: synapse loss is the major correlate of cognitive impairment. Ann Neurol. 1991;30:572–80.
9. Reddy PH, Mani G, Park BS, Jacques J, Murdoch G, Whetsell W, et al. Differential loss of synaptic proteins in Alzheimer's disease: implications for synaptic dysfunction. J Alzheimers Dis. 2005;7:103–17.
10. Kvartsberg H, Portelius E, Andreasson U, Brinkmalm G, Hellwig K, Lelental N, et al. Characterization of the postsynaptic protein neurogranin in paired cerebrospinal fluid and plasma samples from Alzheimer's disease patients and healthy controls. Alzheimers Res Ther. 2015b;7:40.
11. Yang J, Korley FK, Dai M, Everett AD. Serum neurogranin measurement as a biomarker of acute traumatic brain injury. Clin Biochem. 2015;48:843–8.
12. Donnan GA, Fisher M, Macleod M, Davis SM. Stroke. Lancet. 2008;371:1612–23.
13. Brott T, Adams HP, Olinger CP, Marler JR, Barsan WG, Biller J, et al. Measurements of acute cerebral infarction: a clinical examination scale. Stroke. 1989;20:864–70.
14. Duncan PW, Jorgensen HS, Wade DT. Outcome measures in acute stroke trials - a systematic review and some recommendations to improve practice. Stroke. 2000;31:1429–38.
15. Hjalmarsson C, Bjerke M, Andersson B, Blennow K, Zetterberg H, Aberg ND, et al. Neuronal and glia-related biomarkers in cerebrospinal fluid of patients with acute ischemic stroke. J Cent Nerv Syst Dis. 2014;6:54–8.
16. Hesse C, Rosengren L, Vanmechelen E, Vanderstichele H, Jensen C, Davidsson P, Blennow K. Cerebrospinal fluid markers for Alzheimer's disease evaluated after acute ischemic stroke. J Alzheimers Dis. 2000;2:199–206.
17. Hesse C, Rosengren L, Andreasen N, Davidsson P, Vanderstichele H, Vanmechelen E, Blennow K. Transient increase in total tau but not phospho-tau in human cerebrospinal fluid after acute stroke. Neurosci Lett. 2001;297:187–90.
18. Bitsch A, Horn C, Kemmling Y, Seipelt M, Hellenbrand U, Stiefel M, et al. Serum tau protein level as a marker of axonal damage in acute ischemic stroke. Eur Neurol. 2002;47:45–51.
19. Wunderlich MT, Lins H, Skalej M, Wallesch CW, Goertler M. Neuron-specific enolase and tau protein as neurobiochemical markers of neuronal damage are related to early clinical course and long-term outcome in acute ischemic stroke. Clin Neurol Neurosurg. 2006;108:558–63.
20. Bielewicz J, Kurzepa J, Czekajska-Chehab E, Stelmasiak Z, Bartosik-Psujek H. Does serum tau protein predict the outcome of patients with ischemic stroke? J Mol Neurosci. 2011;43:241–5.
21. Adams HP Jr, Bendixen BH, Kappelle LJ, Biller J, Love BB, Gordon DL, Marsh EE 3rd. Classification of subtype of acute ischemic stroke. Definitions for use in a multicenter clinical trial. TOAST. Trial of org 10172 in acute stroke treatment. Stroke. 1993;24:35–41.
22. Albers GW, Caplan LR, Easton JD, Fayad PB, Mohr JP, Saver JL, et al. Transient ischemic attack–proposal for a new definition. N Engl J Med. 2002;347:1713–6.
23. Brouns R, Sheorajpanday R, Wauters A, De Surgeloose D, Mariën P, De Deyn PP. Evaluation of lactate as a marker of metabolic stress and cause of secondary damage in acute ischemic stroke or TIA. Clin Chim Acta. 2008;397:27–31.
24. Willemse JL, Brouns R, Heylen E, De Deyn PP, Hendriks DF. Carboxypeptidase U (TAFIa) activity is induced in vivo in ischemic stroke patients receiving thrombolytic therapy. J Thromb Haemost. 2008;6:200–2.
25. Brouns R, De Vil B, Cras P, De Surgeloose D, Mariën P, De Deyn PP. Neurobiochemical markers of brain damage in cerebrospinal fluid of acute ischemic stroke patients. Clin Chem. 2010;56:451–8.
26. Kehoe K, Brouns R, Verkerk R, Engelborghs S, De Deyn PP, Hendriks D,

De Meester I. Prolyl carboxypeptidase activity decline correlates with severity and short-term outcome in acute ischemic stroke. Neurochem Res. 2015;40:81.

27. Brouns R, Marescau B, Possemiers I, Sheorajpanday R, De Deyn PP. Dimethylarginine levels in cerebrospinal fluid of hyperacute ischemic stroke patients are associated with stroke severity. Neurochem Res. 2009;34:1642–9.
28. Sulter G, Steen C, De Keyser J. Use of the Barthel index and modified Rankin scale in acute stroke trials. Stroke. 1999;30:1538–41.
29. Brouns R, Wauters A, De Surgeloose D, Mariën P, De Deyn PP. Biochemical markers for blood-brain barrier dysfunction in acute ischemic stroke correlate with evolution and outcome. Eur Neurol. 2011;65:23–31.
30. De Vos A, Struyfs H, Jacobs D, Fransen E, Klewansky T, De Roeck E, et al. The cerebrospinal fluid neurogranin/BACE1 ratio is a potential correlate of cognitive decline in Alzheimer's disease. J Alzheimers Dis. 2016;53:1523–38.
31. Mattsson N, Zetterberg H, Janelidze S, Insel PS, Andreasson U, Stomrud E, et al. Plasma tau in Alzheimer disease. Neurology. 2016;87:1827–35.
32. Dage JL, Wennberg AM, Airey DC, Hagen CE, Knopman DS, Machulda MM, et al. Levels of tau protein in plasma are associated with neurodegeneration and cognitive function in a population-based elderly cohort. Alzheimers Dement. 2016;12:1226–34.
33. Yang J, d'Esterre C, Ceruti S, Roversi G, Saletti A, Fainardi E, Lee TY. Temporal changes in blood-brain barrier permeability and cerebral perfusion in lacunar/subcortical ischemic stroke. BMC Neurol. 2015;15:214.
34. Welch RD, Ayaz SI, Lewis LM, Unden J, Chen JY, Mika VH, et al. Ability of serum Glial Fibrillary acidic protein, Ubiquitin C-terminal Hydrolase-L1, and S100B to differentiate normal and abnormal head computed tomography findings in patients with suspected mild or moderate traumatic brain injury. J Neurotrauma. 2016;33:203–14.
35. Bogoslovsky T, Wilson D, Chen Y, Hanlon D, Gill J, Jeromin A, et al. Increases of plasma levels of Glial Fibrillary acidic protein, tau, and Amyloid β up to 90 days after traumatic brain injury. J Neurotrauma. 2016;34:66–73.
36. Strand T, Alling C, Karlsson B, Karlsson I, Winblad B. Brain and plasma proteins in spinal fluid as markers for brain damage and severity of stroke. Stroke. 1984;15:138–44.
37. Kaerst L, Kuhlmann A, Wedekind D, Stoeck K, Lange P, Zerr I. Cerebrospinal fluid biomarkers in Alzheimer's disease, vascular dementia and ischemic stroke patients: a critical analysis. J Neurol. 2013;260:2722–7.

4

Prescription of secondary preventive drugs after ischemic stroke: results from the Malaysian National Stroke Registry

Wen Yea Hwong[1,2*], Zariah Abdul Aziz[3], Norsima Nazifah Sidek[4], Michiel L. Bots[2], Sharmini Selvarajah[2,5], L. Jaap Kappelle[6], Sheamini Sivasampu[1] and Ilonca Vaartjes[2]

Abstract

Background: Evaluation of secondary stroke prevention in low and middle-income countries remains limited. This study assessed the prescription of secondary preventive drugs among ischemic stroke patients upon hospital discharge in Malaysia and identified factors related to the prescribing decisions.

Methods: From Malaysian National Stroke Registry, we included patients with non-fatal ischemic stroke. Prescriptions of antiplatelet, anticoagulants, antihypertensive drugs and lipid-lowering drugs were assessed. Multi-level logistic regressions were performed to determine the relation between potential factors and drug prescriptions.

Results: Of 5292 patients, 48% received antihypertensive drugs, 88.9% antiplatelet and 88.7% lipid-lowering drugs upon discharge. Thirty-three percent of patients with an indication for anticoagulants ($n = 391$) received it. Compared to patients <=50 years, patients above 70 years were less likely to receive antiplatelet (OR: 0.72, 95% CI: 0.50–1.03), lipid-lowering drugs (OR: 0.66, 95% CI: 0.45–0.95) and anticoagulants (OR: 0.27, 95% CI: 0.09–0.83). Patients with moderate to severe disability upon discharge had less odds of receiving secondary preventive drugs; an odds ratio of 0.57 (95% CI: 0.45–0.71) for antiplatelet, 0.86 (95% CI: 0.75–0.98) for antihypertensive drugs and 0.78 (95% CI: 0.63–0.97) for lipid-lowering drugs in comparison to those with minor disability. Having prior specific comorbidities and drug prescriptions significantly increased the odds of receiving these drugs. No differences were found between sexes and ethnicities.

Conclusions: Prescription of antihypertensive drugs and anticoagulants among ischemic stroke patients in Malaysia were suboptimal. Efforts to initiate regular clinical audits to evaluate the uptake and effectiveness of secondary preventive strategies are timely in low and middle-income settings.

Keywords: Brain ischemia, Secondary prevention, Platelet aggregation inhibitors, Anticoagulants, Hydroxymethylglutaryl-CoA reductase inhibitors, Antihypertensive agents

Background

There is a substantial geographical variation for stroke burden between countries of different income levels. The bulk of stroke burden comes from low and middle-income countries (LMIC), accounting for 69% of total incident strokes and 71% of stroke deaths in 2010. The number of disability-adjusted life years (DALYs) for stroke survivors aged below 75 years was 5-times higher in these regions compared to high-income countries [1].

The burden of stroke in LMIC is largely attributable to poor prevention and control of cardiovascular risk factors [2]. Besides primary prevention, part of the burden is potentially modifiable with effective secondary prevention. Stroke patients have a 30% estimated 5-year risk of a recurrent stroke [3]. Regular clinical audits are established to assess control of cardiovascular risk factors for secondary prevention [4] but such structures are particularly lacking in LMIC. Nevertheless, this information is essential because the implementation and uptake of

* Correspondence: w.y.hwong-2@umcutrecht.nl
[1]National Clinical Research Centre, Ministry of Health Malaysia, Kuala Lumpur, Malaysia
[2]Julius Center for Health Sciences and Primary Care, University Medical Center Utrecht, Utrecht, The Netherlands
Full list of author information is available at the end of the article

secondary prevention in LMIC is likely to differ from high-income countries, owing to the disparity in terms of access to health care, average education level and availability of drugs between countries of different income statuses [5].

This study was therefore aimed at evaluating the prescription of secondary preventive drugs upon hospital discharge among ischemic stroke patients in Malaysia, an upper middle-income country. Furthermore, we sought to identify possible factors that influence the likelihood of patients being prescribed with these drugs.

Methods

Participant selection

Participants for this study were selected from cases that were registered in Malaysian National Stroke Registry, a database established under the National Neurology Registry [6]. This database recorded a total of 7592 patients from 14 public hospitals between July 2009 and December 2014. Although the coverage of this registry does not include stroke admissions from private hospitals, this database is the best available representation of the Malaysian stroke population. Moreover, public hospitals cover 66.2% of total hospital admissions for the country in 2014 [7].

For the present study, we included patients who had a diagnosis of non-fatal ischemic stroke upon discharge.

Secondary stroke prevention

We kept to recommendations of the 2012 Malaysian Clinical Practice Guidelines for Management of Ischemic Stroke [8]. The contents are largely similar to the 2011 stroke guidelines published by American Stroke Association [9]. We did not account for evidence from an updated publication for the latter guidelines in 2014. This is to establish a consistency in terms of time frame between dissemination of information from the guidelines and selection of patients for this study.

Prescriptions of three types of drugs were assessed: 1) antithrombotic drugs comprising antiplatelet and anticoagulants; 2) antihypertensive drugs; and 3) lipid-lowering drugs. Indications for long-term anticoagulants in the present analysis included prior history of atrial fibrillation, electrocardiogram showing atrial fibrillation during admission or patients with cardioembolic stroke. Drugs were prescribed upon hospital discharge by treating physicians. Data for the prescription were obtained from medical records. These drugs were coded following the Anatomical Therapeutic Chemical (ATC) Classification, an international classification under the World Health Organization of which drugs are coded based on their active ingredients [10].

Determinant measures

Potential patient-level factors that were studied included 1) demographic characteristics: age, sex, ethnicity and education level; 2) comorbidities and prescriptions recorded prior to the stroke event: previous hypertension, diabetes mellitus, dyslipidemia, atrial fibrillation, ischemic heart disease, previous stroke or transient ischemic attack (TIA) events and prior prescriptions of antiplatelet, anticoagulants, antihypertensive drugs and lipid-lowering drugs; 3) lifestyle factors: obesity and smoking status and 4) status of disability upon discharge that was assessed with Modified Rankin Scale (mRS). A hospital level variable that categorizes hospitals into state and non-state hospitals was also included. State hospitals are classified as hospitals with up to 45 resident specialties or subspecialties and are normally main referral centers for each state. Detailed operationalization of these factors are summarized in Additional file 1: Table S1.

Collection of data for this registry followed local routine clinical practice where it involved collection of existing data that were readily available as part of routine practice. Information on demographic characteristics with the exception of education level was obtained from patient identification cards. Education level was assessed via patient interview. Depending on availability, information on prior co-morbidities, lifestyle factors and drug prescriptions obtained during patient interviews were verified with patients' past medical records from respective general practitioners or availability of drug strips from patients. Clinical diagnosis of an ischemic stroke was confirmed via computed tomographic (CT) imaging where a visible infarct seen on scan confirmed an ischemic stroke. As for disability status, it was measured prior to discharge with mRS. This is a commonly used scale that incorporates both mental and physical adaptations to neurological deficits experienced after a stroke [11, 12]. For the purpose of this study, a score of <3 was considered no or minor disability and a score of $> = 3$ as moderate or severe disability.

Statistical analysis

Proportion of missing data ranged from 0.06% (variable: ischemic heart diseases) to 39% (variable: smoking status). Details on the extent of missingness for each variable are summarized in Additional file 1: Table S1. Missing data were assumed to be missing-at-random and thus, we conducted multiple imputation with $m = 10$ prior to the inclusion of patients for analysis to reduce the extent of bias resulting from missing data [13]. Subsequently, patients who did not fulfil the inclusion criteria were removed from analysis.

As stroke patients were selected within clusters of hospitals, the variable 'Hospital ID' that defines each participating hospital was included as a random effect, to account for variations within and between hospitals. In that respect, multi-level logistic regressions were performed to identify factors that were associated with the likelihood of an ischemic stroke patient being prescribed antiplatelet, antihypertensive drugs and lipid-lowering drugs, respectively. All potential factors were fitted into regression models for the three drugs. Factors with *p*-value <0.05 were considered significant. For anticoagulants, a slightly different model fitting approach was taken as the number of prescriptions (events) were small ($n = 128$). Univariable analysis for each factor was first conducted to assess its possible relation to the outcome. Factors with *p*-value < 0.25 were chosen and subsequently included in a multivariable analysis.

Multiple imputation was conducted with package 'mice' in R version 3.1.1 [14]. Multi-level regression analyses were performed with Stata SE Version 14.3 [15]. Odds ratios with their corresponding 95% confidence intervals were reported.

Results

Patient characteristics

Of 5292 patients, 43% were 60 years old or younger. A majority were of Malay ethnicity and nearly half of the patients had primary education. Table 1 shows that presence of atherosclerotic risk factors was common; 72% had prior hypertension, 47% diabetes mellitus and 32% dyslipidemia. Only 7% had atrial fibrillation. Prior to their hospital admission for ischemic stroke, 40% of patients were receiving antihypertensive drugs, 24% antiplatelet, 28% lipid-lowering drugs and 2%, anticoagulants. Among those with hypertension, 52% ($n = 1960$) were taking antihypertensive drugs. Upon hospital discharge, 62% had moderate to severe disability.

Prescription of secondary preventive drugs

Figure 1 shows that 88.9% (95% CI: 88–90%) were discharged with antiplatelet. Similarly, 88.7% (95% CI: 88–90%) of patients received lipid-lowering drugs. Forty-eight percent (95% CI: 47–49%, $n = 2543$) of patients were discharged with antihypertensive drugs. Of those, 62% of them were on monotherapy. Angiotensin-converting-enzymes inhibitors (ACEIs) recorded the highest number of prescriptions (65%) whereas ACEIs and calcium channel blockers were the most commonly prescribed dual combination.

Among ischemic stroke patients with an indication for long-term anticoagulants ($n = 391$), 33% (95% CI: 28–38%) received it. Figure 2 illustrates the types of antithrombotic drugs prescribed. More than half (52%, 95% CI: 47–57%) were discharged with a single antiplatelet and 4% (95% CI: 2–5%), more than one antiplatelet. There were 12% (95% CI: 8–15%) of the indicated patients who did not receive any antithrombotic drugs.

Table 1 Patient characteristics

Characteristics	Patients Included ($N = 5292$) n (%)
Age category (years)	
< =50	855 (16)
51–60	1413 (27)
61–70	1544 (29)
> 70	1480 (28)
Sex	
Men	2913 (55)
Women	2379 (45)
Ethnic group	
Malay	4392 (83)
Non-Malay	900 (17)
Education level	
Nil	936 (18)
Primary	2455 (46)
Secondary	1685 (32)
Tertiary	216 (4)
Co-morbidities prior to admission	
Hypertension	3798 (72)
Diabetes mellitus	2462 (47)
Dyslipidemia	1665 (32)
Atrial fibrillation[a]	346 (7)
Ischemic heart disease	686 (13)
Previous stroke/TIA[b] events	1166 (22)
Life-style factors	
Smoking	
Never smoked	2634 (50)
Previous smoker (quit >30 days)	1024 (19)
Current smoker	1634 (31)
Obesity	343 (7)
Drug use prior to admission	
Antiplatelet	1283 (24)
Anticoagulants	96 (2)
Antihypertensive drugs	2117 (40)
Lipid-lowering drugs	1490 (28)
Disability scale at discharge (mRS[b])	
< 3	2028 (38)
> =3	3264 (62)

[a]includes patients with documented history of atrial fibrillation and patients with electrocardiogram showing atrial fibrillation during admission for ischemic stroke
[b]TIA = transient ischemic attack; mRS = Modified Rankin Scale

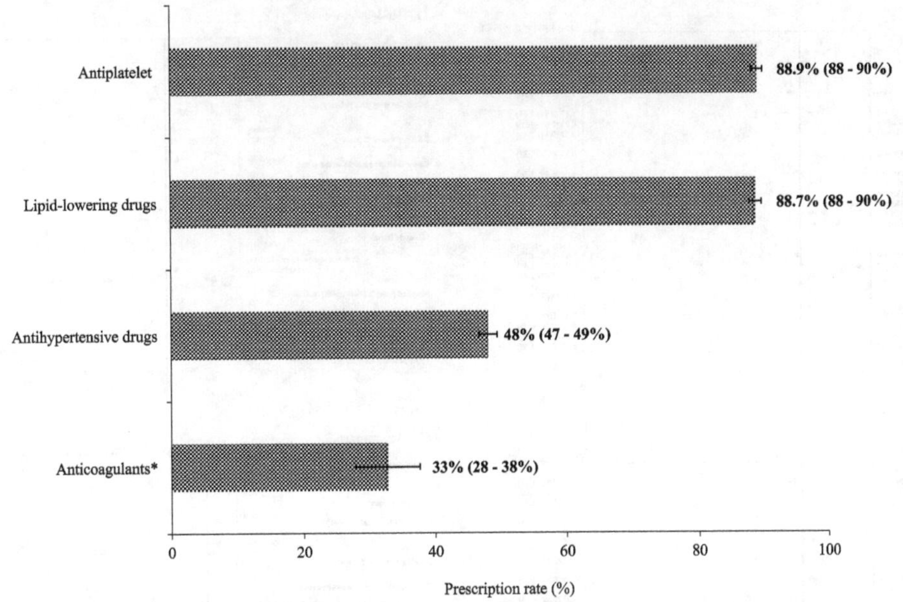

Fig. 1 Prescription of secondary preventive drugs. *for ischemic stroke patients with indications to receive anticoagulants ($n = 391$)

Factors associated with the prescription of secondary preventive drugs (Fig. 3a–d and Additional file 2: Table S2)

Increasing age was associated with less odds of receiving secondary preventive drugs (Fig. 3a–d). Patients above 70 years old were less likely to be discharged with secondary preventive drugs when compared to those aged 50 years and below; an odds ratio of 0.72 (95% CI: 0.50–1.03) for antiplatelet, 0.66 (95% CI: 0.45–0.95) for lipid-lowering drugs and 0.27 (95% CI:0.09–0.83) for anticoagulants. Contrastingly, this association was not observed for the prescription of antihypertensive drugs.

Figure 3a–d displays no differences in the odds of receiving secondary preventive drugs between men and women or their ethnicities. In contrast, patients with moderate to severe disability (mRS > =3) were less likely to be discharged with antiplatelet (OR: 0.57, 95% CI: 0.45–0.71), antihypertensive drugs (OR: 0.86, 95% CI: 0.75–0.98) and lipid-lowering drugs (OR: 0.78, 95% CI:

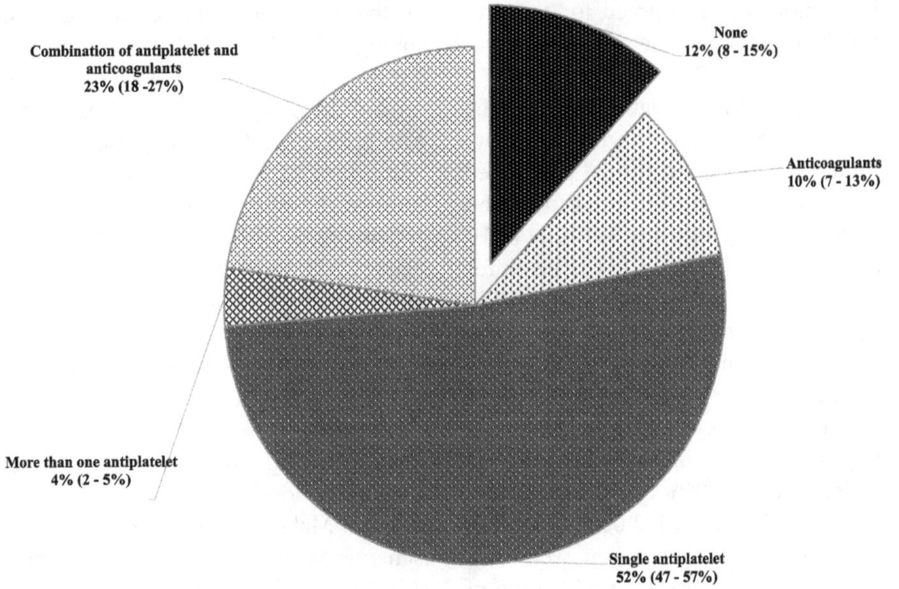

Fig. 2 Types of antithrombotic drugs prescribed among ischemic stroke patients with indications for anticoagulation. ($n = 391$). *exploded slice from the pie chart indicates the proportion of patients who were not prescribed with any antithrombotic drugs

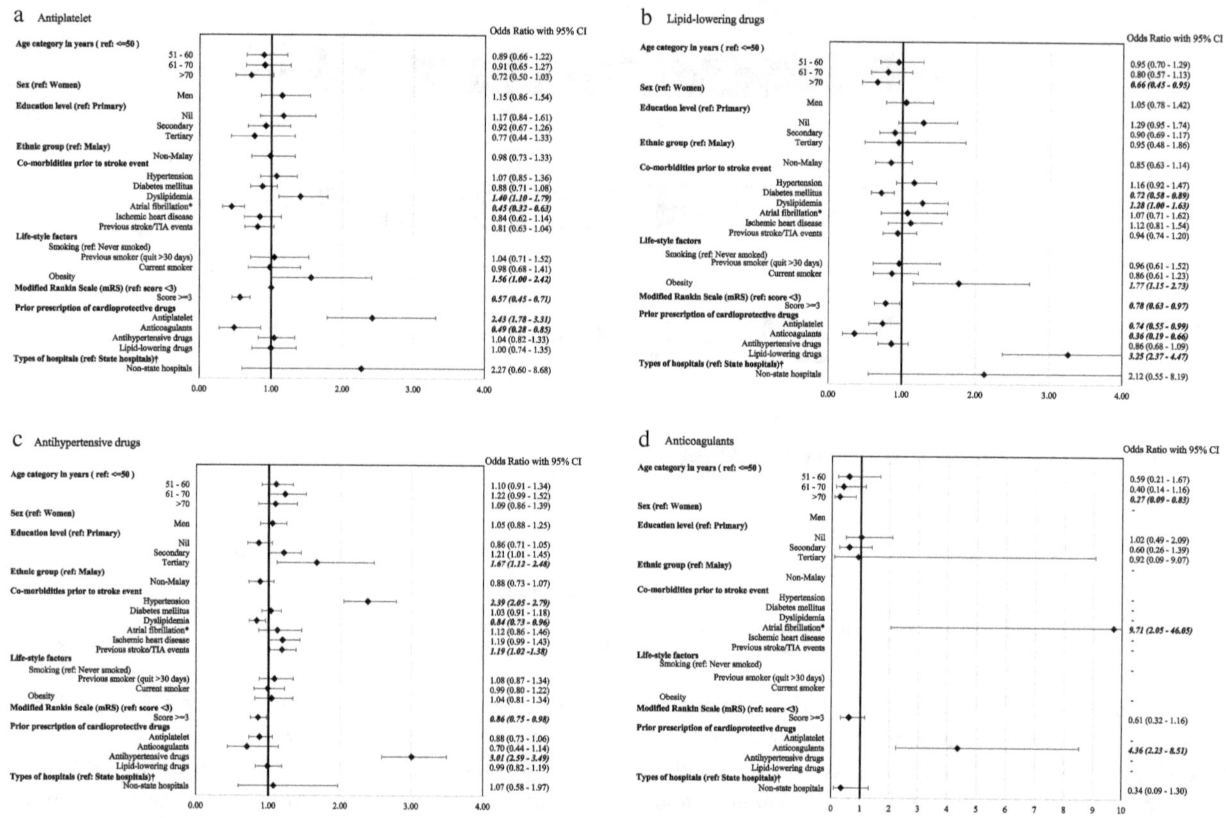

Fig. 3 Factors related to the prescription of secondary preventive drugs among ischemic stroke patients. (Fig. 3 **a**–**d** are results from multivariable analyses, ref. = reference groups, TIA = transient ischemic attack, mRS = Modified Rankin Scale, – = factors were not included in multivariable analysis). *atrial fibrillation includes patients with documented history of atrial fibrillation and patients with electrocardiogram showing atrial fibrillation during admission for ischemic stroke. †state hospitals refer to hospitals with up to 45 resident specialties or subspecialties and are normally main referral centers for each state

0.63–0.97) in comparison to those with minor disability (mRS < 3). This observation was also noted for the prescription of anticoagulants although the association was not significant (OR: 0.61, 95% CI: 0.32–1.16).

Some factors were found to be associated with specific to respective drug prescriptions. Patients with secondary and tertiary education were more likely to be prescribed antihypertensive drugs when compared to those who completed primary education (OR: 1.21, 95% CI: 1.01–1.45 for the former and OR: 1.67, 95% CI: 1.12–2.48 for the latter). There was a 2.4-fold increase (95% CI: 2.05–2.79) in the prescription of antihypertensive drugs in patients with prior hypertension and similarly in those with previous TIA or ischemic stroke, a 19% increase (95% CI: 1.02–1.38) was noted (Fig. 3c).

Patients with dyslipidemia had significantly higher odds of receiving antiplatelet (OR: 1.40, 95% CI: 1.10–1.79) and lipid-lowering drugs (OR: 1.28, 95% CI: 1.00–1.63). Likewise, patients who were obese at admission were also more likely to be prescribed these drugs; an odds ratio of 1.56 (95% CI: 1.00–2.42) for antiplatelet and OR: 1.77 (95% CI: 1.15–2.73) for lipid-lowering drugs. Besides, our findings revealed a 9.7-fold increase (95% CI: 2.05–46.05) in the odds of being discharged with anticoagulants among ischemic stroke patients with atrial fibrillation. Figure 3a–d shows that the odds of receiving secondary preventive drugs significantly increased between 2 to 4-fold with prior respective drug prescription.

In addition, we found a 16% decrease (95% CI: 0.73–0.96) in the odds of receiving antihypertensive drugs in patients with dyslipidemia and similarly, a 28% decrease (95% CI: 0.58–0.89) in the odds of receiving lipid-lowering drugs in diabetic patients. Patients with prior antithrombotic drugs were also less likely to be prescribed with lipid-lowering drugs.

Discussion

Prescription of antihypertensive drugs and anticoagulants upon hospital discharge among ischemic stroke patients in Malaysia were suboptimal. Less than half of the ischemic stroke patients were prescribed antihypertensive drugs and only 1 out of 3 ischemic stroke patients with an indication for long-term anticoagulants received the drug. Increasing age and poorer disability status consistently decreased the odds of receiving secondary preventive drugs upon hospital discharge whereas patients with specific comorbidities prior to admission and who were previously taking the respective drugs were more likely to be treated for secondary prevention. Importantly, prescription of these secondary preventive drugs was not influenced by different sexes and ethnicities.

The high proportion of patients receiving antiplatelet was consistent with previous studies [16–19]. In contrast, a majority of studies reported low prescriptions of lipid-lowering drugs with a range between 31 and 45% [16, 17, 19], with the exception of Thailand [18]. Inclusion of statin prescription as a key performance indicator for stroke management in the country and similarly, in Thailand may explain the larger proportions observed [8, 18].

The low rate of in-hospital initiation of antihypertensive drugs after an ischemic stroke event however, warrants crucial attention. Comparatively, the proportion of antihypertensive drugs received varied within LMIC regions; from 31% in Thailand [18] to 63% in China [19] whereas a higher range between 69 and 77% were observed in high-income countries [17, 20]. While fluctuations in the measurement of blood pressure during hospital admission may had possibly led to a delay in prescription among some patients, there were potentially other contributing factors to the fact that more than half of the patients in our cohort were discharged without an antihypertensive drug. Of importance is the uncertainty to prescribe these drugs to normotensive patients after an ischemic stroke and the extent of lowering their blood pressure levels [21]. Despite this contentious issue, the local guidelines, supported by the international guidelines on secondary stroke prevention in 2011 have recommended the use of antihypertensive drugs, in particular ACE inhibitors as part of secondary preventive therapy in both hypertensive and normotensive patients [8, 9]. Moreover, Thompson et al. [22] showed a significant reduction in the risk of recurrent stroke for non-hypertensive patients who were prescribed antihypertensive drugs (RR: 0.77; 95%CI: 0.61–0.98). It is essential to be aware that initiation of secondary stroke prevention goes beyond solely treating specific risk factors. In addition, despite an increase in the prevalence of hypertension in Malaysia, treatment, awareness and control of the condition remains alarmingly low [23]. This is clearly observed from our findings where only half of the hypertensive patients received antihypertensive drugs prior to admission.

Besides that, the influence of education level on the likelihood of being prescribed antihypertensive drugs upon hospital discharge is of particular interest. The decision to prescribe is often a complex interplay between the prescriber, patient and resources available. Used as a proxy for socioeconomic status and literacy level, patients of higher education levels are more likely to understand the benefits attained with secondary prevention and thus, showed more acceptance towards treatment [24].

Parallel to our findings, a range between 19 and 40% for the prescription of anticoagulants was reported among Asian cohorts in LMIC [18, 25]. Fear of intracranial bleeding as well as difficulties in achieving optimal anticoagulation with warfarin especially among elderly Asians might play a role in the suboptimal prescription of long-term anticoagulants [26]. This is reflected in our findings where younger patients with lower risk of bleeding and those who received the drugs before, were more likely to receive anticoagulants. Locally, the current delivery of stroke care is fragmented, in particular between the points of transfer of care. Besides a lack of post-discharge stroke care guidelines in primary care, resources are restricted especially in rural areas. Follow-up services for post-stroke patients therefore, largely remain within the settings of tertiary centres that are located in the main cities [27]. Nonetheless, this poses several challenges in terms of distance, logistics and convenience for patients. Initiation of treatment such as warfarin that requires frequent monitoring of prothrombin time and dose readjustments are often not possible.

Increase in age and higher mRS score are predictors of recurrent vascular events [28]. While rightfully patients with higher risks of stroke recurrence should be more optimally treated, we found that older patients and those with worse disability were less likely to receive secondary preventive drugs. Although previous studies reported conflicting results on prescription of secondary preventive drugs in older patients, under prescription in older patients could be attributed to issues on increased adverse effects [16]. Comparatively, findings on the relation between disability status and drug prescription were similar to other studies [19, 25]. Restrictions in drug availability within some LMIC may explain such practice but more importantly, this is a reflection of the difficulties faced by physicians in providing the best 'do no harm' care to patients. Patients with poor independence status are generally those with a higher number of co-morbidities. Pill burden may cause non-adherence and an increase risk of adverse drug reactions [29]. Moreover, secondary prevention is perhaps viewed as of little value for these patients because they are perceived to have less to lose with future recurrent events.

Furthermore, we found no differences in the odds of receiving secondary preventive drugs between sexes and ethnicities of the patients. In developing countries where issues of gender and ethnic discriminations ranging from job choices, societal expectations to limited access to education and healthcare are often raised [30], absence of such associations are reassuring facts that these social determinants do not influence a prescriber's decision to treat.

Exact reasons remain to be ascertained so as to why there were less odds in prescribing antihypertensive drugs among patients with prior dyslipidemia and similarly, lipid-lowering drugs for diabetic patients and patients with prior antithrombotic drugs. We postulate the probability of variations in blood pressure and lipid levels after an acute ischemic stroke that can potentially delay the prescription of antihypertensive drugs [31]. Statin precautions such as fear of increased risk for intracranial bleed or raised liver enzymes in diabetic patients with fatty liver disease are among possible reasons [32, 33] Nevertheless, recent evidences are increasingly proving the greater benefits of these drugs over their minimal risks [34]. Thus, unless for absolute contraindications, there is no reason to withhold secondary preventive drugs from these indicated patients.

To the best of our knowledge, we are among the few LMIC regions within Southeast Asia to initiate evaluation of secondary stroke prevention. Our large study sample is of advantage. In addition, we performed multiple imputations to reduce possible bias from missing data. It was not possible, however to identify patients with absolute contraindications to the drugs because reasons for non-prescription were unknown. Comorbidities upon hospital discharge or its proxy measurements were unavailable. Besides, this study is not designed to be nationally representative. Caution should be taken when generalizing the findings to the whole Malaysian stroke population.

Fundamentally, this study sets a benchmark of the current status of secondary stroke care among ischemic stroke patients in Malaysia. These findings imply that it is timely to establish regular assessment on the uptake and effectiveness of these preventive strategies. Establishing collaborations with other countries will allow initiation of such evaluation to be carried out. Among the few examples are the conduct of EUROASPIRE and Survey of Risk Factors audit (SURF) where a standardized method of assessing secondary prevention for cardiovascular diseases is implemented across participating countries to enable comparisons and benchmarking [4, 35]. Findings from the assessment should subsequently be put into use by initiating a continuous feedback system to relevant healthcare professionals and stakeholders. Besides, the need for an improved stroke care model in the country with an emphasis on continuity of care for post-stroke patients at various levels of care should be made a priority. Other targeted plans include organizing regular continuous medical updates to increase prescribers' awareness on the impact of in-hospital initiation of secondary preventive drugs on subsequent improvement in patient adherence and overall survival [36].

Conclusions

In summary, the prescription of antihypertensive drugs and anticoagulants upon hospital discharge among ischemic stroke patients in Malaysia were suboptimal. Our findings revealed a treatment pattern that was influenced by age, disability upon discharge, specific comorbidities and prior drug prescriptions. No differences were found between sexes and ethnicities. Continuous efforts from relevant aspects of healthcare stakeholders are essential to allow better cardiovascular preventive actions to be put into place.

Abbreviations

ATC: Anatomical Therapeutic Chemical; CT: Computed tomographic; DALYs: Disability-adjusted-life-years; LMIC: Low and middle-income countries; mRS: Modified Rankin Scale; TIA: Transient ischemic attack

Acknowledgements

We thank the Director General of Health, Ministry of Health, Malaysia for his permission to publish this manuscript. Our sincere thanks also go to personnel from all participating hospitals for their contribution in the data collection.

Funding

The registry is funded by Ministry of Health Malaysia. Ministry of Health Malaysia had no role in the study design, analysis and preparation of the manuscript. WYH is funded by Julius Center for Health Sciences and Primary Care, University Medical Center Utrecht under the Netherlands Organization for Scientific Research grant (Grant number: 022.005.021). IV is funded by the Dutch Heart Foundation for project Facts and Figures. The Julius Center and the Dutch Heart Foundation had no role in study design, data collection and analysis, decision to publish, or preparation of the manuscript.

Authors' contributions

WYH, MLB and IV were involved in the conception, design, analysis and interpretation of the data as well as drafting of the manuscript. ZAA, NNS, LJK, SS[1] (Sharmini Selvarajah) and SS[2] (Sheamini Sivasampu) were involved in interpretation of the data and revising the manuscript for important intellectual contents. All authors read and approved the final manuscript.

Authors' information

Not applicable.

Competing interests

The authors declare that they have no competing interests.

Author details

[1]National Clinical Research Centre, Ministry of Health Malaysia, Kuala Lumpur, Malaysia. [2]Julius Center for Health Sciences and Primary Care, University Medical Center Utrecht, Utrecht, The Netherlands. [3]Department of Neurology, Hospital Sultanah Nur Zahirah, Kuala Terengganu, Terengganu, Malaysia. [4]Clinical Research Centre, Hospital Sultanah Nur Zahirah, Kuala Terengganu, Terengganu, Malaysia. [5]Sharmini Selvarajah Consulting, Selangor, Malaysia. [6]Department of Neurology and Neurosurgery, Brain Center Rudolf Magnus, University Medical Center Utrecht, Utrecht, The Netherlands.

References

1. Feigin VL, Forouzanfar MH, Krishnamurthi R, Mensah GA, Connor M, Bennett DA, et al. Global and regional burden of stroke during 1990-2010: findings from the global burden of disease study 2010. Lancet. 2014;383:245–54.
2. Who | Cardiovascular Diseases (Cvds): World Health Organization; 2016 [cited 2016 4th October]. Available from: http://www.who.int/mediacentre/factsheets/fs317/en/.
3. Burn J, Dennis M, Bamford J, Sandercock P, Wade D, Warlow C. Long-term risk of recurrent stroke after a first-ever stroke. The Oxfordshire community stroke project. Stroke. 1994;25:333–7.
4. Zhao M, Cooney MT, Klipstein-Grobusch K, Vaartjes I, De Bacquer D, De Sutter J, et al. Simplifying the audit of risk factor recording and control: a report from an international study in 11 countries. Eur J Prev Cardiol. 2016; 23:1202–10.
5. Yusuf S, Islam S, Chow CK, Rangarajan S, Dagenais G, Diaz R, et al. Use of secondary prevention drugs for cardiovascular disease in the Community in High-Income, middle-income, and low-income countries (the pure study): a prospective epidemiological survey. Lancet. 2011;378:1231–43.
6. Nneur: National Neurology Registry: Ministry of Health Malaysia; 2009 [cited 2016 4th October]. Available from: http://acrm.org.my/nneur/.
7. Ministry of Health Virtual Library. Health Facts 2014. Ministry of Health Malaysia; 2014. [cited 2016 4th October]. Available from: http://vlib.moh.gov.my/cms/content.jsp?id=com.tms.cms.document.Document_2e8e997f-a0188549-d5315d00-2d9464b7.
8. Clinical Practice Guidelines. Management of Ischemic Stroke. 2nd Edition ed. Malaysia: Ministry of Health Malaysia; 2012.
9. Furie KL, Kasner SE, Adams RJ, Albers GW, Bush RL, Fagan SC, et al. Guidelines for the prevention of stroke in patients with stroke or transient ischemic attack: a guideline for healthcare professionals from the American Heart Association/American Stroke Association. Stroke. 2010;42:227–76.
10. Whocc - Atc/Ddd Index: WHO Collaborating Centre for Drug Statistics Methodology; 2016 [cited 2016 4th October]. Available from: http://www.whocc.no/atc_ddd_index/.
11. Rankin J. Cerebral vascular accidents in patients over the age of 60. Ii Prognosis Scott Med J. 1957;2:200–15.
12. Sulter G, Steen C, De Keyser J. Use of the Barthel index and modified Rankin scale in acute stroke trials. Stroke. 1999;30:1538–41.
13. McCleary L. Using multiple imputation for analysis of incomplete data in clinical research. Nurs Res. 2002;51:339–43.
14. R Core Team. R: A Language and Environment for statistical computing. Vienna: R Foundation for Statistical Computing; 2014.
15. Corp S. Stata statistical software: release 14.3. College Station: Stata Corp LP; 2013.
16. Asberg S, Henriksson KM, Farahmand B, Asplund K, Norrving B, Appelros P, et al. Ischemic stroke and secondary prevention in clinical practice: a cohort study of 14,529 patients in the Swedish stroke register. Stroke. 2010;41:1338–42.
17. Niewada M, Sarzynska-Dlugosz IM, Skowronska M, Kaminski B, Kobayashi A, Czlonkowska A. Pharmacotherapy prior to and in acute Ischaemic stroke. The use of pharmacotherapy and drug-associated outcomes in real world practice - findings from the polish hospital stroke registry. Neurol Neurochir Pol. 2013;47:509–16.
18. Nilanont Y, Nidhinandana S, Suwanwela NC, Hanchaiphiboolkul S, Pimpak T, Tatsanavivat P, et al. Quality of acute ischemic stroke Care in Thailand: a prospective multicenter countrywide cohort study. J Stroke Cerebrovasc Dis. 2014;23:213–9.
19. Wei JW, Wang JG, Huang Y, Liu M, Wu Y, Wong LK, et al. Secondary prevention of ischemic stroke in urban China. Stroke. 2010;41:967–74.
20. Ovbiagele B, Hills NK, Saver JL, Johnston SC. Antihypertensive medications prescribed at discharge after an acute ischemic cerebrovascular event. Stroke. 2005;36:1944–7.
21. Boan AD, Lackland DT, Ovbiagele B. Lowering of blood pressure for recurrent stroke prevention: topical review. Stroke. 2014;45:2506–13.
22. Thompson AM, Hu T, Eshelbrenner CL, Reynolds K, He J, Bazzano LA. Antihypertensive treatment and secondary prevention of cardiovascular disease events among persons without hypertension: a meta-analysis. JAMA. 2011;305:913–22.
23. Abdul-Razak S, Daher AM, Ramli AS, Ariffin F, Mazapuspavina MY, Ambigga KS, et al. Prevalence, awareness, treatment, control and socio demographic determinants of hypertension in Malaysian adults. BMC Public Health. 2016; 16:351.
24. Dusing R. Overcoming barriers to effective blood pressure control in patients with hypertension. Curr Med Res Opin. 2006;22:1545–53.
25. Yang X, Li Z, Zhao X, Wang C, Liu L, Wang C, et al. Use of warfarin at discharge among acute ischemic stroke patients with Nonvalvular atrial fibrillation in China. Stroke. 2016;47:464–70.
26. Chen CH, Chen MC, Gibbs H, Kwon SU, Lo S, On YK, et al. Antithrombotic treatment for stroke prevention in atrial fibrillation: the Asian agenda. Int J Cardiol. 2015;191:244–53.
27. Abdul Aziz AF, Mohd Nordin NA, Abd Aziz N, Abdullah S, Sulong S, Aljunid SM. Care for Post-Stroke Patients at Malaysian public health Centres: self-reported practices of family medicine specialists. BMC Fam Pract. 2014;15:40.
28. Park JH, Ovbiagele B. Relationship of functional disability after a recent stroke with recurrent stroke risk. Eur J Neurol. 2016;23:361–7.
29. Farrell B, French Merkley V, Ingar N. Reducing pill burden and helping with medication awareness to improve adherence. Can Pharm J (Ott). 2013;146:262–9.
30. Sultana AM, Mohd Zulkefli NE. Discrimination against women in the developing countries: a comparative study. International Journal of Social Science and Humanity. 2012;2
31. Krone W, Nagele H. Effects of Antihypertensives on plasma lipids and lipoprotein metabolism. Am Heart J. 1988;116:1729–34.
32. Amarenco P, Bogousslavsky J, Callahan A, 3rd, Goldstein LB, Hennerici M, Rudolph AE, et al. High-dose atorvastatin after stroke or transient ischemic attack. N Engl J Med 2006;355:549–559.
33. Rzouq FS, Volk ML, Hatoum HH, Talluri SK, Mummadi RR, Sood GK. Hepatotoxicity fears contribute to underutilization of statin medications by primary care physicians. Am J Med Sci. 2010;340:89–93.
34. Flint AC, Conell C, Ren X, Kamel H, Chan SL, Rao VA, et al. Statin adherence is associated with reduced recurrent stroke risk in patients with or without atrial fibrillation. Stroke. 2017;48:1788–94.
35. Euroaspire. A European Society of Cardiology Survey of Secondary Prevention of Coronary Heart Disease: Principal Results. Euroaspire Study Group. European Action on Secondary Prevention through Intervention to Reduce Events. Eur Heart J. 1997;18:1569–82.
36. Fonarow GC. The role of in-hospital initiation of cardiovascular protective therapies to improve treatment rates and clinical outcomes. Rev Cardiovasc Med. 2003;4(Suppl 3):S37–46.
37. Hwong WY, Bots ML, Selvarajah S, Kappelle LJ, Aziz ZA, Sidek NN, et al. Factors Influencing the Prescription of Secondary Preventive Drugs among Ischaemic Stroke Patients in Malaysia European. J Preventive Cardiology. 2017;24(1_suppl):S140–S8.

5

Reperfusion therapy in acute ischemic stroke: dawn of a new era?

Sonu Bhaskar[1,2,3,4,6,7*], Peter Stanwell[7], Dennis Cordato[2,4,5], John Attia[7,8] and Christopher Levi[1,2,3,4,5,6*]

Abstract

Following the success of recent endovascular trials, endovascular therapy has emerged as an exciting addition to the arsenal of clinical management of patients with acute ischemic stroke (AIS). In this paper, we present an extensive overview of intravenous and endovascular reperfusion strategies, recent advances in AIS neurointervention, limitations of various treatment paradigms, and provide insights on imaging-guided reperfusion therapies. A roadmap for imaging guided reperfusion treatment workflow in AIS is also proposed. Both systemic thrombolysis and endovascular treatment have been incorporated into the standard of care in stroke therapy. Further research on advanced imaging-based approaches to select appropriate patients, may widen the time-window for patient selection and would contribute immensely to early thrombolytic strategies, better recanalization rates, and improved clinical outcomes.

Keywords: Stroke, Reperfusion therapy, Prognosis, Endovascular treatment, Neurointervention

Background

An overwhelming number of studies and clinical trials confirm the efficacy of thrombolytic therapy, in a given therapeutic window, in improving the clinical outcome and recovery of acute ischemic stroke (AIS) patients [1–5]. The primary therapeutic goal for patients with AIS is the timely restoration of blood flow to salvageable ischemic brain tissue that is not already infarcted [6]. Reperfusion therapy using thrombolysis, including intravenous (IV) tissue plasminogen activator (tPA) and endovascular interventions such as mechanical thrombectomy (MT), are the only approved treatments for AIS. Both these treatment options have limitations when used as monotherapies. The only pharmaceutical agent approved for the treatment of AIS is IV-rtPA; however, it is not effective in patients with AIS due to large artery occlusion, where the clot burden is very high. In such patients, MT has proven more effective. Currently, the primary criterion for candidate selection in reperfusion is the time from stroke symptom onset. Reperfusion therapy must be administered within a narrow window time of up to 4.5 h after symptom onset for IV-tPA, and up to 6–8 h for endovascular MT. The restriction on IV-tPA treatment beyond 4.5 h disqualifies the majority of stroke patients admitted beyond this time-window (around 85%), thereby drastically limiting the eligible population [7–10].

In this article, we review the literature on the various reperfusion strategies available for AIS patients, and provide insights on potential applications, limitations of various reperfusion strategies and role of imaging in guiding therapy.

Evolution of reperfusion therapy

Thrombolysis, commonly known as “clot-busting”, is a pharmacological treatment using an infusion of analogues of tPA which leads to the breakdown (lysis) of the culprit blood-clot. Thrombolytic drugs dissolve blood clots by activating a proteolytic enzyme, plasminogen, to plasmin. Fibrin molecules provide the structural scaffold for blood clots, and plasmin cleaves cross-linkages between fibrin molecules. Subsequently, the clot becomes soluble and undergoes further degradation through proteolysis by other enzymes, eventually restoring blood flow. Due to their mechanism of action, thrombolytic

* Correspondence: Sonu.Bhaskar@health.nsw.gov.au; Christopher.Levi@unsw.edu.au
[1]Western Sydney University (WSU), School of Medicine, South West Sydney Clinical School, Sydney, NSW 2170, Australia
Full list of author information is available at the end of the article

drugs are also referred to as "plasminogen activators" or "fibrinolytic drugs". The three major classes of plasminogen activators are (i) tPA, (ii) streptokinase (SK), and (iii) urokinase (UK). Thrombolytic drugs differ in the mechanism by which they act on fibrin clots. The sequence that leads to the breakdown of the clot or fibrinolysis by tPA is shown in Fig. 1. At first, tPA binds to clot-bound fibrin. This activates fibrin-bound plasminogen from an inactive form to plasmin, the active form. The enzyme plasmin acts on the fibrin mesh, leading to the breakdown of the fibrin scaffold. Subsequently, the dissolution of the fibrin clot produces circulating fibrin fragments called fibrin degradation products. These products prevent the conversion of fibrinogen to fibrin, which slows down clot formation. The liver and kidney, ultimately clear these products, as well as other proteases. Two serine protease inhibitors, namely plasminogen activator inhibitor-1 and 2 (PAI-1 and PAI-2), endogenously inhibit tPA and UK. Alpha 2-antiplasmin and alpha 2-macroglobulin also act as inhibitors of plasmin. Factors XII, XIIa, and Kallikrein stimulate the process of plasmin formation from plasminogen. On the other hand, another factor called thrombin-activatable fibrinolysis inhibitor (TAFI) alters the fibrin to make it more resistant to plasminogen activated by tPA. Efficacy of thrombolytic drugs depends on the size, location, and age of the clot because of the increased density of fibrin cross-linking which make clots more compact and harder to dissolve the older they are.

Some of the known tPA analogues are Alteplase (Activase®; recombinant tPA (rtPA)), Retaplase (Retavase®) and Tenecteplase (TNK-tPA). Alteplase, the most commonly used thrombolytic drug, is a fibrin-selective analogue of tPA administered intravenously or intra-arterially. It is the only Food and Drug Administration (FDA)-approved thrombolytic agent for the treatment of AIS. rtPA causes lysis of fibrin; thereby dissolving the thrombus and resulting in recanalization of the occluded artery [6]. It has a short half-life (~5 min) and is therefore administered as an IV bolus followed by an infusion. Several trials including the National Institute of Neurological Disorders and Stroke (NINDS) [11] and European Collaborative Acute Stroke Study (ECASS) have demonstrated evidence for the benefit of rtPA for a select group of AIS patients. In comparison to rtPA, TNK-tPA has a greater binding affinity for fibrin, higher resistance to inactivation by PAI-1, and a longer half-life.

Urokinase, also known as urinary-type plasminogen activator (uPA), is found in urine. Clinically, UK is used as a thrombolytic drug in conditions such as pulmonary embolism, myocardial infarction, and severe deep venous thrombosis (DVT). In comparison to rtPA, SK and UK lack fibrin specificity and bind equally to circulating plasminogen and clot-bound plasminogen. On binding with plasminogen, SK forms a complex that activates plasmin, triggering a proteolytic cascade. The proteolytic cascade leads to thrombolysis (clot degradation in AIS) or extracellular matrix degradation (e.g., tissue

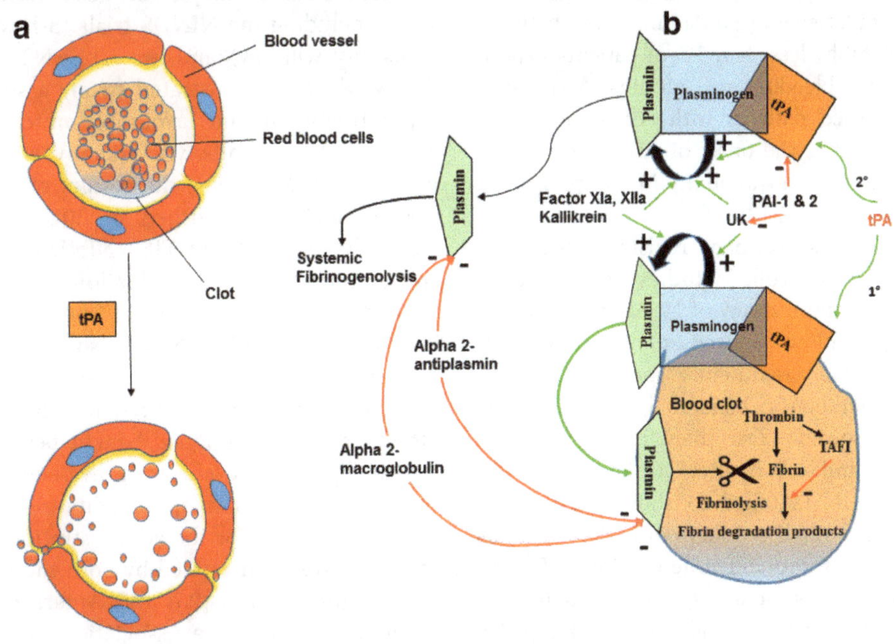

Fig. 1 The illustration of the fibrinolytic mechanisms: (**a**) tissue plasminogen activator (tPA) causes breakdown of the clot, and (**b**) detailed mechanism of fibrinolysis. Green arrow denotes activation/stimulation, and the red arrow indicates inhibition. tPA = tissue plasminogen activator; UK = Urokinase; PAI = plasminogen activator inhibitor

degradation causing tissue invasion and metastasis in tumour malignancy) depending upon the physiological environment. Therefore, SK and UK have less favourable adverse event profiles than rtPA. Thrombolytic drugs can be used as (a) Intravenous, and (b) Intra-arterial. Next, we will discuss the important aspects of these thrombolytic procedures.

Intravenous thrombolysis

Table 1 gives a detailed overview of clinical trials that evaluated the "time is brain" paradigm. The selection of patients for IV thrombolysis was based mainly on time since stroke onset. All of these trials used non-contrast CT (NCCT) for assessment of parenchymal injury. The exclusion criteria were the presence of a large infarct occupying more than one-third of the MCA territory or causing severe oedema or mass effect visible on NCCT [7].

The field of acute ischemic treatment using thrombolytic therapy before 1995 was despairing given the high rates of intracerebral haemorrhage in early clinical trials, which changed dramatically after the publication of results of NINDS stroke trial, showing benefit for IV Alteplase within 3 h of symptom onset [4]. The trial recruited 624 patients who were randomly assigned to treatment with IV Alteplase (0.9 mg/kg up to 90 mg; 10% as a bolus followed by a 60-min infusion [12]) or placebo. A significantly greater proportion of patients (38 (Alteplase) vs. 21% (placebo)) who received Alteplase showed a favourable clinical recovery at 90 days after stroke. However, the Alteplase group showed a dramatic 10-fold increase in symptomatic intracerebral haemorrhage. There was no significant difference in 90-day mortality between the two groups. Notably, less than 1% of patients experienced severe systemic bleeding at 3 months. A one-year follow-up study showed patients with AIS treated with Alteplase within 3 h after the onset of stroke were more likely to have minimal or no disability in comparison to patients receiving placebo [5, 13].

Subsequent serial observational registries and prospective randomised controlled studies conducted to investigate the safety and efficacy of IV Alteplase within the eligible time window showed a time-dependent relationship, with earlier treatment associated with larger proportional therapeutic benefits [3, 14, 15]. The ECASS-III trial showed clear benefit for patients treated between 3 and 4.5 h after stroke onset [16], which the previous RCTs failed to show because the earlier trials recruited small numbers of patients in this time window, and had treatment time windows of up to 6 h [17–19]. Other studies including the Canadian Alteplase for Stroke Effectiveness Study (CASES) registry [20], and Safe Implementation of Thrombolysis in Stroke-International Stroke Thrombolysis Register (SITS-ISTR) [21] provided further evidence of benefit for the administration of IV-rtPA therapy in the 3–4.5 h treatment window. These registries, CASES and SITS-ISTR, found comparable rates of mortality, functional independence, and incidence of symptomatic ICH within 24 h [22]. The extension of the time-window up to 4.5 h obviously offers an opportunity for treatment for more patients [21]. With regard to the treatment beyond 4.5 and up to 6 h, three trials including the Alteplase Thrombolysis for Acute Noninterventional Therapy in Ischemic Stroke (ATLANTIS-A for up to 6 h [19], and ATLANTIS-B for 3 to 5 h [18]), ECASS-II (for 0–6 h) [17], and the third International Stroke Thrombolysis Trial (IST-3) (for 0–6 h) [15] failed to demonstrate a treatment benefit for rtPA. However, a recent meta-analysis of 12 trials including 7012 patients, who received Alteplase within 6 h of onset of AIS, found significant improvement in the favourable outcome (mRS 0–1), functional independence (mRS 0–2), and survival rates at the end of final follow-up [23]. On the one hand, this analysis reinforces the need to treat patients as early as possible, though, it also suggested that some patients might benefit from Alteplase up to 6 h after stroke [15]. However, subgroup analysis for the treatment window between 4.5 and 6 h was not presented. Moreover, no significant trend toward a favourable outcome was found in a subset of patients ($n = 4971$) who received Alteplase between 3 and 6 h. The overall trend towards a beneficial outcome in 0–6-h window may have been influenced by the dominant trend observed in 0–3-h window. Pooled analysis of three trials, published in 2004, including the NINDS trials (3-h window), ECASS trials (6-h window), and two ATLANTIS trials (6-h and 5-h window), demonstrated strong association between rapid treatment and favourable outcome for patients receiving IV thrombolytic therapy within a 3 h time window [2]. Moreover, the results of two other recent pooled analyses published in 2010 ($n = 2775$ pooled from ECASS, ATLANTIS, NINDS, and Echoplanar Imaging Thrombolysis Evaluation Trial (EPITHET) trials and 2014 ($n = 6756$ pooled from IST-3, ECASS, EPITHET, ATLANTIS, NINDS) also indicated modest, yet clinically relevant, benefits to a select group in the therapeutic window of three to 4.5 h [2, 3, 14, 24]. However, risk outweighed benefit beyond 4.5 h [3, 14, 15]. In light of the emerging evidence and to provide more patients with an opportunity to receive tPA, acute stroke guidelines for the administration of rtPA following AIS have been revised by both the European Stroke Organization (ESO) [25] and American Heart Association/American Stroke Association (AHA/ASA) [26] by expanding the window of treatment from 3 h to 4.5 h. Interestingly, the Federal Drugs Agency (FDA) has not yet approved this extended indication.

Table 1 List of thrombolytic trials in acute ischemic stroke based on time-window

Trial (n)	Remarks
	TIME WINDOW 0–3 HOURS
NINDS [4, 231] (*n* = 624)	Time window: 0–3 h, 3–6 h Endpoints: A favourable outcome was defined as recovery with minimal or no deficit 3 months after treatment using four outcome measures: the BI ≥95, mRS seven ≤1, Glasgow Outcome Scale 8 of 1, and NIHSS score ≤ 1. Results: Treatment with tPA within 3 h of the onset led to the improved clinical outcome at 3 months, and increase in the incidence of symptomatic ICH.
SITS-MOST [232] (*n* = 6483)	Time window: 0–3 h Endpoints: Primary outcomes were symptomatic (a deterioration in NIHSS score of ≥4) ICH type 2 within 24 h and mortality at 3 months. Functional independence (defined by an mRS score of 0–2 at 90 days) was a secondary outcome. Results: Treatment with Alteplase is safe and effective when used within 3 h of stroke onset.
TESPI [64, 233] (*n* = 248)	Time window: 0–3 h Endpoints: Primary endpoint for efficacy was the disability at day 90, dichotomized as a favourable outcome (mRS 0–2) or unfavourable outcome (mRS 3–6) [64]. The end-point for safety is symptomatic ICH radiologically confirmed on the 22–36 h post-treatment scan combined with neurological deterioration leading to an increase of ≥1 point/s on the NIHSS scale. Results: Higher mortality in patients aged >80 years than younger patients treated with IV-rtPA. No significant differences in symptomatic ICH nor for a favourable outcome. Thrombolytic therapy should not be a priori denied for appropriately selected >80-year old patients [233].
SITS-NEW [234] (*n* = 591)	Time window: 0–3 h Endpoints: Primary endpoints were symptomatic (deterioration in NIHSS score ≥ 4 or death within the first 24 h) intracerebral haemorrhage type 2 22–36 h after the thrombolysis, and mortality at 90 days follow-up. The secondary outcome was functional independence (mRS 0–2) at three-months [234]. Results: IV alteplase is safe and efficient in the treatment of ischaemic stroke in Asian population in congruence to the observations of SITS trials performed on European population.
	TIME WINDOW 3–4.5 HOURS
ECASS-III [11] (*n* = 821)	Time window: 3–4.5 h Endpoints: Primary outcome was a disability at 3 months, assessed by the mRS as either favourable (score of 0 or 1) or unfavourable (score of 2 to 6). Secondary end-points included combined BI and RS, Scandinavian Stroke Scale (SSS) at 90 days, and 30 day mortality. Tertiary outcomes included early neurologic recovery (SSS) and duration of in-hospital stay. Results: Significant benefit of IV-rtPA when administered up to 4·5 h. Symptomatic ICH is significantly more likely with alteplase than with placebo. No difference in mortality between the groups.
CASES [20] (*n* = 1112)	Time window: 3–4.5 h, 0–3 h Endpoints: The primary endpoints were mRS at 90 days, mortality and symptomatic ICH. An mRS 0–1 at 90 days was defined as a favourable outcome. Results: IV alteplase is efficacious in treating AIS patients in 3–4.5 h window; however, there is a tendency towards increased risk of symptomatic ICH in the later time window.
SITS-ISTR [21] (*n* = 23,942)	Time window: 3–4.5 h Endpoints: Primary endpoints were functional independence at 3 months, and incidence of symptomatic ICH. Results: Safety and the functional outcome less favourable after 3 h.
	TIME WINDOW 4.5–6 HOURS
ATLANTIS-B [18] (*n* = 613)	Time window: 3–5 h Endpoints: Primary efficacy endpoint was an excellent neurologic recovery at day 90 (NIHSS ≤1); Secondary endpoints included remarkable recovery on functional outcome measures (BI, mRS, and Glasgow Outcome Scale) at days 30 and 90. Serious adverse events such as symptomatic ICH were also assessed. Results: No significant rtPA benefit on the 90 day efficacy endpoints in patients treated between 3 and 5 h. A significant increase in the risk of symptomatic ICH with treatment using IV-rtPA.
ECASS-II [17] (*n* = 800)	Time window: 0–3 h and 3–6 h Endpoints: The primary outcome was the mRS at 90 days, dichotomised for favourable (score 0–1) and unfavourable (score 2–6) outcome. Results: Trend towards benefit for alteplase, though not statistically significant. Increased risk of symptomatic ICH (8.6% alteplase-group vs. 3.4% placebo-group).
ATLANTIS-A [19] (*n* = 142)	Time window: 0–6 h Endpoints: Primary efficacy endpoints were the number of patients with a decrease of ≥ points on the NIHSS scale at 24 h and day 30, along with infarct volume at day 30. Secondary outcomes included mortality and functional status on the BI and mRS scales at days 30 and 90. Results: Significantly higher proportion of 4-point NIHSS improvement at 24 h for rtPA groups (40%) vs. placebo (21%). The trend reversed at 30 days with more improvement observed in placebo (75%) vs. rtPA patients (60%). rtPA is strongly correlated with an increased risk of ICH, especially in patients treated between 5 and 6 h after onset.
IST-3 [15] (*n* = 3035)	Time window: 0–6 h Endpoints: Primary outcome was the proportion of patients who were alive and independent (defined by an Oxford Handicap Score (OHS) of 0–2) at 6 months. Symptomatic ICH recorded at 7 days, and at 6 months. Results: Higher proportion of symptomatic ICH at 7 days in the rtPA group (7%) vs. control group (1%), and deaths at 7 days in rtPA (11%) vs. control group (7%). A similar number of fatalities in either rtPA or control groups (27% each). Despite early hazards, IV alteplase improved functional outcome.

IV Intravenous; *rtPA* Recombinant tissue plasminogen activator; *NINDS* National Institute of Neurological Disorders and Stroke; *mRS* Modified Rankin Score; *BI* Barthel Index; *SITS-MOST* Safe Implementation of Thrombolysis in Stroke-Monitoring Study; *NIHSS* National Institute of Health Stroke Scale; *ICH* Intracerebral haemorrhage; *TESPI* Thrombolysis in Elderly Stroke Patients in Italy; *SITS-NEW* Safe Implementation of Thrombolysis in Stroke-Non-European Union World; *ECASS* European Cooperative Acute Stroke Study; *ATLANTIS* The Alteplase ThromboLysis for Acute Noninterventional Therapy in Ischemic Stroke; *CASES* Canadian Alteplase for Stroke Effectiveness Study; *IST-3* third international stroke trial

Some contraindications limit the use of IV-rtPA in AIS (see Table 2) [27]. Moreover, the narrow time window of 4.5 h along with the multitude of contraindications prevent many patients from receiving treatment; indeed, less than 3% of patients presenting with AIS receive IV-rtPA [28]. Other limitations of IV-rtPA are: (a) increased rate of mortality and intracranial bleeding in internal carotid artery occlusion (ICA) [29–32] or other disabling strokes such as those with no detectable residual flow signals [33–35], (b) low recanalization rate ranging from 13 to 50% in large artery occlusion such as the proximal middle cerebral artery (MCA), the ICA, or the basilar artery [27, 35–41], and (c) unresponsiveness to large thrombi (especially when the thrombus length exceeds 8 mm [42–45], or location is proximal, such as terminal carotid artery occlusion [34, 46]. One study found only 10 and 25% of ICA and proximal MCA occlusions are recanalizable by IV-rtPA [47]. Incomplete recanalization is often observed in patients treated with IV-rtPA. For instance, 70% of patients who received IV-rtPA were found to have angiographically confirmed residual thrombus requiring complimentary intra-arterial treatment such as clot angioplasty [48].

Table 2 Contraindications for intravenous recombinant tissue plasminogen activator (rtPA) in acute ischemic stroke

Contraindications applicable to use of intravenous rtPA in acute ischemic stroke (AIS)
Onset of stroke symptoms more than 4.5 h.[Ψ]
History of stroke or significant head trauma in previous 3 months
Previous intracranial haemorrhage.
Symptoms are suggestive of subarachnoid haemorrhage.
Prolonged blood pressure elevation (systolic ≥185 mmHg or diastolic ≥110 mmHg).
Hypoglycemia (serum glucose <50 mg/dL (<2.8 mmol/L)).
Active internal bleeding, acute bleeding diathesis, including platelet count <100, 000/mm^3, current anticoagulant use with an INR > 1.7, or PT > 15 s.
Heparin use within 48 h with an abnormally elevated aPTT.
Arterial puncture at noncompressible site in previous 7 days.
History of gastrointestinal tract haemorrhage within 21 days.
The recent history of major surgery intracranial or intraspinal surgery within 14 days.
Previous history of a previous aneurysm, arteriovenous malformation, or intracranial neoplasm.
Current use of a direct thrombin inhibitor or direct factor Xa inhibitors with an evidence of anticoagulation effect by laboratory tests such as aPTT, INR < ECT, TT, or relevant factor Xa activity assays.
Early ischemic changes are visible on CT in more than one-third of MCA artery vascular territory consistent with irreversible injury or evidence of haemorrhage on CT scan.

[Ψ]Additional criteria applicable for IV-rtPA between 3 to 4.5 h: patient older than 80 years, severe stroke (baseline NIHSS >25), no prior history of diabetes mellitus and AIS (both), and not currently on any oral anticoagulants regardless of INR.

CT Computed tomography; *INR* International normalised ratio; *IV-rtPA* Intravenous recombinant tissue plasminogen activator; *MCA* Middle cerebral artery; *NIHSS* National Institute of Health Stroke Scale; *PT* Prothrombin time; *aPTT* Activated partial thromboplastin time; *ECT* Ecarin clotting time

Novel therapies are being currently investigated to overcome the limitations of IV thrombolysis or to extend the time window of treatment, for example: (i) use of alternative fibrinolytic agents such as desmoteplase [49–53], argatroban [54], tenecteplase [19, 55], albumin [56], and plasmin [57], (ii) mixed approaches that involve combination of rtPA and other agents or therapies such as GP IIb/IIIa antagonists [58–60], antiplatelet agents (e.g., acetylsalicylic acid [61–63]), low-molecular-weight heparin [64, 65], and sonothrombolysis [66–69] to enhance microcirculatory flow, reduce residual thrombus, and boost lytic efficacy, (iii) use of non-invasive or minimally invasive methods such ventilator support [70], and pterygopalatine ganglion and petrosal nerve stimulation [71] to augment cerebral blood flow by cerebral vasodilation and alleviate blood flow steal, and (iv) endovascular procedures such as intra-arterial thrombolysis, stenting, and angioplasty to achieve greater clot manipulation and significantly higher rates of arterial recanalization [46, 72].

Endovascular treatment

Intra-arterial thrombolysis

Intra-arterial (IA) thrombolysis has emerged as a promising intervention, especially for AIS patients with contraindications for IV-tPA [73–75]. Intra-arterial procedures are performed under direct visualisation; therefore, one can limit the dose of the fibrinolytic agent, mechanically manipulate the clot if required and deliver higher concentrations of the agent to the clot target (local delivery) with reduced systemic effects [76, 77]. IA can also deliver higher recanalization rates. However, IA therapy also has its unique set of challenges and disadvantages. Mechanical manipulation of a clot during IA may also increase the risk of injuring adjacent blood vessels. Moreover, advanced training is required for neuro interventionists or neuroradiologists to gain expertise in IA procedures which can be demanding [74, 78–80]. As such, endovascular treatment is only available in a limited number of specialised stroke centres.

Prolyse in Acute Cerebral Thromboembolism (PROACT) was the first randomized trial (phase II study; $n = 46$) of 6 mg recombinant pro-urokinase (rpro-UK) versus placebo undertaken in patients with angiographically documented proximal MCA occlusion to test the safety, recanalization frequency, and clinical efficacy of intra-arterial local infusion of plasminogen activators in AIS patients with symptomatic MCA occlusion of less than 6 h' duration [81]. Investigators found a significant association of intra-arterial local rpro-UK infusion with greater frequency of recanalization in acute stroke patients with M1 or M2 occlusions compared with placebo (57.7% vs. 14.3%, $P = 0.017$). However, an increased, though not significant, symptomatic haemorrhage rate was also reported. Subsequently, a phase III, PROACT II study was undertaken, involving fifty-four stroke centers in the United States and Canada, with an increased 9 mg dosage of r-pro-UK administered over 2 h infusion while using heparin in low dose (from PROACT I) to improve the recanalization in addition to containing symptomatic brain haemorrhages [82]. Out of 180 randomied patients with AIS, treatment with IA r-pro UK within 6 h of the onset of AIS caused by MCA occlusion was significantly associated with improved clinical outcome at 90 days. The IA r-pro-UK group demonstrated significantly higher recanalization rates (66% vs. 18%, $P < 0.001$), and increased favourable independent outcome (60% vs. 18%, $P < 0.001$) than the IA heparin alone. However, higher frequency of early symptomatic intra-cerebral haemorrhage (ICH) was also observed in the intervention group (10% vs. 2%). Overall, the proportion of ICH was relatively higher in PROACT II than previous IV thrombolysis trials [81], perhaps due to greater baseline National Institutes of Health Stroke Scale (NIHSS) in PROACT II in comparison to other trials. The median baseline stroke severity in PROACT was 17, in contrast to 14 and 11 in the NINDS and ECASS II trials respectively. Contrary to the positive findings of PROACT II, another large open-label trial, Local Versus Systemic Thrombolysis for Acute Ischemic Stroke (SYNTHESIS) Expansion, found that IA thrombolytic therapy was not superior to standard treatment with IV-rtPA [83]. Disability-free outcome at 90 days was not significantly different between the IA thrombolytic and IV-rtPA groups (30.4% vs. 34.8%; adjusted odds ratio = 0.71, 95% CI 0.44–1.14). Another randomized trial, the Middle Cerebral Artery Embolism Local Fibrinolytic Intervention Trial (MELT), conducted in Japan, to investigate the safety and clinical efficacy of intra-arterial urokinase (UK) in patients within 6 h of onset of stroke with angiographically documented M1 or M2 occlusion, found a trend towards favourable outcome (defined by Modified Rankin Score (mRS) 0–2) at 90 days, and a substantial increase in likelihood of excellent outcome (defined by mRS 0–1) [84]. However, the primary endpoint (good outcome; mRS 0–2) did not reach statistical significance as the trial was aborted prematurely. A meta-analysis of five RCTs with 395 AIS patients with MCA occlusion compared IA thrombolysis with control (IV heparin) [85]. The study concluded that IA thrombolysis was significantly associated with substantial increases in recanalization rates and good (odds ratio = 2.05; 95% CI, 1.33 to 3.14; $P = 0.001$) and excellent outcomes (odds ratio = 2.14; 95% CI, 1.31 to 3.51; $P = 0.003$) in AIS. Intra-arterial thrombolytic treatment is gaining traction at some comprehensive stroke facilities at tertiary hospitals. It is often administered as an off-label therapy within 6 h of onset of stroke in patients with anterior circulation and up to 12–24 h after onset in the posterior circulation [74]. As per the guidelines of the AHA issued in 2005, and again in 2013, IA thrombolysis has been recommended in appropriately selected AIS patients with MCA occlusions within 6 h provided they were not candidates for IV-rtPA (Class I, Level of Evidence: B) [86]. The FDA has not approved IA-pro-UK.

Mechanical Thrombectomy (MT)

MT involves a minimally invasive surgical procedure using a microcatheter and other thrombectomy devices to trap and remove the blood clot from an occluded artery. MT, delivered as a stand-alone treatment or in conjunction with systemic thrombolysis (IV-rtPA or IA thrombolysis), is currently the standard of care for AIS therapy [87]. MT devices can be classified into different subtypes based on their mechanism of action: (a) coil retriever, (b) aspiration, (c) stent-retriever, and (d) mechanical clot disruption, using laser or ultrasound. A comprehensive list of past and current MT devices is given in Table 3. Coil retriever devices and the early Penumbra aspiration system [88, 89] were the first generation of MT devices; they failed to show long-term improvements in clinical outcomes despite satisfactory revascularization efficacy (up to 50%) [90]. Coil retrievers such as MERCI [91–94], Phenox [95, 96] and Catch retrievers [97–99] use microcatheter to deliver a coiled wire across the targeted clot in the occluded artery [91–94]. Once the coil is deployed, the neuro interventionist pulls both the coil and the clot towards the catheter leading to the removal of the clot [100]. Aspiration devices such as Penumbra (Penumbra Inc., US) use vacuum aspiration to remove target clot in the occluded artery. The early generation of aspiration devices was often subject to clogging of the aspiration tips; this has been overcome in the later models by the addition of a separator wire with a bulbous tip inside the bore, which can be pushed in and pulled out by the neurointerventionist. The continual back and forth motion cleave the clot detaching it from the lumen. Eventually, the clot is sucked in, without clogging the tip, ahead of the catheter [101]. The second generation of MT devices used self-expanding stents to trap the clot by deploying them in the occluded artery [101]. They were originally conceived for stent-assisted coiling and retraction of aberrant coils dislodged during the endovascular procedures. These self-expanding stents are first lodged across the thrombus within the vessel wall, following which, once the clot is entrapped, the stent-clot combination is subsequently retracted back under constant aspiration into the delivery guide microcatheter. Some clinical trials using

Table 3 List of mechanical thrombectomy (MT) devices

MT device	Vendor	Mechanism of action	References
Merci Clot Retriever	Concentric Medical	Coil retriever	[91–94]
Phenox	Phenox, Bochum, Germany	Coil retriever/Aspiration	[95, 96]
Catch	Balt, Montmorency, France	Coil retriever	[97–99]
Distal Access Catheter (DAC)	DAC; Concentric Medical, US	Coil retriever	[129]
Early Penumbra	Penumbra Inc., US	Aspiration	[88, 89, 235–237]
AngioJet	Possis Medical, MN, USA	Aspiration/Rheolytic thrombectomy[a]	[238–241]
EKOS Primo	EKOS, Bothell, WA	Ultrasound-based on mechanical clot disruption	[242]
Neuroform	Stryker Neurovascular, US	Stent Retriever	[243, 244]
Enterprise	Codman, Raynham, MA, US	Stent Retriever	[245–247]
Solitaire	Covidien/Medtronic, Dublin, Ireland	Stent retriever	[126, 223, 248–254]
Trevo	Stryker, Kalamazoo, Michigan, US	Stent Retriever	[92, 255–259]
ReVive™	Micrus Endovascular, CA, US	Stent Retriever	[260, 261]
APERIO	Acandis, Pfzorheim, Germany	Stent Retriever	[261–263]
Embotrap Revascularization system	Neuravi, Ireland	Stent Retriever	[264]
pREset	Phenox, Bochum, Germany	Stent Retriever	[265]
The Mindframe Capture LP	Medtronic, Minneapolis, Minnesota, USA	Stent Retriever	[266, 267]
ERIC	MicroVention, CA, US	Stent Retriever	[268]
SOFIA	MicroVention, CA, US	Stent Retriever	[269–271]
Penumbra 5MAX ACE	Penumbra Inc., California, US	Aspiration	[103, 104, 106, 107, 272]
Penumbra ACE 64	Penumbra Inc., California, US	Aspiration	[105, 107, 273, 274]
Penumbra 3D separator	Penumbra Inc., California, US	Aspiration	[108, 109]
LaTIS Neurolaser laser	Latis Inc., Minneapolis, Minn	Laser recanalization based mechanical clot disruption	[275]
EPAR laser	EndoVasix, Belmont, CA	Laser recanalization based mechanical clot disruption	[130]
MicroLysUS catheter	EKOS, Bothell, WA, US	Ultrasound-based mechanical clot disruption	[276]
Wingspan	Stryker Neurovascular, Fremont, CA, US	Ultrasound-based mechanical clot disruption	[277–284]

ERIC Embolus Retriever with Interlinked Cage; *SOFIA* Soft Torqueable Catheter Optimized For Intracranial Access
[a]Rheolytic thrombectomy refers to the mechanical procedure of removing thrombus using multiple high-velocity, high-pressure saline jets of saline from the tip of a catheter using an AngioJet system [285]

the new generation stent retrievers, such as Solitaire, Trevo Pro, and ReVive, have yielded recanalization rates as high as 85% in AIS with large vessel occlusion [93, 100–102].

Combined interventions, using both suction embolectomy with large bore catheters and mechanical retrieval using stent retrievers, have shown promise in recent studies [103]. In this technique, aspiration of the clot, a cheaper alternative, is attempted first using a large bore microcatheter such as the Penumbra MAX systems [104–107]. If the aspiration fails, mechanical retrieval is attempted by inserting the stent retrievers via the aspiration catheter. Using this sequential combination, phenomenal recanalization rates of up to 95% have been achieved [103], compared with stand-alone direct aspiration rates of 78%. Another application of combined approach is the latest generation Penumbra device called Penumbra 3D separator, which incorporates lesional aspiration technology coupled with an advanced stent retriever device, allowing the breakdown of a clot in addition to radial direction using stent struts [100, 108]. Penumbra 3D separators have demonstrated good revascularization of large vessel occlusions and a greater rate of functional independence at 90 days [108, 109].

A detailed comparative overview of successful clinical trials concerning endovascular treatment for AIS along with the imaging and clinical selection criteria, and the outcome measures are presented in Table 4.

Following the success of five multicentre, open-label, randomized controlled endovascular acute stroke trials including MR CLEAN (Multicenter Randomized Clinical Trial of Endovascular Treatment for Acute Ischemic Stroke in the Netherlands) [110], ESCAPE (Endovascular Treatment for Small Core and Anterior Circulation Proximal Occlusion with Emphasis on Minimizing CT to Recanalization Times) [111], SWIFT PRIME (Solitaire

Table 4 Comparison of baseline characteristics and outcome measures of the recent endovascular trials [27, 194, 286]

Trials	MR CLEAN [110]	ESCAPE [111]	EXTEND-IA [76]	SWIFT PRIME [112]	REVASCAT [113]	THERAPY [128]	THRACE [127]
Region	Netherlands	United States, Canada, South Korea, Ireland, United Kingdom	Australia and New Zealand	United States and Europe	Spain	United States	France
Number of centres	16	22	10	39	4	4	26
Number of patients; n (CG/IA)	500 (267/233)	315 (150/165)	70 (35/35)	196 (98/98)	206 (103/103)	108 (54/54)	412 (208/204)
BASELINE CHARACTERISTICS							
Age Range	≥ 18	≥ 18	≥ 18	18–80 years	18–80 years	18–85	18–80
NIHSS Range	≥ 2	> 5	N.R.	8–29	≥ 6	≥8	10–25
Control group	Standard medical therapy (+/− IV tPA)	Standard medical therapy (+/− IV tPA)	IV-tPA only	IV-tPA only	Standard medical therapy (+/− IV tPA)	IV-tPA only	IV-tPA only
Intervention group	IAT	IAT	ET with Solitaire FR stentriever	ET with Solitaire FR stentriever	ET with Solitaire FR stentriever	ET with Penumbra aspiration system	Endovascular MT
Intervention using Stent retriever in IA arm	81.5%	86.1%	100%	100%	100%	0%	N.R.
Time window	0–6 h	0–12 h	0–6 h	0–6 h	0–8 h	0–4.5 h	0–5 h
Neurologic inclusion criteria	N.A.	Barthel Index of ≥90	mRS scores of 0–2	mRS scores of 0–1	mRS scores of 0–1		
Neuroimaging techniques	CT/CTA	CT/CTA/CTA Multiphase (for collaterals)	CT/CTA/CTP (for mismatch)	CT/CTA/MRA/ MRP/CTP (for infarct core)	CT/ CTA(MRA/DSA)	CT/CTA	CT/CTA
Large artery occlusion	CTA	CTA	CTA or MRA	CTA or MRA	CTA or MRA	CTA	CTA or MRA
Affected arteries	TICA, M1, M2, A1, A2	TICA, M1	TICA, M1, M2	TICA, M1, M2	TICA, M1	MCA	ICA, M1, TB, M2
Infarct core/perfusion	N.R.	NCCT, CBV or CBF ASPECTS ≥6	Core$^{\Psi}$ < 70 ml (>1.2)$^{¥}$	CoreΦ< 50 ml (>1.8)$^{¥}$ NCCT ASPECTS ≥6	NCCT ASPECTS ≥7 DWI ASPECTS ≥6	Clot length ≥ 8 mm	N.R.
Collateral status	N.R.	Good/Moderate	N.R.	N.R.	N.R.	N.R.	N.R.
Median stroke onset to groin puncture	260 min	241 min	210 min	224 min	269 min	226 min	255 min
Baseline NIHSS [Median (IQR)]; CG vs IA	18 (14–22) vs17 (14–21)	17 (12–20) vs 16 (13–20)	13 (9–19) vs 17 (13–20)	17 (13–19) vs 17 (13–20)	17 (12–19) vs 17 (14–20)	N.R.	17 (13–20) vs 18 (15–21)
Median ASPECTS (%); CG/IA	9/9	9/9	NR/NR	9/9	8/7	N.R.	N.R.
Patients Receiving IV-rtPA (%); CG/IA	91/87	79/73	100/100	100/100	78/68	100/100	100/100
STUDY OUTCOMES							
Primary Outcomes	Shift in mRS at 90 days	Shift in mRS at 90 days	Reduction in perfusion lesion volume; NIHSS reduction ≥8 pointsor mRS score of 0–1 at day 3	Distribution of mRS at 90 days; % mRS 0–2 at 90 days	Shift in mRS at 90 days	Shift in mRS at 90 days	Shift in mRS at 90 days
mRS (0–2) at 90 days %; CG vs IA	19.1 vs 32.6, $P < 0.05$	29.3 vs 53, $P < 0.001$	40 vs 70, $P = 0.001$	35.5 vs 60.2, $P < 0.001$	28.2 vs 43.7	30.4 vs 38	42.1 vs 54.2
Improvement in mRS 0–2 at 90 days	13.5%	23.7%	31.4%	24.7%	15.5%	7.6%	12.1%
sICH risk (%); CG vs IA, P	6.4 vs 7.7, $P > 0.05$	2.7 vs 3.6, $P > 0.05$	5.7 vs 0, $P > 0.05$	3.1 vs 0, $P = 0.12$	1.9 vs 1.9, $P > 0.05$	11.3 vs 10.9	2 vs 2, $P = 0.71$.
Parenchymal Hematoma Risk (%); CG/IA	6 vs 6	2.0 vs 4.8	8.6 vs 11.4	N.R. vs N.R.	5.8 vs 5.8	N.A.	9.45 vs 13.8, $P = 0.53$

Table 4 Comparison of baseline characteristics and outcome measures of the recent endovascular trials [27, 194, 286] *(Continued)*

Trials	MR CLEAN [110]	ESCAPE [111]	EXTEND-IA [76]	SWIFT PRIME [112]	REVASCAT [113]	THERAPY [128]	THRACE [127]
Mortality (%); CG vs IA, P	22.1 vs 21, $P > 0.05$	19 vs10.4, $P = 0.04$	20 vs 8.6, $P > 0.05$	12.4 vs 9.2, $P > 0.05$	15.5 vs 18.4, $P = 0.06$	23.9 vs 12	13 vs 12; $P = 0.70$
Decrease in mortality at 90 days	1.1%	8.6%	11.4%	3.2%	−2.9%	11.9%	1%
Complete recanalization rates							
mTICI Score 2b/3	58.7%	72.4%	86.2%	88.0%	65.7%	N.R.	N.R.
Complete recanalization based on neuroimaging 24–27 h later; CG vs IA	68/207 (33%)[a] vs 141/187 (75%)[a]	N.A. vs N.A.	15/35 (43%)[a] vs 33/35 (94%)[a]	21/52 (40%)[b] vs 53/64 (83%)[b]	N.A. vs N.A.	N.A.	N.A.
Brain infarction volume at 24 hc (mean, 95% CI); CG vs IA, P	79 mL (34–125) vs 49 mL (22–96), $P < 0.01$	N.A. vs N.A.	N.A. vs N.A.	35 mL (0–407) vs 32 mL (0–503), $P = 0.09$	39 mL (12–87) vs 16 mL (8–59), $P = 0.02$	N.A.	N.A.
NNT	7.1	4.2	3.2	4.0	6.3	13.2	8.3

IQR Interquartile range; *TICA* Terminal internal carotid artery (Carotid T/L); *M1* and *M2* Branches of the MCA; *A1* and *A2* Branches of the ACA; *mTICI* Modified Thrombolysis in Cerebral Infarction; *mRS* Modified Rankin Scale; *N.R.* Not required; *N.S.* Not significant; *N.A.* Not available; *CTA* Computed tomography angiography; *NCCT* Non-contract computed tomography; *CBV* Cerebral blood volume; *CBF* Cerebral blood flow; *MRA* Magnetic resonance angiography; *ASPECTS* Alberta Stroke Program Early CT score; *CG* Control group; *IA* Intervention arm; *IAT* Intra-arterial therapy; *TB* Upper third of the basilar artery; *MCA* Middle cerebral artery; *M2* Insular portion of the MCA; *M1* Proximal portion of the MCA; *ET* Endovascular Thrombectomy; *MT* Mechanical thrombectomy; *ESCAPE* Endovascular Treatment for Small Core and Anterior Circulation Proximal Occlusion With Emphasis on Minimizing CT to Recanalization Times; *EXTEND-IA* Extending the Time for Thrombolysis in Emergency Neurological Deficits—Intra-Arterial; *MR CLEAN* Multicentre Randomized Clinical Trial of Endovascular Treatment for Acute Ischemic Stroke in the Netherlands; *NIHSS* National Institutes of Health Stroke Scale; *REVASCAT* Randomized Trial of Revascularization with Solitaire FR Device Versus Best Medical Therapy in the Treatment of Acute Stroke Due to Anterior Circulation LVO Presenting within 8 h of Symptom Onset; *SWIFT PRIME* Solitaire with the Intention for Thrombectomy as Primary Endovascular Treatment; *NNT* Number needed to treat for benefit (mRS score 0–2); *THRACE* Mechanical thrombectomy after intravenous alteplase versus alteplase alone after stroke

[¥]Target mismatch ratio; [λ] Sum of median of parameters; [Φ]The ischemic core was assessed by MRI or CT; [Ψ]The ischemic core was defined by regional cerebral blood flow on CT perfusion or diffusion-weighted imaging; [a]Recanalization shown in brain CTA/MRA at 24 h; [b]Reperfusion shown in brain CT perfusion/MR perfusion at 27 h; [c]Brain infarction volume at 24 h after treatment measured with CT in MR CLEAN trial and with CT or MRI in SWIFT PRIME and REVASCAT trials

With the Intention for Thrombectomy as Primary Endovascular Treatment of Acute Ischemic Stroke) [112], EXTEND-IA (Extending the Time for Thrombolysis in Emergency Neurological Deficits–Intra-arterial) [76], and REVASCAT (Randomized Trial of Revascularization with Solitaire FR Device vs Best Medical Therapy in the Treatment of Acute Stroke Due to Anterior Circulation Large Vessel Occlusion Presenting within 8 h of Symptom Onset) [113], it is now accepted that the combined treatment with second-generation stent retriever MT devices and IV-rtPA within 6 h after stroke onset is superior to standard medical therapy (with IV-rtPA alone) for AIS caused by a proximal large artery occlusion of the anterior circulation [114].

Immediately after the announcement of the MR CLEAN results [110], the other four trials were terminated prematurely for interim analysis. The results of these trials were then published in quick succession in late 2014 and early 2015. The number needed to treat (NNT) for these five trials ranged from a minimum of three (EXTEND-IA) to a maximum of 7.4 (MR CLEAN). The success of these trials has revolutionised stroke therapy. However, given that only trained neuro-interventionists can perform the MT procedures, stroke care facilities should expeditiously work on integrating MT with standard care, to minimise the time required for imaging and preoperative preparation needed for this therapy [115]. A recent meta-analysis, based on a pooled analysis of 1287 patients, published by the Highly Effective Reperfusion evaluated in Multiple Endovascular Stroke Trials (HERMES) collaboration, showed that endovascular MT added to the best medical therapy more than doubles the odds of a higher rate of (a) functional independence (mRS score at 90 days of 0 to 2) (46% vs. 27%, odds ratio 2.35, 95% CI 1.85–2.98) [116], and (b) significantly reduced disability (improvement of ≥1 points on the mRS at 90 days) (adjusted OR 2.49, 95% CI 1.76–3.53) compared with best medical therapy alone in AIS patients with large vessel occlusion in the anterior circulation. The rates of symptomatic ICH or 90-day mortality were also not significantly different between the endovascular MT and control groups [117]. Another recent meta-analysis by the same HERMES collaboration has suggested that the endovascular MT plus medical therapy is beneficial up to 7.3 h after the onset of stroke [118]. Recently published DAWN trial has shown benefit of MT for an extended time window of 6–24 h [119]. To sum up, these studies make a convincing case for the administration of early thrombectomy using second-generation stent retrievers for limiting post-stroke disability in patients with large vessel occlusion in the anterior circulation. They also reinforce the importance of early treatment based on an inverse association between time to endovascular reperfusion and better functional outcome [118].

Clinical trials with first-generation devices

Prior to MR CLEAN trial, three endovascular trials, using mainly first generation MT devices during 2004 and 2012, including MR RESCUE (Mechanical Retrieval and Recanalization of Stroke Clots Using Embolectomy) [120], the IMS (Interventional Management of Stroke) III [121], and the SYNTHESIS Expansion (Intra-arterial vs. Systemic Thrombolysis for Acute Ischemic Stroke) [83] failed to demonstrate any functional benefit for intra-arterial treatment in AIS. The results of these trials, which were published in 2013, raised concerns regarding the efficacy of endovascular MT in large vessel occlusion. Potential causes for this lack of effect were suggested including: (a) the three trials used old-generation devices with reduced recanalization efficacy in comparison to the later generation devices which were used in the MR CLEAN trial, and (b) previous trials did not use vessel occlusion as an eligibility criterion because radiological confirmation of large artery occlusion was lacking due to limited availability of CTA at that time [122–124].

Phase 2 clinical trials with second-generation devices

The second-generation MT devices, Solitaire flow restoration device and Trevo retriever, are based on stent retrievers, which are very effective in capturing thrombus and produce excellent vessel recanalization. Two phase 2 clinical trials, SWIFT (Solitaire Flow Restoration Device Versus the Merci Retriever in Patients with Acute Ischemic Stroke) and TREVO 2 (Trevo Versus Merci Retrievers for Thrombectomy Revascularization of large vessel occlusion in Acute Ischemic Stroke), demonstrated that stent retrievers achieved better clinical outcomes by increasing recanalization of large artery occlusions, than the first-generation Merci Retriever and Penumbra System devices [93, 94, 125, 126]. The SWIFT study assigned eligible patients to receive MT treatment with either MERCI device ($n = 55$) or Solitaire stent retriever ($n = 58$). The Solitaire group showed significantly improved recanalization, as defined by a Thrombolysis in Myocardial Infarction (TIMI) Score of two (partial recanalization) or three (total recanalization) (61% vs. 24%, $P < 0.0001$), and better functional outcomes (58% vs. 33%, $P < 0.0001$) than the MERCI group. The TREVO trial produced similar outcomes, with the TREVO device achieving better recanalization (86% vs. 60%, $P < 0.0001$), defined by Thrombolysis in Cerebral Infarction (TICI) score of 2 or 3, and improved long-term clinical outcomes (40% vs. 22%, $P < 0.013$) in comparison to the first generation Merci retriever. No difference in the incidence of symptomatic intracerebral haemorrhage (sICH) was reported between TREVO and Merci groups.

Phase 3 clinical trials with second-generation devices

MR CLEAN was a Dutch endovascular trial that assigned 500 patients to the intervention arm (IAT with standard therapy; $n = 233$) and the control arm (standard therapy; $n = 267$) alone [110]. All patients in the control arm received IV-rtPA. Endovascular procedures were performed using second-generation stent retrievers. Stent retrievers were used in 81.5% (190/233) of patients who received IA treatment. MR CLEAN included patients presenting within 6 h of stroke onset, aged 18 and above, with a minimum NIHSS score of two, and large artery occlusion confirmed on CTA. MR CLEAN trial did not have an upper age threshold for eligibility unlike previous trials, where patients above 80 years were excluded. Moreover, an Alberta Stroke Program Early CT Score (ASPECTS) score was not used in the randomization of patients. Patients who received MT and standard treatment (intervention arm) showed good recanalization (defined by TICI score of 2b (>50% recanalization) or 3) in 59% (115/196) of the patients. This arm also demonstrated improvement in good outcome at 90 days (32.6% vs. 19.1%; OR = 1.67 [95% CI 1.21 to 2.3]), and a significant decrease in brain infarct at 24 h (49 mL vs. 79 mL, $P < 0.01$) in comparison to the standard medical therapy group. The number need to treat (NNT) was 7.1. No significant difference in the occurrence of sICH or death was found in between the two groups.

The Endovascular Treatment for Small Core and Proximal Occlusion Ischemic Stroke (ESCAPE) trial randomised 315 patients, 150 in the control arm and 160 in the MT arm, for an extended therapeutic time window of 0–12 h [111]. Strict inclusion criteria including NIHSS > 5, pre-morbid Barthel index of 90 and above, large artery occlusion confirmed on CT angiography (CTA), ASPECTS score of ≥6, and good or moderate leptomeningeal collateral status on CTA was applied. In comparison to previous trials, ESCAPE used CTA, preferably multiphase CTA, to select patients based on the neuroimaging assessment of the site of occlusion and collateral status. The trial was unique given the pioneering enrollment goals, including door to puncture times of less than 60 min, and door to recanalization time of fewer than 90 min. Given the trial was stopped following the announcement of MR CLEAN results, an interim analysis showed good recanalization rates (72%), defined by TICI score of 2b or 3, and significantly better functional outcomes in the MT group vs. the standard therapy (53% vs. 29%, $P < 0.001$). Concerning safety endpoints, MT showed reduced mortality rate (10% vs.

19%, $P = 0.04$), and comparable sICH rates (3.6% vs. 2.7%, $P > 0.05$) vs. the control group.

The SWIFT-PRIME trial boasted the maximum number ($n = 39$) of recruitment centres spanning the United States and Europe [112]. Between 2012 and 2014, 196 patients presenting within 6 h of stroke onset were enrolled and assigned to treatment groups: MT (using Solitaire FR stentriever) plus standard therapy, IV-rtPA ($n = 98$), or standard therapy alone (n = 98). For randomization, patients with NIHSS scores between 8 and 30, aged between 18 and 80 years, and a premorbid score of mRS < 1 were considered. The SWIFT-PRIME study used neurovascular angiography imaging (CTA/ magnetic resonance angiography (MRA)) to identify patients with large artery occlusion prior to randomization. SWIFT PRIME introduced an automated post-processing imaging pipeline software for penumbra profiling (RAPID), although its use was not mandatory or part of the inclusion criteria. Infarct core volume was estimated from CT Perfusion (CTP) using RAPID. A cut-off of infarct core volume of >50 mL on CTP was used to exclude patients. The ischemic core was defined by regional cerebral blood volume (CBV) or delayed time to peak (TTP) of the residual function. Moreover, patients with baseline ASPECTS score of less than six were excluded. The SWIFT PRIME study achieved the highest recanalization (defined by modified TICI score of 2b or 3) rate of 88% for the MT arm in comparison to the other four contemporary endovascular trials. The MT group showed 24.7% improvement in the functional outcome at 90 days (mRS 0–2: MT 60.2% vs standard therapy 35.5%, $P < 0.001$). Efficacy of MT in SWIFT-PRIME (60.2%) was higher than MR CLEAN (32.6%) and ESCAPE (53%) trials. No significant group differences in sICH risk (0% vs 3%, $P = 0.12$), or 90-day mortality (9% vs 12%, $P > 0.05$) were found.

EXTEND-IA was an Australasian trial involving 10 centres across Australia and New Zealand that enrolled 70 patients who were randomised to receive IV-rtPA alone, or MT using Solitaire FR stentriever plus IV-rtPA [76]. Like the SWIFT PRIME, EXTEND-IA also required administration of MT and IV-rtPA within 6 and 4.5 h of onset of stroke symptom, respectively. However, unlike other trials, there was no restriction on stroke severity as a criterion for patient inclusion. Moreover, age or ASPECTS score was not part of criteria for randomization. Premorbid functional status of mRS 0 to 2 was required for inclusion in the study. With regards to neuroimaging selection criteria, CTP for detection of favourable penumbra using RAPID software similar to SWIFT PRIME (CTP core volume less than 70 mL or mismatch ratio greater than 1.2), and CTA for large artery occlusion diagnosis were used to randomise patients. The primary outcome for the EXTEND-IA study was a reduction in the NIHSS score of 8 or higher, a score of 0 or 1 on mRS at 90 days, or reduction in perfusion lesion volume. EXTEND-IA showed the highest improvement in functional outcome at 90 days in comparison to the other four-endovascular trials (31.4%), and recanalization rate (86.2%) comparable to SWIFT PRIME. The number needed to treat (NNT) was the lowest for EXTEND-IA (NNT: 3.2 (EXTEND-IA) vs. 7.1 (MR PRIME) vs. 4.2 (ESCAPE) vs. 4 (SWIFT-PRIME) vs. 6.3 (REVASCAT)). The MT arm showed significantly improved functional outcome compared to the standard therapy arm (70% vs. 40%, $P = 0.001$). The investigators reported no significant differences in risk of sICH and mortality between the two groups.

REVASCAT was a Spanish trial involving four tertiary hospitals that enrolled 206 AIS patients presenting within 8 h of the symptom onset randomised to receive MT with the Solitaire FR plus standard medical therapy ($n = 103$) or standard medical therapy including IV-rtPA for eligible patients (n = 103) [113]. Clinical inclusion criteria included age between 18 and 80 years, NIHSS of 6 or more, and a pre-treatment mRS score of 0 to 1. Neuroimaging with CTA or MRA was used to select patients with large vessel occlusion. Moreover, only patients with ASPECTS scores of seven and above on NCCT or six and above on DWI MRI were included. Interestingly, the inclusion criteria were revised to age < 85 years and ASPECTS score of eight or above on NCCT after the enrollment of 160 patients. The REVASCAT trial showed 65.7% recanalization for patients in MT arm, and a significant reduction in brain infarction volume at 24 h (16 mL vs. 39 mL, $P = 0.02$) vs. standard medical therapy. No significant differences were noted in the rates of sICH (1.9% vs. 1.9%, $P > 0.05$) or mortality (18.4 vs. 15.5, $P = 0.06$) between the two groups. Patients in the MT arm were more likely to have a better functional outcome at 90 days (43.7% vs. 28.2%; OR 2.1, 95% CI 1.1 to 4).

In summary, these five-endovascular randomised controlled trials have consistently shown that MT significantly improves reperfusion and functional outcome at 90 days without an increase in mortality compared to patients receiving standard medical therapy. Use of advanced imaging features such as ASPECTS scale or perfusion imaging may assist in selecting patients who are most likely to benefit from a combined approach. Advanced imaging helps to differentiate between salvageable tissue and irreversibly dead core. Unfortunately, selection of patients using advanced imaging excludes many patients who may otherwise have received intra-arterial treatment.

Two new clinical trials, the Trial and Cost-Effectiveness Evaluation of Intra-arterial Thrombectomy in Acute Ischemic Stroke (THRACE) [127] and the Assess the Penumbra System in the Treatment of Acute Stroke (THERAPY) [128], have addressed these shortcomings by keeping selection criteria to a minimum except for the use of angiographic technique such as CTA or MRA to localize and confirm the arterial occlusion. The THRACE trial, conducted across 26 centres in France, included 336 patients, aged 18 to 80 years and NIHSS score ranging between 10 and 25, presenting within 5 h of symptom onset with moderate to a severe stroke caused by the large artery occlusion of the anterior circulation (radiologically confirmed on CTA), out of which 195 received IVT, and 141 received combined IVT and MT treatment, without a selection based on advanced imaging-based criteria. Combined IV-rtPA and MT provided a higher rate of functional outcome at 90 days (54.2% vs. 42.1%). No significant differences in mortality and sICH risks were noted between the MT and control arms. The THERAPY trial, undertaken across four centres in the United States, selected patients with AIS presenting within 4.5 h of symptom onset who have evidence of large clot burden (clot length ≥ 8 mm) in the anterior circulation [128]. CTA was used to identify patients with large vessel occlusion. Patients with NIHSS score of eight and above and age between 18 and 85 years were included for randomization. Patients were then treated with both combined IV-rtPA and IAT with the Penumbra aspiration system (a new technique of aspiration thrombectomy) or with the IV-rtPA alone. The results showed a positive trend, though not significant, of aspiration thrombectomy towards better functional outcomes (38% vs. 30.4%). Interestingly, the intervention arm showed a considerable reduction (11.9%) in mortality (mortality in intervention arm vs. control arm: 12% vs. 23.9%). No significant difference in sICH risk was observed (10.9% vs. 11.3%).

To sum up, MT has a number of advantages over systemic thrombolysis [87]: (a) MT yields higher rates of revascularization, and reduced rates of long-term functional dependence, in a select group of AIS patients with large vessel occlusion, compared to IVT alone [78, 79, 129–131], (b) MT extends the therapeutic time-window for acute intervention up to 24 h from stroke onset, beyond the 4.5 h restricted time window for IVT, which is applicable to only a small number of AIS patients [74, 119, 132–134], (c) MT presents a viable alternative to patients with large vessel occlusion who respond poorly, vis a vis poor recanalization rates and risk of haemorrhage, with systemic therapy [134], or those who have contraindications to the use of systemic thrombolysis, and (d) MT is efficient in dissolving clots which are resistant to enzymatic degradation, such as old and large clots with hardened fibrin and cross-linked thrombi containing calcium and cholesterol crystals, which have poor recanalization yields with systemic thrombolysis [93, 133, 135].

Combined intravenous and endovascular therapy: A multimodal reperfusion therapy (MMRT) approach

The idea behind combining intravenous and endovascular approaches, also called bridge therapy [136–141] or multimodal reperfusion therapy (MMRT), is to take advantage of best of both approaches by allowing fast and early access to IV-rtPA within the first 4.5 h of stroke onset, and superior recanalization rates even for delayed time windows beyond 4.5 h using endovascular therapy [142]. Notably, the Interventional Management of Stroke (IMS) I [143] and II [144] trials were conducted to investigate the feasibility and safety of combined interventions: low dose, 0.6 mg/kg, IV-rtPA followed by intra-arterial rtPA within 3 h since stroke onset, to recanalization of AIS. The bridge IV and IA therapy were not significantly different from the IV-rtPA alone as both yielded similar proportions of ICH, rates of mortality and mRS at 90 days. The subsequent IMS III trial also found no additional benefit of bridge therapy compared with IV-rtPA alone [145]. One of the important factors that may have played a role in these results is the time delay (approximately 32 min) between the IV-rtPA and initiation of intra-arterial therapy [121, 143]. Unlike the neutral results of IMS III trial, a recent meta-analysis reported a significantly strong association of combined intravenous-IA thrombolysis over IV fibrinolysis alone with favourable outcome, reduced mortality, and improved recanalization rates [146].

The Stent-Assisted Recanalization in Acute Ischemic Stroke (SARIS) trial, conducted to investigate the safety of intracranial stent deployment within 8 h of stroke onset, demonstrated expeditious recanalization, and favourable outcomes at 30 and 180 days clinical follow-up [147, 148]. Stent deployment averts arterial reocclusion and thrombus reformation in cases with partial embolectomy or arterial stenosis. The utility of self-expanding stents (SES) has been explored. The SES yields dramatically high recanalization rate of up to 90% by a combination of balloon angioplasty and stent implantation [147]. Undoubtedly, the bridge endovascular therapy using MT, intracranial stent deployment, and IV thrombolysis allows an extended time window, and therefore a higher proportion of revascularisations and improved clinical outcomes in AIS patients with large artery occlusion of anterior circulation [22].

A number of MMRT approaches including combined IV-rtPA and IA-tPA [136–138, 140, 141, 149], IV-tPA followed by multimodal endovascular therapy [150], combined IA thrombolytics and glycoprotein IIb/IIIa inhibitors [151], IA administration of microbubbles and continuous 2-MHz ultrasound insonation [139], IA-tPA followed by stenting [152, 153] or angioplasty or both [154, 155], IA urokinase and mechanical clot disruption following failed IV-tPA [156], MT using balloon angioplasty and adjuvant systemic thrombolysis (IV-tPA, IA urokinase, both IV-tPA and IA-urokinase, and IV and/or IA eptifibatide) [157], MT (MERCI retrieval, angioplasty/stent) with or without adjunctive IA-tPA/ Urokinase [158], MT using clot retrievers and angioplasty with intracranial or extracranial stenting [151], have demonstrated considerably improved recanalization, reperfusion and clinical outcomes [140, 150, 151, 154, 155, 159, 160]. Gupta et al. (2011) reported significantly higher recanalization rates for multimodal therapy (MT using intracranial stenting in conjunction with IV/ IA thrombolysis) (74% [435/584]) in comparison to pharmacologic treatment only (61% [160/264]), or MT only (63% [173/274]) in a large retrospective cohort of 1122 AIS patients involving the anterior circulation who received IAT within 8 h of stroke onset [153].

Drawing from the success of these studies, an endovascular MMRT approach using pharmacological thrombolytics (IA lytic drugs), in conjunction with MT using mechanical devices such as clot retrievers, angioplasty with stenting, aspiration devices, and stent retrievers is being increasingly adopted as the treatment of choice for stroke due to large vessel occlusion [153, 159]. Endovascular MMRT or bridge therapy offers a safe alternative for AIS patients, with large intracranial vessel occlusion, who fail to reperfuse with systemic thrombolytic drugs.

Role of collaterals in penumbral sustenance and recanalization

Recanalization is positively associated with favourable clinical outcome and increased survival rates in acute ischemic stroke [39, 40, 161–165]. A meta-analysis of 53 studies encompassing 2066 patients reported strong association of recanalization with the good functional outcome (OR 4.43, 95% CI 3.32 to 5.91), and reduced mortality (OR 0.24, 95% CI 0.16 to 0.35) at 3 months in AIS [146]. The rate of recanalization classified based on intervention: spontaneous, IV fibrinolytic, intra-arterial fibrinolytic, combined IV and IA thrombolysis or MT was 24.1, 46.2, 63.2, 67.5, 83.6%, respectively. Early recanalization is associated with rapid clinical improvement in some patients [166]. However, despite early recanalization, some patients who are otherwise unresponsive to treatment over short-time follow-up, may show delayed recovery or favourable long-term outcome suggesting the possibility of an "ischemic stunning" or "stunned brain" syndrome [167]. Recanalization enables restoration of cerebral blood flow to the hypoperfused brain region surrounding the infarcted 'core'. This area of the brain with reversible ischemia surrounding the infarcted core is called ischemic penumbra [168]. Animal studies have indicated that considerable salvage of penumbral tissue is possible on the restoration of blood flow to the hypoperfused brain area, even after 24 h, irrespective of time of reperfusion [169, 170]. From a pathophysiological standpoint, the survival of penumbra, independent of time, for up to 48 h has been reported using a ligand that selectively binds to hypoxic but viable tissue ([(18)F]fluoromisonidazole), and positron emission tomography (PET) on consecutive patients presenting within 48 h of AIS [171]. As expected, the penumbra reduces over time; it is observed in 90–100% of stroke patients in the first 3 h after stroke onset [172], 75–80% of patients 6 h after stroke onset, and approximately 33% of patients 18 h after stroke onset [173].

Despite the success of endovascular procedures, a number of patient-specific factors may determine the response to treatment such as (a) collateral circulation [174–176], (b) site of vessel occlusion [48], (c) onset to angiographic reperfusion time [177–179], (d) hyperglycemia [180–182], and (c) location of cerebral ischemia [174, 183]. In the case of cerebral ischemia, collaterals compensate for the sudden drop in CBF in the hypoperfused area by the maintenance of a continual blood supply to ischemic penumbra. For recanalization to translate into positive outcomes, adequate collaterals must delay the infarction of tissue until recanalization is achieved [184]. Collaterals can sustain the penumbra even in the absence of reperfusion or recanalization. According to a meta-analysis, good baseline collaterals were associated with favourable outcome at 90 days, decrease in the risk of symptomatic ICH, and decrease in risk of death at 90 days in patients with AIS receiving endovascular treatment [176]. Good baseline collaterals have been found to be associated with 24 h perilesional hyperperfusion [185], good clinical outcome [176, 186–189], lower rates of symptomatic ICH and mortality [176], improved radiologic outcome [188], cortical infarct volume [190], good reperfusion [191], and stroke severity [191]. On the other hand, delayed-cortical vein filling was independently associated with reduced baseline collateral status in AIS [185]. Collateral grading is used to determine recanalization rate after endovascular reperfusion therapy [175, 192]. Collateral pathophysiology may have predictive value, and patent collaterals may help boost reperfusion [193]. Some scales and grading tools are available for reliable and quick assessment of the patency of collaterals by visual examination of multiphase CTA [189].

Limitations and unresolved questions of endovascular reperfusion therapy

Despite the substantial advantages of MT, this is only offered to a limited number (5–10%) of AIS patients [131]. Currently, vascular imaging such as CTA or MRA is not routinely performed at the time of presentation. The treating physician needs to make a rapid decision based on the vascular imaging (whether or not angiography shows a large vessel occlusion), assessment of ischemic penumbra (based on CT or MR perfusion imaging), time since the onset of stroke symptoms, along with other baseline clinical factors and previous history (such as significant past trauma, haemorrhage or stroke) [90, 127, 194]. The need for advanced imaging, especially CTA, implies that only a few select AIS patients would be suitable for MT. MT with current devices is not well suited for AIS with occlusions in distal locations and with penetrator occlusions due to difficulty in navigating with the catheter, increased risk of intraprocedural vessel perforation, and a higher risk of mortality [101, 195]. Also, patients with in situ intracranial atherothrombi (in situ atherosclerotic plaque with supervening thrombosis), may be more suited for balloon angioplasty and stenting over MT [101]. MT yields superior recanalization rates with occlusions of cardioembolic origin [196] or proximal aortocervical arterial source [101]. Delayed treatment may lead to further shrinking of salvageable penumbral tissue due to absence or insufficient reperfusion. MT is a highly specialized interventional procedure; as such, it is strongly recommended that MT be performed in a comprehensive stroke unit with a well-equipped neurointervention suite by an interventional neuroradiologist or an endovascular specialist with experience in the procedure, or a credentialed neurointerventionist along with a team of stroke neurologists, and nursing staff [197]. Lack of experienced practitioners (such as credentialed neuro interventionist, endovascular specialists) [197], along with logistic difficulties such as prehospital delays (e.g., prolonged transfer time to and from rural hospitals), and inter-facility transfers, make MT unlikely to be widely implemented. A comprehensive national and international stroke care policy needs to be adopted to address these logistical and other systemic deficiencies within the relevant healthcare systems.

In addition to the limitations of present reperfusion therapies in AIS settings, a number of unresolved questions or issues need to be addressed.

Extending the time window of MT beyond 6 h

Evidence for efficacy and safety of endovascular reperfusion beyond 6 h is still insufficient given that no randomised trial has used this as an inclusion criterion. However, a recent meta-analysis has indicated the benefit of endovascular MT plus medical therapy up to 7.3 h after the symptom onset [118]. Some trials including the premise of the Diffusion and Perfusion Imaging Evaluation for Understanding Stroke Evolution (DEFUSE 3), the DWI or CTP Assessment With Clinical Mismatch in the Triage of Wake-Up and Late Presenting Strokes Undergoing Neurointervention (DAWN), the Perfusion Imaging Selection of Ischemic Stroke Patients for Endovascular Therapy (POSITIVE) and Imaging-Guided Patient Selection for Interventional Revascularization Therapy (START) trials seek to extend the time to endovascular reperfusion. DEFUSE 3 selects AIS patients using penumbral mismatch on CTP or MRI who may benefit from MT between 6 h and 16 h post onset [198]. Similarly, the goal of the POSITIVE trial is to use appropriate imaging selection to improve stroke-related disability, and functional outcome in AIS patients treated with MT presenting between 6 to 12 h who are either ineligible for or refractory to IV-tPA treatment [199]. DAWN, which recruited patients in which treatment with Trevo MT was initiated within 6–24 h after stroke onset [200] [201], was terminated early after an interim analysis of the first 200 patients demonstrated a 73% relative risk reduction in disability (48.6% in MT group vs. 13.6% in control group). DAWN study has confirmed that advanced imaging based patient selection outweighs time-based decision making in acute ischemic stroke [119]. This has major implications for treatment in acute ischemic stroke given that DAWN showed efficacy over an extended time window from 6 to 24 h [202].

General anaesthesia vs. conscious sedation

The type of anaesthesia, whether general anaesthesia (GA) or conscious sedation, has implications for outcomes in AIS patients during and after endovascular treatment [203]. This has been a subject of ongoing debate given that several retrospective studies have hypothesised that GA may be associated with periprocedural hypotension that may cause poorer clinical outcome, despite the procedural advantages of GA [203–205]. A consensus is still missing over the anaesthetic management of AIS patients during IAT [206]. The MR CLEAN pre-trial study group found that non-GA was significantly associated with good clinical outcomes in AIS patients undergoing IAT [206]. Three randomized trials, Sedation vs Intubation for Endovascular Stroke Treatment (SIESTA) [207], the General or Local Anaesthesia in Intra-arterial Therapy (GOLIATH) [208], and the Sedation Versus General Anaesthesia for Endovascular Therapy in Acute Stroke (ANSTROKE) [209], aimed to investigate the impact of anaesthesia type on neurological outcome in IAT, and whether conscious sedation is the optimal anaesthesiologic management modality in endovascular stroke therapy [122, 210]. ANSTROKE [211] and SIESTA [212, 213] have both recently demonstrated no advantage in neurological status at 24 h or 3 months for patients undergoing MT with conscious sedation.

Posterior circulation stroke

AIS in the posterior circulation is associated with poor prognosis with standard medical therapy (IV-tPA) [214, 215]. Basilar artery occlusion (BAO) is a form of posterior circulation stroke that results in higher rates of poor functional outcome and mortality if not recanalized [214, 216]. A systematic analysis of 420 BAO patients treated with IVT (76) and IAT (344) found that without recanalization only 2% patients were likely to have good outcome [216]. Recanalization was more common in IAT-treated patients than those who received IVT (65% (225/344) vs. 53% (40/76). The success of recanalization of acute BAO following IVT depends on thrombus length [45]. Another analysis on 592 BAO patients drawn from a prospective register also challenged the notion of unequivocal superiority of IAT over IV-tPA in BAO patients [217]. Interestingly, bridge therapies combining IAT using modern MT devices and IV-tPA have yielded good recanalization and improved survival rates for acute BAO [218–220]. Based on these findings, a multicenter randomized controlled trial, Basilar Artery International Cooperation Study (BASICS), was conceived, and is currently underway, to evaluate the efficacy of IAT plus standard medical treatment versus standard therapy alone in patients with acute BAO stroke [221, 222]. Recent studies have shown MT with the Solitaire FR device is associated with high recanalization rates and favourable outcome [223, 224].

Minimising the delay to endovascular reperfusion

Direct Transfer to an Endovascular Center Compared to Transfer to the Closest Stroke Centre in Acute Stroke Patients With Suspected Large Vessel Occlusion (RACECAT) is a prospective, randomized controlled trial which aims to evaluate the effectiveness of direct transfer to an endovascular stroke center based on identification of suspected large vessel occlusion in AIS patients using a prehospital screening tool, rapid artery occlusion evaluation (RACE) scale, in comparison to the transfer to the closest local stroke center [225]. The motivation behind this trial is to minimise the time to endovascular reperfusion. Triaging of AIS patients for their eligibility to IAT requires CT for determination of the presence of large artery occlusion. However, it may be possible to select patients based on non-imaging scales that can be easily applied without extensive training. Staff with emergency medical services (EMS) could be trained to use these scales (e.g., NIHSS, RACE) in screening AIS patients for their eligibility to receive reperfusion therapy.

In addition to the above issues, other treatment options such as the use of antithrombotic medications along with reperfusion therapy are also being explored. A phase III trial, Multi-Arm Optimisation of Stroke Thrombolysis [226], is investigating the efficacy of IV delivery of Argatroban and Eptifibatide in combination with rtPA in AIS. This strategy may be extended to patients who undergo MT. Some trials are currently underway or are in the planning phase to address the issues that limit the efficacy of endovascular reperfusion. A comprehensive list of ongoing and future trials is shown in Table 5.

Conclusions, discussions, and future recommendations

The approved treatment for acute ischemic stroke is reperfusion therapy using systemic thrombolysis or endovascular mechanical thrombectomy. The recent success of endovascular trials has revolutionised the way large artery occlusion stroke patients are managed. AHA/ASA has accordingly updated its guidelines for stroke care. The recommendation is to use MT with stent retriever in combination with standard therapy (IV-rtPA) in AIS patients, aged ≥18 years; baseline ASPECTS score ≥ 6, baseline NIHSS score ≥ 6 with angiographically confirmed large vessel occlusion presenting within 6 h of symptom onset (Level 1A evidence) [227, 228]. The workflow algorithm detailing the standard of care for IV-tPA and mechanical thrombectomy in AIS patients is shown in Fig. 2 (algorithm has been updated keeping in consideration recently published DAWN study [119, 202]).

Endovascular therapy also provides an alternative to systemic thrombolysis for patients who fail to reperfuse with IV-rtPA or those who are not eligible for IVT due to restricted time-window, or those with unknown onset or "wake-up" stroke, or contraindications [153, 159, 215]. However, due to a shortage of neurointerventionists or endovascular specialists experienced in the procedure [197], procedural complexity, high costs, pre-hospital delays, inter-facility transfers, and a limited number of institutions that offer endovascular treatment, only a select number of patients will likely be offered this therapy [229]. Future efforts to shorten the endovascular procedural time, build infrastructure to provide MT, and increase access to endovascular facilities are required [27]. Comprehensive stroke centers with access to IV and IA techniques, trained stroke neurointerventionists, imaging-guided treatment workflow, and access to advanced neurosurgical support will pave the way for high-end stroke care delivery. Meanwhile, given the present limitations, careful selection of patients is crucial to maximize the gain for appropriate patients. It has been suggested that patients with angiographically confirmed proximal large vessel occlusion with a viable penumbra on MRI and NIHSS > 18, within 8 and 24 h of stroke onset in the anterior and posterior circulation respectively, should be given endovascular MMRT [159]. Other authors

Table 5 List of ongoing and upcoming trials aimed to address the issues concerning the endovascular treatment of acute ischemic stroke

Trial	Time window	Purpose	Inclusion criteria	Outcome measure
RACECAT [225]	0-8 h	Triage of the acute LVO on direct transfer to EVT-SC bypassing LSC vs. transfer to the LSC according to the current stroke protocol.	Premorbid mRS 0–2 Age ≥ 18 Suspected LVO AIS identified by a RACE scale score > 4 evaluated by EMS professional Time to arrival at EVT-SC <7 h from symptom onset	mRS at 90 days (shift analysis) Mortality at 90 days Mortality in haemorrhagic stroke patients Clinical deterioration (≥4 points on the NIHSS) Clinical benefit of direct vs. local transfer Dramatic early favourable response (NIHSS improvement ≥8 or NIHSS score of 0–2 at 24 h)
DEFUSE 3 [198]	6-16 h	Benefit of carefully selected patients with target mismatch and MCA (M1 segment) or ICA occlusion using CT/MR within 6–16 h treated with MT plus standard therapy vs. standard therapy alone.	Age 18–90 years Baseline NIHSSS is ≥6 Time to endovascular treatment since symptom onset = 6–16 h Premorbid mRS 0–2 ICA or MCA-M1 occlusion by MRA or CTA and target mismatch profile on CTP or MRI (ischemic core volume < 70 mL, mismatch ratio >/= 1.8, and mismatch volume >/= 15 mL) ASPECT on NCCT >/=6 No evidence of tumour, mass effect with midline shift, ICA or aortic dissection No occlusions in multiple vascular territories	Distribution of mRS scores at 90 days Proportion of patients with mRS 0–2 Infarct growth within 24 h Reperfusion rates at 24 h Ischemic lesion growth at 24 h
DAWN [119, 200]	6-24 h	MT using the Trevo Retriever with medical management is superior to medical management alone in improving clinical outcomes at 90 days in appropriately selected wake up and late presenting AIS within 6–24 h after symptom onset [119]	Subjects with failed IV-tPA or contraindicated for IV-tPA Age ≥ 18 Baseline NIHSS ≥ 10 Can be randomised within 6–24 h of stroke onset Pre-stroke mRS 0 or 1 <1/3 MCA territory involved, as evidenced by CT or MRI Intracranial ICA and/or MCA-M1 occlusion on MRA/CTA CIM defined on MR-DWI or CTP-rCBF maps: (a) 0- < 21 cm^3 core infarct and NIHSS ≥10 (and age ≥ 80 years old), (b) 0- < 31 cm^3 core infarct and NIHSS ≥10 (and age < 80 years old), or (c) 31 cm^3 to <51 cm^3 core infarct and NIHSS ≥20 (and age < 80 years old) ICH or differential diagnosis on CT/MRI	Weighted mRS at 90 days Mortality at 90 days Good functional outcome (mRS 0–2) Revascularization rate at 24 h on CTA/MRA Neurological deterioration defined by as ≥4-point increase in the NIHSS score from the baseline score at 5–7 days or at discharge.
POSITIVE [199]	6-12 h	To determine the safety and efficacy of IAT in AIS patients Ineligible for or refractory to IV-rtPA as selected by physiologic imaging	Age ≥ 18 NIHSS ≥8 at the time of neuroimaging Time to the groin puncture 6–12 h Large vessel proximal occlusion (distal ICA through MCA M1 bifurcation) Patients who have had IV-tPA without improvement in symptoms Pre-stroke morbidity mRS 0–1 Presence of large penumbra No evidence of SAH or ICH or mass effect with midline shift <1/3 MCA territory involved, as evidenced by baseline CT or ASPECTS of >7	90 day mRS Good functional outcome mRS 0–2 at 90 days Mortality at 30 and 90 days ICH with neurological deterioration (NIHSS worsening >4) within 24 h Arterial revascularization measured by TICI 2b or 3 following MT
ENDOSTROKE [287]	NR	Predictors of the good or poor clinical outcome following MT in AIS	Age ≥ 18 years Proximal arterial vessel occlusion No evidence of venous occlusion	mRS at 90 days Complete recanalization defined by TIMI grade two or 3. Periprocedural complication rate (sICH defined by ECASS PH1 and PH2, SAH and thromboembolic events).
START [288]	0-8 h	Efficacy of the Penumbra System in AIS with a known core infarct volume at admission presenting within 8 h of onset. To study the correlation between infarct-volume and functional outcome at 90 days in MT treated patients	Age 18 to 85 years NIHSS ≥10 at admission Evidence of proximal large vessel occlusion (supra clinoid segment of ICA through the M1 segment of MCA) Patients presenting within 8 h, and those within 3 h must be ineligible or refractory to IV-rtPA Core infarct volume assessed by CTP, CTA or DWI scans within 60 min to arterial puncture. No history of stroke within 3 months No evidence of mass effect with midline shift or ICH on NCCT No evidence of arterial stenosis proximal to the occlusion that could prevent thrombectomy No evidence of preexisting arterial injury Life expectancy <90 days	Good functional outcome mRS 0–2 at 90 days Recanalization assessment using TIMI and mTICI immediately after MT Periprocedural serious events Good neurological recovery (NIHSS ≥10) at discharge Incidence of sICH and asymptomatic haemorrhage defined by ECASS criteria and patient neurological status within 24 h of the procedure.

Table 5 List of ongoing and upcoming trials aimed to address the issues concerning the endovascular treatment of acute ischemic stroke *(Continued)*

Trial	Time window	Purpose	Inclusion criteria	Outcome measure
EASI [289]	0-5 h	To evaluate the efficacy of IV-rtPA vs combined (MT plus IV-rtPA) treatment in AIS	Age ≥ 18 NIHSS ≥8 Onset to treatment less than 5 h or symptom/ imaging mismatch Occlusion of MCA (m1 or M2), supraclinoid ICA or basilar trunk No evidence of haemorrhagic transformation of the infarcted territory	Favourable clinical outcome (mRS 0–2 at 90 days) sICH on CT at 24 h Infarct evolution on CT between pre-treatment and 24 h using the ASPECT score Recanalization using TICI scale after thrombectomy Procedural complication within 3 months ICH on NCCT at 24 h
BASICS [221, 222]	0-6 h	Efficacy and safety of IAT plus standard medical therapy vs. standard medical alone in patients with an acute symptomatic basilar artery occlusion (BAO)	Symptoms of BAO stroke BAO confirmed by CTA or MRA Age ≥ 18 NIHSS ≥8 at the time of neuroimaging IAT initiated within 6 h of onset of symptoms Premorbid score of 0–2 No ICH or mass effect on CT	Favourable outcome mRS 0–2 Excellent outcome mRS 0–3 Recanalization at 24 ± 6 h on CTA Volume of infarction on NCCT and CTA source images at 24 ± 6 h sICH at 24 ± 6 h on CTA Mortality at 90 days NIHSS pre, and port IV-tPA and at 24 h EQ-5D – Quality of life at 90 and 120 days
SIESTA [207, 213]	NR	Efficacy of conscious sedation vs. general anaesthesia during IAT. Update: No advantage for the use of conscious sedation recently reported [213].	Age ≥ 18 years Acute stroke in anterior circulation ICA or MCA occlusion on CTA No evidence of ICH	Higher NIHSS of >10 at 24 h NIHSS improvement mRS at 90 days Mortality before discharge or at 90 days Duration of hospital stay Recanalization status on TICI Periinterventional complications
GOLIATH [208]	NR	Efficacy of general vs. local anaesthesia during IAT	Age ≥ 18 years NIHSS > 10 mRS = <2 groin puncture < 6 h from stroke onset occlusion of ICA, ICA-T, M1, M2 GCS > 9 No evidence of posterior circulation stroke	Growth of DWI lesion (48–72 h] mRS score at 90 days Blood pressure during intervention (1–2 h) Time from arrival to the groin puncture and recanalization (1–2 h)
ANSTROKE [209]	NR	To study the efficacy of general anaesthesia vs sedation technique during embolectomy for AIS stroke (systolic pressure 140–180 mmHg)	Age ≥ 18 years CTA confirmed occlusion in ICA, ACA (A1 segment), MCA (M1 or M2 segments) NIHSS ≥14 for patients with embolus in left hemisphere or NIHSS ≥10 for embolus in right hemisphere No evidence of posterior circulation embolus No evidence of ICH on CT Pre-stroke mRS of ≤3 No evidence of spontaneous recanalization	90 day mRS Change in NIHSS score compared to admission (Day 3, 7 and 90) Degree of recanalization and reperfusion (1 day after embolectomy) Periprocedural complications Infarction magnitude CT day 1 including CTP MR on day 3 (2–4) and 3 months Brain markers (GFAP, Tau, S-100B) before, 2, 24, 48, 72 h and 3 months after the embolectomy Quantitative EEG 1, 2 and 90 days after onset Length of hospital stay Preprocedural time consumption (stroke onset to CTA, CTA to start of anaesthesia/ sedation, stroke onset to start of embolectomy and duration of embolectomy.
MOST [226]	NR	Phase III trial to explore the efficacy of IV delivery of antithrombotic medications Argatroban and Eptifibatide in combination with rtPA in AIS.	NIHSS > 6	mRS at 90 days longitudinal model relating 30 day mRS to 90 days mRS

RACECAT Direct Transfer to an Endovascular Centre Compared to Transfer to the Closest Stroke Centre in Acute Stroke Patients With Suspected Large Vessel Occlusion; *RACE* scale Rapid Arterial occlusion Evaluation; *mRS* Modified Rankin score; *EMS* Emergency medical service; *LVO* Large vessel occlusion; *AIS* Acute ischemic stroke; *LSC* Local stroke centre; *EVT-LSC* Endovascular stroke centre; *DEFUSE-3* Endovascular Therapy Following Imaging Evaluation for Ischemic Stroke 3; *DAWN* Trevo and Medical Management Versus Medical Management Alone in Wake Up and Late Presenting Strokes; *BASICS* Basilar Artery International Cooperation Study; *IAT* Intra-arterial therapy; *IV-rtPA* Intra venous tissue plasminogen activator; *NCCT* Non-contrast computed tomography; *CTA CT* angiography; *sICH* Symptomatic intracranial haemorrhage; *SAH* Sub-arachnoid haemorrhage; *BAO* Basilar artery occlusion; *SIESTA* Sedation vs. Intubation for Endovascular Stroke Treatment; *GOLIATH* The General or Local Anaesthesia in Intra-arterial Therapy; *MOST* The Multi-Arm Optimization of Stroke Thrombolysis; *NR* Not required; *ANSTROKE* Sedation Versus General Anaesthesia for Endovascular Therapy in Acute Stroke - Impact on Neurological Outcome; *ENDOSTROKE* International Multicenter Registry for Mechanical Recanalization Procedures in Acute Stroke; *TIMI* Thrombolysis in Myocardial Infarction; *START* Imaging Guided Patient Selection for Interventional Revascularization Therapy; *EASI* Endovascular Acute Stroke Intervention Trial

recommend a lower threshold of NIHSS ≥7 on the addition of advanced neuroimaging parameters including ASPECTS ≥6 or 7, and angiographically confirmed large vessel occlusion with moderate-to-good collaterals on multiphase CT to select candidates for endovascular MT using stent retriever [230]. With regards to MRI led patient selection based on infarct volume, endovascular therapy is also preferred for large artery occluded AIS patients with small infarct defined by early DWI volume < 70 mL, and an

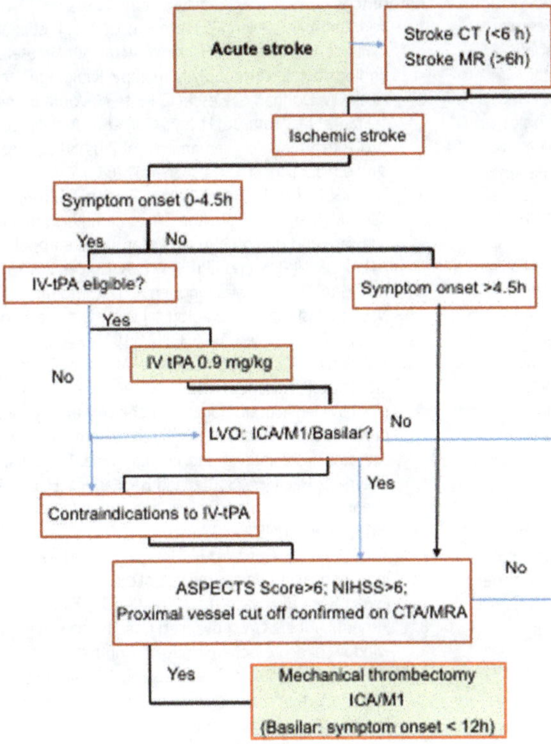

Fig. 2 Workflow diagram detailing the algorithm to select AIS patients with or without large artery occlusion for IV-tPA, MT, or IV-tPA followed by MT. CT = computed tomography; MRI = magnetic resonance imaging; IV-tPA = intravenous trans-plasminogen activator; ICU = intensive care unit; CTA = CT angiography; MRA = MR angiography; LVO = large vessel occlusion; NIHSS = National Institutes of Health Stroke Scale; ICA = internal carotid artery

accessible proximal occlusion. Endovascular MMRT or standalone MT is not suitable with distal occlusion or lacunar stroke. High revascularization yields obtained using (a) MMRT or combinational approaches that include IA/IV thrombolytic agents, stenting, angioplasty, aspiration, clot retrieval, (b) second generation MT devices such as Solitaire and Trevo, (c) combined MT interventions using suction embolectomy with large bore microcatheters such as Penumbra MAX [104–107] and stent retrievers, and (d) with latest generation Penumbra 3D separator [100, 108, 109] are encouraging.

In conclusion, both IV thrombolysis and endovascular treatment have been incorporated into the standard of care in stroke therapy. In light of recent studies in favour of imaging based selection of AIS patients for reperfusion therapy, the time window of MT may extend to 24 h (or beyond) since symptom onset [119, 202]. However, further research, exploring bridge therapy or MMRT in addition to advanced imaging-based approaches to select appropriate patients, may also widen the time-window for patient selection and would contribute immensely to early thrombolytic strategies, better recanalization rates, and improved clinical outcomes.

Abbreviations

AHA/ASA: American Heart Association/American Stroke Association; AIS: Acute Ischemic Stroke; ANSTROKE: Sedation Versus General Anaesthesia for Endovascular Therapy in Acute Stroke; ASPECTS: Alberta Stroke Program Early CT Score; ATLANTIS: Alteplase Thrombolysis for Acute Noninterventional Therapy in Ischemic Stroke; BAO: Basilar artery occlusion; BASICS: Basilar Artery International Cooperation Study; CASES: Canadian Alteplase for Stroke Effectiveness Study; CBV: Cerebral blood volume; CTA: CT angiography; CTP: CT Perfusion; DAWN: DWI or CTP Assessment with Clinical Mismatch in the Triage of Wake-Up and Late Presenting Strokes Undergoing Neurointervention; DEFUSE: Diffusion and Perfusion Imaging Evaluation for Understanding Stroke Evolution; DVT: deep venous thrombosis; ECASS: European Collaborative Acute Stroke Study; EMS: Emergency medical services; EPITHET: Echoplanar Imaging Thrombolysis Evaluation Trial; ESCAPE: Endovascular Treatment for Small Core and Anterior Circulation Proximal Occlusion with Emphasis on Minimizing CT to Recanalization Times; ESCAPE: Endovascular Treatment for Small Core and Proximal Occlusion Ischemic Stroke; ESO: European Stroke Organisation; EXTEND-IA: Extending the Time for Thrombolysis in Emergency Neurological Deficits–Intra-arterial; FDA: Federal Drugs Agency; GA: General anaesthesia; GOLIATH: General or Local Anaesthesia in Intra-arterial Therapy; HERMES: Highly Effective Reperfusion evaluated in Multiple Endovascular Stroke Trials; IAT: Intra-arterial thrombolysis; ICA: Internal carotid artery occlusion; ICH: Intra-cerebral hemorrhage; IMS: Interventional Management of Stroke; IST: International Stroke Thrombolysis; IV rtPA: Intravenous recombinant tissue plasminogen activator; MCA: Middle cerebral artery; MELT: Middle Cerebral Artery

Embolism Local Fibrinolytic Intervention Trial; MMRT: Multimodal reperfusion therapy; MR CLEAN: Multicenter Randomized Clinical Trial of Endovascular Treatment for Acute Ischemic Stroke in the Netherlands; MRA: Magnetic resonance angiography; mRS: Modified Rankin Score; MT: Mechanical thrombectomy; NCCT: non-contrast computed tomography; NIHSS: National Institutes of Health Stroke Scale; NINDS: National Institute of Neurological Disorders and Stroke; NNT: Number need to treat; PAI: Plasminogen activator inhibitor; POSITIVE: Perfusion Imaging Selection of Ischemic Stroke Patients for Endovascular Therapy; PROACT: Prolyse in Acute Cerebral Thromboembolism; RACE: Rapid artery occlusion evaluation; RACECAT: Direct Transfer to an Endovascular Centre Compared to Transfer to the Closest Stroke Centre in Acute Stroke Patients with Suspected Large Vessel Occlusion; REVASCAT: Randomized Trial of Revascularization with Solitaire FR Device vs Best Medical Therapy in the Treatment of Acute Stroke Due to Anterior Circulation Large Vessel Occlusion Presenting within 8 h of Symptom Onset; SARIS: Stent-Assisted Recanalization in Acute Ischemic Stroke; SES: Self-expanding stents; sICH: Symptomatic intracerebral haemorrhage; SIESTA: Sedation vs Intubation for Endovascular Stroke Treatment; SITS-ISTR: Safe Implementation of Thrombolysis in Stroke-International Stroke Thrombolysis Register; SK: Streptokinase; START: Imaging-Guided Patient Selection for Interventional Revascularization Therapy; SWIFT PRIME: Solitaire with the Intention for Thrombectomy as Primary Endovascular Treatment of Acute Ischemic Stroke; SYNTHESIS: Local Versus Systemic Thrombolysis for Acute Ischemic Stroke; TAFI: Thrombin-activatable fibrinolysis inhibitor; THERAPY: Assess the Penumbra System in the Treatment of Acute Stroke; THRACE: Trial and Cost-Effectiveness Evaluation of Intra-arterial Thrombectomy in Acute Ischemic Stroke; TICI: Thrombolysis in Cerebral Infarction; TIMI: Thrombolysis in Myocardial Infarction; TK: Tenecteplase; TTP: Time to peak; UK: Urokinase; uPA: urinary-type plasminogen activator

Acknowledgements
We would like to acknowledge Prof Mark Parsons for his critical feedback.

Funding
Hunter Medical Research Institute, National Health & Medical Research Council, & the University of Newcastle.

Authors' contributions
SB and CL conceptualised the original draft. PS, JRA and DC contributed to the revision of the manuscript. All authors read and approved the final manuscript.

Competing interests
The authors declare that they have no competing interests.

Author details
[1]Western Sydney University (WSU), School of Medicine, South West Sydney Clinical School, Sydney, NSW 2170, Australia. [2]Liverpool Hospital, Department of Neurology & Neurophysiology, Liverpool 2170, NSW, Australia. [3]The Sydney Partnership for Health, Education, Research & Enterprise (SPHERE), Liverpool, NSW, Australia. [4]Stroke & Neurology Research Group, Ingham Institute for Applied Medical Research, 1 Campbell Street, Liverpool, NSW 2170, Australia. [5]School of Medicine, University of New South Wales (UNSW), Sydney, NSW, Australia. [6]Department of Neurology, John Hunter Hospital, Newcastle, NSW, Australia. [7]Priority Research Centre for Stroke & Brain Injury, Faculty of Health & Medicine, Hunter Medical Research institute (HMRI) and School of Medicine & Public Health, University of Newcastle, Newcastle, NSW, Australia. [8]Centre for Clinical Epidemiology & Biostatistics, Hunter Medical Research Institute, University of Newcastle, Newcastle, NSW, Australia.

References

1. von Kummer R, Allen KL, Holle R, Bozzao L, Bastianello S, Manelfe C, Bluhmki E, Ringleb P, Meier DH, Hacke W. Acute stroke: usefulness of early CT findings before thrombolytic therapy. Radiology. 1997;205(2):327–33.
2. Hacke W, Donnan G, Fieschi C, Kaste M, von Kummer R, Broderick JP, Brott T, Frankel M, Grotta JC, Haley EC Jr, et al. Association of outcome with early stroke treatment: pooled analysis of ATLANTIS, ECASS, and NINDS rt-PA stroke trials. Lancet. 2004;363(9411):768–74.
3. Lees KR, Bluhmki E, von Kummer R, Brott TG, Toni D, Grotta JC, Albers GW, Kaste M, Marler JR, Hamilton SA, et al. Time to treatment with intravenous alteplase and outcome in stroke: an updated pooled analysis of ECASS, ATLANTIS, NINDS, and EPITHET trials. Lancet. 2010;375(9727):1695–703.
4. NINDS-rtPA: Tissue plasminogen activator for acute ischemic stroke. The National Institute of Neurological Disorders and Stroke rt-PA stroke study group. N Engl J Med. 1995;333(24):1581–7.
5. Kwiatkowski TG, Libman RB, Frankel M, Tilley BC, Morgenstern LB, Lu M, Broderick JP, Lewandowski CA, Marler JR, Levine SR, et al. Effects of tissue plasminogen activator for acute ischemic stroke at one year. National Institute of Neurological Disorders and Stroke recombinant tissue Plasminogen activator stroke study group. N Engl J Med. 1999;340(23):1781–7.
6. Balami JS, Hadley G, Sutherland BA, Karbalai H, Buchan AM. The exact science of stroke thrombolysis and the quiet art of patient selection. Brain. 2013;136(Pt 12):3528–53.
7. Yoo AJ, Pulli B, Gonzalez RG. Imaging-based treatment selection for intravenous and intra-arterial stroke therapies: a comprehensive review. Expert Rev Cardiovasc Ther. 2011;9(7):857–76.
8. Fisher M, Albers GW. Advanced imaging to extend the therapeutic time window of acute ischemic stroke. Ann Neurol. 2013;73(1):4–9.
9. Duffis EJ, Al-Qudah Z, Prestigiacomo CJ, Gandhi C. Advanced neuroimaging in acute ischemic stroke: extending the time window for treatment. Neurosurg Focus. 2011;30(6):E5.
10. Sandhu GS, Sunshine JL. Advanced neuroimaging to guide acute stroke therapy. Curr Cardiol Rep. 2012;14(6):741–53.
11. Hacke W, Kaste M, Fieschi C, Toni D, Lesaffre E, von Kummer R, Boysen G, Bluhmki E, Hoxter G, Mahagne MH, et al. Intravenous thrombolysis with recombinant tissue plasminogen activator for acute hemispheric stroke. The European cooperative acute stroke study (ECASS). JAMA. 1995;274(13):1017–25.
12. Glauser J. Will EPs' reluctance to embrace Thrombolysis for stroke lead to lawsuits? Emerg Med News. 2006;28(7):23–5.
13. Schmulling S, Grond M, Rudolf J, Heiss WD. One-year follow-up in acute stroke patients treated with rtPA in clinical routine. Stroke. 2000;31(7):1552–4.
14. Emberson J, Lees KR, Lyden P, Blackwell L, Albers G, Bluhmki E, Brott T, Cohen G, Davis S, Donnan G, et al. Effect of treatment delay, age, and stroke severity on the effects of intravenous thrombolysis with alteplase for acute ischaemic stroke: a meta-analysis of individual patient data from randomised trials. Lancet. 2014;384(9958):1929–35.
15. Sandercock P, Wardlaw JM, Lindley RI, Dennis M, Cohen G, Murray G, Innes K, Venables G, Czlonkowska A, Kobayashi A, et al. The benefits and harms of intravenous thrombolysis with recombinant tissue plasminogen activator within 6 h of acute ischaemic stroke (the third international stroke trial [IST-3]): a randomised controlled trial. Lancet. 2012;379(9834):2352–63.
16. Hacke W, Kaste M, Bluhmki E, Brozman M, Davalos A, Guidetti D, Larrue V, Lees KR, Medeghri Z, Machnig T, et al. Thrombolysis with alteplase 3 to 4.5 hours after acute ischemic stroke. N Engl J Med. 2008;359(13):1317–29.
17. Hacke W, Kaste M, Fieschi C, von Kummer R, Davalos A, Meier D, Larrue V, Bluhmki E, Davis S, Donnan G, et al. Randomised double-blind placebo-controlled trial of thrombolytic therapy with intravenous alteplase in acute ischaemic stroke (ECASS II). Second European-Australasian acute stroke study investigators. Lancet. 1998;352(9136):1245–51.
18. Clark WM, Wissman S, Albers GW, Jhamandas JH, Madden KP, Hamilton S. Recombinant tissue-type plasminogen activator (Alteplase) for ischemic stroke 3 to 5 hours after symptom onset. The ATLANTIS study: a randomized controlled trial. Alteplase Thrombolysis for acute noninterventional therapy in ischemic stroke. JAMA. 1999;282(21):2019–26.
19. Clark WM, Albers GW, Madden KP, Hamilton S. The rtPA (alteplase) 0- to 6-hour acute stroke trial, part a (A0276g) : results of a double-blind, placebo-controlled, multicenter study. Thromblytic therapy in acute ischemic stroke study investigators. Stroke. 2000;31(4):811–6.

20. Shobha N, Buchan AM, Hill MD. Thrombolysis at 3-4.5 hours after acute ischemic stroke onset–evidence from the Canadian Alteplase for stroke effectiveness study (CASES) registry. Cerebrovasc Dis. 2011; 31(3):223–8.
21. Ahmed N, Wahlgren N, Grond M, Hennerici M, Lees KR, Mikulik R, Parsons M, Roine RO, Toni D, Ringleb P. Implementation and outcome of thrombolysis with alteplase 3-4.5 h after an acute stroke: an updated analysis from SITS-ISTR. Lancet Neurol. 2010;9(9):866–74.
22. Zhang D, Zou X, Sy C, Qin H, Wang Y, Liao X, Liu L. Thrombolysis and reperfusion: advanced understanding of early management strategies in acute ischemic stroke. Neurol Res. 2014;36(5):391–6.
23. Wardlaw JM, Murray V, Berge E, del Zoppo G, Sandercock P, Lindley RL, Cohen G. Recombinant tissue plasminogen activator for acute ischaemic stroke: an updated systematic review and meta-analysis. Lancet. 2012; 379(9834):2364–72.
24. Whiteley WN, Emberson J, Lees KR, Blackwell L, Albers G, Bluhmki E, Brott T, Cohen G, Davis S, Donnan G, et al. Risk of intracerebral haemorrhage with alteplase after acute ischaemic stroke: a secondary analysis of an individual patient data meta-analysis. Lancet Neurol. 2016;15(9):925–33.
25. The European Stroke Organisation (ESO) Executive Committee and the ESO Writing Committee. Guidelines for management of ischaemic stroke and transient ischaemic attack 2008. Cerebrovasc Dis. 2008;25(5):457–507.
26. Del Zoppo GJ, Saver JL, Jauch EC, Adams HP Jr. Expansion of the time window for treatment of acute ischemic stroke with intravenous tissue plasminogen activator: a science advisory from the American Heart Association/American Stroke Association. Stroke. 2009;40(8):2945–8.
27. Khandelwal P, Yavagal DR, Sacco RL. Acute ischemic stroke intervention. J Am Coll Cardiol. 2016;67(22):2631–44.
28. Albers GW, Olivot JM. Intravenous alteplase for ischaemic stroke. Lancet. 2007;369(9558):249–50.
29. Medlin F, Amiguet M, Vanacker P, Michel P. Influence of arterial occlusion on outcome after intravenous thrombolysis for acute ischemic stroke. Stroke. 2015;46(1):126–31.
30. Hong JH, Kang J, Jang MU, Kim BJ, Han MK, Park TH, Park SS, Lee KB, Lee BC, Yu KH, et al. Recanalization therapy for internal carotid artery occlusion presenting as acute ischemic stroke. J Stroke Cerebrovasc Dis. 2014;23(8): 2183–9.
31. Paciaroni M, Balucani C, Agnelli G, Caso V, Silvestrelli G, Grotta JC, Demchuk AM, Sohn SI, Orlandi G, Leys D, et al. Systemic thrombolysis in patients with acute ischemic stroke and internal carotid ARtery occlusion: the ICARO study. Stroke. 2012;43(1):125–30.
32. Paciaroni M, Agnelli G, Caso V, Pieroni A, Bovi P, Cappellari M, Zini A, Nichelli P, Inzitari D, Nesi M, et al. Intravenous thrombolysis for acute ischemic stroke associated to extracranial internal carotid artery occlusion: the ICARO-2 study. Cerebrovasc Dis. 2012;34(5–6):430–5.
33. Saqqur M, Tsivgoulis G, Molina CA, Demchuk AM, Shuaib A, Alexandrov AV, Investigators C. Residual flow at the site of intracranial occlusion on transcranial Doppler predicts response to intravenous thrombolysis: a multi-center study. Cerebrovasc Dis. 2009;27(1):5–12.
34. Saqqur M, Uchino K, Demchuk AM, Molina CA, Garami Z, Calleja S, Akhtar N, Orouk FO, Salam A, Shuaib A, et al. Site of arterial occlusion identified by transcranial Doppler predicts the response to intravenous thrombolysis for stroke. Stroke. 2007;38(3):948–54.
35. Rubiera M, Ribo M, Delgado-Mederos R, Santamarina E, Delgado P, Montaner J, Alvarez-Sabin J, Molina CA. Tandem internal carotid artery/ middle cerebral artery occlusion: an independent predictor of poor outcome after systemic thrombolysis. Stroke. 2006;37(9):2301–5.
36. Zhu W, Xiao L, Lin M, Liu X, Yan B. Large-vessel occlusion is associated with poor outcome in stroke patients aged 80 years or older who underwent intravenous Thrombolysis. J Stroke Cerebrovasc Dis. 2016;25(11):2712–6.
37. Rai A, Cline B, Williams E, Carpenter J, Roberts T. Intravenous thrombolysis outcomes in patients presenting with large vessel acute ischemic strokes–CT angiography-based prognosis. J Neuroimaging. 2015;25(2):238–42.
38. Zhu W, Churilov L, Campbell BC, Lin M, Liu X, Davis SM, Yan B. Does large vessel occlusion affect clinical outcome in stroke with mild neurologic deficits after intravenous thrombolysis? J Stroke Cerebrovasc Dis. 2014; 23(10):2888–93.
39. Linfante I, Llinas RH, Selim M, Chaves C, Kumar S, Parker RA, Caplan LR, Schlaug G. Clinical and vascular outcome in internal carotid artery versus middle cerebral artery occlusions after intravenous tissue plasminogen activator. Stroke. 2002;33(8):2066–71.
40. Lee KY, Han SW, Kim SH, Nam HS, Ahn SW, Kim DJ, Seo SH, Kim DI, Heo JH. Early recanalization after intravenous administration of recombinant tissue plasminogen activator as assessed by pre- and post-thrombolytic angiography in acute ischemic stroke patients. Stroke. 2007;38(1):192–3.
41. von Kummer R, Hacke W. Safety and efficacy of intravenous tissue plasminogen activator and heparin in acute middle cerebral artery stroke. Stroke. 1992;23(5):646–52.
42. Riedel CH, Zimmermann P, Jensen-Kondering U, Stingele R, Deuschl G, Jansen O. The importance of size: successful recanalization by intravenous thrombolysis in acute anterior stroke depends on thrombus length. Stroke. 2011;42(6):1775–7.
43. Friedrich B, Gawlitza M, Schob S, Hobohm C, Raviolo M, Hoffmann KT, Lobsien D. Distance to thrombus in acute middle cerebral artery occlusion: a predictor of outcome after intravenous thrombolysis for acute ischemic stroke. Stroke. 2015;46(3):692–6.
44. Riedel CH, Jensen U, Rohr A, Tietke M, Alfke K, Ulmer S, Jansen O. Assessment of thrombus in acute middle cerebral artery occlusion using thin-slice nonenhanced computed tomography reconstructions. Stroke. 2010;41(8):1659–64.
45. Strbian D, Sairanen T, Silvennoinen H, Salonen O, Lindsberg PJ. Intravenous thrombolysis of basilar artery occlusion: thrombus length versus recanalization success. Stroke. 2014;45(6):1733–8.
46. Liu X. Beyond the time window of intravenous thrombolysis: standing by or by stenting? Interv Neurol. 2012;1(1):3–15.
47. Wolpert SM, Bruckmann H, Greenlee R, Wechsler L, Pessin MS, del Zoppo GJ. Neuroradiologic evaluation of patients with acute stroke treated with recombinant tissue plasminogen activator. The rt-PA acute stroke study group. AJNR Am J Neuroradiol. 1993;14(1):3–13.
48. Lum C, Stys PK, Hogan MJ, Nguyen TB, Srinivasan A, Goyal M. Acute anterior circulation stroke: recanalization using clot angioplasty. Can J Neurol Sci. 2006;33(2):217–22.
49. Albers GW, von Kummer R, Truelsen T, Jensen JK, Ravn GM, Gronning BA, Chabriat H, Chang KC, Davalos AE, Ford GA, et al. Safety and efficacy of desmoteplase given 3-9 h after ischaemic stroke in patients with occlusion or high-grade stenosis in major cerebral arteries (DIAS-3): a double-blind, randomised, placebo-controlled phase 3 trial. Lancet Neurol. 2015;14(6):575–84.
50. Furlan AJ, Eyding D, Albers GW, Al-Rawi Y, Lees KR, Rowley HA, Sachara C, Soehngen M, Warach S, Hacke W. Dose escalation of Desmoteplase for acute ischemic stroke (DEDAS): evidence of safety and efficacy 3 to 9 hours after stroke onset. Stroke. 2006;37(5):1227–31.
51. Hacke W, Albers G, Al-Rawi Y, Bogousslavsky J, Davalos A, Eliasziw M, Fischer M, Furlan A, Kaste M, Lees KR, et al. The Desmoteplase in acute ischemic stroke trial (DIAS): a phase II MRI-based 9-hour window acute stroke thrombolysis trial with intravenous desmoteplase. Stroke. 2005;36(1):66–73.
52. Hacke W, Furlan AJ, Al-Rawi Y, Davalos A, Fiebach JB, Gruber F, Kaste M, Lipka LJ, Pedraza S, Ringleb PA, et al. Intravenous desmoteplase in patients with acute ischaemic stroke selected by MRI perfusion-diffusion weighted imaging or perfusion CT (DIAS-2): a prospective, randomised, double-blind, placebo-controlled study. Lancet Neurol. 2009;8(2):141–50.
53. Mori E, Minematsu K, Nakagawara J, Hasegawa Y, Nagahiro S, Okada Y, Truelsen T, Lindsten A, Ogawa A, Yamaguchi T. Safety and tolerability of Desmoteplase within 3 to 9 hours after symptoms onset in Japanese patients with ischemic stroke. Stroke. 2015;46(9):2549–54.
54. Sugg RM, Pary JK, Uchino K, Baraniuk S, Shaltoni HM, Gonzales NR, Mikulik R, Garami Z, Shaw SG, Matherne DE, et al. Argatroban tPA stroke study: study design and results in the first treated cohort. Arch Neurol. 2006;63(8):1057–62.
55. Haley EC Jr, Lyden PD, Johnston KC, Hemmen TM. A pilot dose-escalation safety study of tenecteplase in acute ischemic stroke. Stroke. 2005;36(3): 607–12.
56. Ginsberg MD, Hill MD, Palesch YY, Ryckborst KJ, Tamariz D. The ALIAS pilot trial: a dose-escalation and safety study of albumin therapy for acute ischemic stroke–I: physiological responses and safety results. Stroke. 2006; 37(8):2100–6.
57. Marder VJ, Jahan R, Gruber T, Goyal A, Arora V. Thrombolysis with plasmin: implications for stroke treatment. Stroke. 2010;41(10 Suppl):S45–9.
58. Gurm HS, Lincoff AM, Lee D, Tang WH, Jia G, Booth JE, Califf RM, Ohman EM, Van de Werf F, Armstrong PW, et al. Outcome of acute ST-segment elevation myocardial infarction in diabetics treated with fibrinolytic or combination reduced fibrinolytic therapy and platelet glycoprotein IIb/IIIa inhibition: lessons from the GUSTO V trial. J Am Coll Cardiol. 2004;43(4):542–8.

59. Lincoff AM, Califf RM, Van de Werf F, Willerson JT, White HD, Armstrong PW, Guetta V, Gibler WB, Hochman JS, Bode C, et al. Mortality at 1 year with combination platelet glycoprotein IIb/IIIa inhibition and reduced-dose fibrinolytic therapy vs conventional fibrinolytic therapy for acute myocardial infarction: GUSTO V randomized trial. JAMA. 2002;288(17):2130–5.
60. Topol EJ. Reperfusion therapy for acute myocardial infarction with fibrinolytic therapy or combination reduced fibrinolytic therapy and platelet glycoprotein IIb/IIIa inhibition: the GUSTO V randomised trial. Lancet. 2001; 357(9272):1905–14.
61. Uyttenboogaart M, Koch MW, Koopman K, Vroomen PC, De Keyser J, Luijckx GJ. Safety of antiplatelet therapy prior to intravenous thrombolysis in acute ischemic stroke. Arch Neurol. 2008;65(5):607–11.
62. Zinkstok SM, Vermeulen M, Stam J, de Haan RJ, Roos YB. Antiplatelet therapy in combination with rt-PA thrombolysis in ischemic stroke (ARTIS): rationale and design of a randomized controlled trial. Cerebrovasc Dis. 2010; 29(1):79–81.
63. Zinkstok SM, Vermeulen M, Stam J, de Haan RJ, Roos YB. A randomised controlled trial of antiplatelet therapy in combination with Rt-PA thrombolysis in ischemic stroke: rationale and design of the ARTIS-trial. Trials. 2010;11:51.
64. Lorenzano S, Toni D. TESPI (Thrombolysis in elderly stroke patients in Italy): a randomized controlled trial of alteplase (rt-PA) versus standard treatment in acute ischaemic stroke in patients aged more than 80 years where thrombolysis is initiated within three hours after stroke onset. Int J Stroke. 2012;7(3):250–7.
65. Mikulik R, Dufek M, Goldemund D, Reif M. A pilot study on systemic thrombolysis followed by low molecular weight heparin in ischemic stroke. Eur J Neurol. 2006;13(10):1106–11.
66. Alexandrov AV, Molina CA, Grotta JC, Garami Z, Ford SR, Alvarez-Sabin J, Montaner J, Saqqur M, Demchuk AM, Moye LA, et al. Ultrasound-enhanced systemic thrombolysis for acute ischemic stroke. N Engl J Med. 2004;351(21): 2170–8.
67. Alexandrov AV, Wojner AW, Grotta JC. CLOTBUST: design of a randomized trial of ultrasound-enhanced thrombolysis for acute ischemic stroke. J Neuroimaging. 2004;14(2):108–12.
68. Eggers J, Konig IR, Koch B, Handler G, Seidel G. Sonothrombolysis with transcranial color-coded sonography and recombinant tissue-type plasminogen activator in acute middle cerebral artery main stem occlusion: results from a randomized study. Stroke. 2008;39(5):1470–5.
69. Saqqur M, Shuaib A, Alexandrov AV, Sebastian J, Khan K, Uchino K. The correlation between admission blood glucose and intravenous rt-PA-induced arterial recanalization in acute ischemic stroke: a multi-Centre TCD study. Int J Stroke. 2015;10(7):1087–92.
70. Tsivgoulis G, Zhang Y, Alexandrov AW, Harrigan MR, Sisson A, Zhao L, Brethour M, Cava L, Balucani C, Barlinn K, et al. Safety and tolerability of early noninvasive ventilatory correction using bilevel positive airway pressure in acute ischemic stroke. Stroke. 2011;42(4):1030–4.
71. Toda N, Tanaka T, Ayajiki K, Okamura T. Cerebral vasodilatation induced by stimulation of the pterygopalatine ganglion and greater petrosal nerve in anesthetized monkeys. Neuroscience. 2000;96(2):393–8.
72. Barreto AD, Alexandrov AV. Adjunctive and alternative approaches to current reperfusion therapy. Stroke. 2012;43(2):591–8.
73. Martin PJ, Enevoldson TP, Humphrey PR. Causes of ischaemic stroke in the young. Postgrad Med J. 1997;73(855):8–16.
74. Gobin YP, Starkman S, Duckwiler GR, Grobelny T, Kidwell CS, Jahan R, Pile-Spellman J, Segal A, Vinuela F, Saver JL. MERCI 1: a phase 1 study of mechanical embolus removal in cerebral ischemia. Stroke. 2004;35(12):2848–54.
75. Meyers PM, Schumacher HC, Connolly ES Jr, Heyer EJ, Gray WA, Higashida RT. Current status of endovascular stroke treatment. Circulation. 2011; 123(22):2591–601.
76. Campbell BC, Mitchell PJ, Kleinig TJ, Dewey HM, Churilov L, Yassi N, Yan B, Dowling RJ, Parsons MW, Oxley TJ, et al. Endovascular therapy for ischemic stroke with perfusion-imaging selection. N Engl J Med. 2015;372(11):1009–18.
77. Novakovic R, Toth G, Purdy PD. Review of current and emerging therapies in acute ischemic stroke. J Neurointerv Surg. 2009;1(1):13–26.
78. Smith WS, Sung G, Starkman S, Saver JL, Kidwell CS, Gobin YP, Lutsep HL, Nesbit GM, Grobelny T, Rymer MM, et al. Safety and efficacy of mechanical embolectomy in acute ischemic stroke: results of the MERCI trial. Stroke. 2005;36(7):1432–8.
79. Smith WS. Safety of mechanical thrombectomy and intravenous tissue plasminogen activator in acute ischemic stroke. Results of the multi mechanical embolus removal in cerebral ischemia (MERCI) trial, part I. AJNR Am J Neuroradiol. 2006;27(6):1177–82.
80. Asadi H, Dowling R, Yan B, Wong S, Mitchell P. Advances in endovascular treatment of acute ischaemic stroke. Intern Med J. 2015;45(8):798–805.
81. del Zoppo GJ, Higashida RT, Furlan AJ, Pessin MS, Rowley HA, Gent M. PROACT: a phase II randomized trial of recombinant pro-urokinase by direct arterial delivery in acute middle cerebral artery stroke. PROACT investigators. Prolyse in acute cerebral Thromboembolism. Stroke. 1998;29(1):4–11.
82. Furlan A, Higashida R, Wechsler L, Gent M, Rowley H, Kase C, Pessin M, Ahuja A, Callahan F, Clark WM, et al. Intra-arterial prourokinase for acute ischemic stroke. The PROACT II study: a randomized controlled trial. Prolyse in acute cerebral Thromboembolism. JAMA. 1999;282(21):2003–11.
83. Ciccone A, Valvassori L, Nichelatti M, Sgoifo A, Ponzio M, Sterzi R, Boccardi E. Endovascular treatment for acute ischemic stroke. N Engl J Med. 2013; 368(10):904–13.
84. Ogawa A, Mori E, Minematsu K, Taki W, Takahashi A, Nemoto S, Miyamoto S, Sasaki M, Inoue T. Randomized trial of Intraarterial infusion of Urokinase within 6 hours of middle cerebral artery stroke. Stroke. 2007;38(10):2633.
85. Lee M, Hong KS, Saver JL. Efficacy of intra-arterial fibrinolysis for acute ischemic stroke: meta-analysis of randomized controlled trials. Stroke. 2010; 41(5):932–7.
86. Adams H, Adams R, Del Zoppo G, Goldstein LB. Guidelines for the early management of patients with ischemic stroke: 2005 guidelines update a scientific statement from the stroke Council of the American Heart Association/American Stroke Association. Stroke. 2005;36(4):916–23.
87. Fanous AA, Siddiqui AH. Mechanical thrombectomy: stent retrievers vs. aspiration catheters. Cor et Vasa. 2016;58(2):e193–203.
88. The Penumbra Pivotal Stroke Trial Investigators. The penumbra pivotal stroke trial: safety and effectiveness of a new generation of mechanical devices for clot removal in intracranial large vessel occlusive disease. Stroke. 2009;40(8):2761–8.
89. Bose A, Henkes H, Alfke K, Reith W, Mayer TE, Berlis A, Branca V, Sit SP. The penumbra system: a mechanical device for the treatment of acute stroke due to thromboembolism. AJNR Am J Neuroradiol. 2008;29(7):1409–13.
90. Pereira VM, Yilmaz H, Pellaton A, Slater LA, Krings T, Lovblad KO. Current status of mechanical thrombectomy for acute stroke treatment. J Neuroradiol. 2015;42(1):12–20.
91. Almekhlafi MA, Menon BK, Freiheit EA, Demchuk AM, Goyal M. A meta-analysis of observational intra-arterial stroke therapy studies using the merci device, penumbra system, and retrievable stents. AJNR Am J Neuroradiol. 2013;34(1):140–5.
92. Gupta R, Xiang B, Ge S, Sun CH, Yoo AJ, Mehta BP. Stagnation of treatment times over a decade: results of a pooled analysis from the MERCI registry, MERCI, TREVO, and TREVO 2 trials. J Neurointerv Surg. 2016;8(5):453–6.
93. Nogueira RG, Lutsep HL, Gupta R, Jovin TG, Albers GW, Walker GA, Liebeskind DS, Smith WS. Trevo versus merci retrievers for thrombectomy revascularisation of large vessel occlusions in acute ischaemic stroke (TREVO 2): a randomised trial. Lancet. 2012;380(9849):1231–40.
94. Saver JL, Jahan R, Levy EI, Jovin TG, Baxter B, Nogueira R, Clark W, Budzik R, Zaidat OO. SOLITAIRE with the intention for thrombectomy (SWIFT) trial: design of a randomized, controlled, multicenter study comparing the SOLITAIRE flow restoration device and the MERCI retriever in acute ischaemic stroke. Int J Stroke. 2014;9(5):658–68.
95. Mordasini P, Hiller M, Brekenfeld C, Schroth G, Fischer U, Slotboom J, Arnold M, Gralla J. In vivo evaluation of the Phenox CRC mechanical thrombectomy device in a swine model of acute vessel occlusion. AJNR Am J Neuroradiol. 2010;31(5):972–8.
96. Prothmann S, Lockau H, Dorn F, Poppert H, Forschler A, Zimmer C, Liebig T: The phenox clot retriever as part of a multimodal mechanical thrombectomy approach in acute ischemic stroke: single center experience in 56 patients. TheScientificWorldJOURNAL 2012, 2012:190763.
97. Brekenfeld C, Schroth G, El-Koussy M, Nedeltchev K, Reinert M, Slotboom J, Gralla J. Mechanical thromboembolectomy for acute ischemic stroke: comparison of the catch thrombectomy device and the merci retriever in vivo. Stroke. 2008;39(4):1213–9.
98. Mourand I, Brunel H, Costalat V, Riquelme C, Lobotesis K, Milhaud D, Heroum C, Arquizan C, Moynier M, Bonafe A. Mechanical thrombectomy in acute ischemic stroke: catch device. AJNR Am J Neuroradiol. 2011;32(8):1381–5.
99. Peker A, Arsava EM, Topcuoglu MA, Arat A. Catch plus thrombectomy device in acute stroke: initial evaluation. J Neurointerv Surg. 2016;9(12): 1214–18.

100. Przybylowski CJ, Ding D, Starke RM, Durst CR, Crowley RW, Liu KC. Evolution of endovascular mechanical thrombectomy for acute ischemic stroke. World J Clin Cases. 2014;2(11):614–22.
101. Raychev R, Saver JL. Mechanical thrombectomy devices for treatment of stroke. Neurol Clin Pract. 2012;2(3):231–5.
102. Fargen KM, Meyers PM, Khatri P, Mocco J. Improvements in recanalization with modern stroke therapy: a review of prospective ischemic stroke trials during the last two decades. J Neurointerv Surg. 2013;5(6):506–11.
103. Hu YC, Stiefel MF. Force and aspiration analysis of the ADAPT technique in acute ischemic stroke treatment. J Neurointerv Surg. 2016;8(3):244–6.
104. John S, Hussain MS, Toth G, Bain M, Uchino K, Hui FK. Initial experience using the 5MAX ACE reperfusion catheter in intra-arterial therapy for acute ischemic stroke. J Cerebrovasc Endovasc Neurosurg. 2014;16(4):350–7.
105. Navia P, Larrea JA, Pardo E, Arce A, Martinez-Zabaleta M, Diez-Gonzalez N, Murias E, Arraez-Aybar LA, Masso J. Initial experience using the 3MAX cerebral reperfusion catheter in the endovascular treatment of acute ischemic stroke of distal arteries. J Neurointerv Surg. 2016;8(8):787–90.
106. Suzuki K, Aoki J, Sakamoto Y, Kanamaru T, Abe A, Suda S, Okubo S, Kimura K. Efficiency of the penumbra 5MAX ACE reperfusion catheter in acute ischemic stroke patients. J Stroke Cerebrovasc Dis. 2016;25(12):2981–6.
107. Vidal GA, Milburn JM. The penumbra 5MAX ACE catheter is safe, efficient, and cost saving as a primary mechanical Thrombectomy device for large vessel occlusions in acute ischemic stroke. Ochsner J. 2016;16(4):486–91.
108. Mpotsaris A, Bussmeyer M, Weber W. Mechanical thrombectomy with the penumbra 3D separator and lesional aspiration: technical feasibility and clinical outcome. Clin Neuroradiol. 2014;24(3):245–50.
109. Behme D, Kowoll A, Mpotsaris A, Hader C, Hechelhammer L, Weber J, Weber W. Multicenter clinical experience in over 125 patients with the penumbra separator 3D for mechanical thrombectomy in acute ischemic stroke. J Neurointerv Surg. 2016;8(1):8–12.
110. Berkhemer OA, Fransen PS, Beumer D, van den Berg LA, Lingsma HF, Yoo AJ, Schonewille WJ, Vos JA, Nederkoorn PJ, Wermer MJ, et al. A randomized trial of intraarterial treatment for acute ischemic stroke. N Engl J Med. 2015; 372(1):11–20.
111. Goyal M, Demchuk AM, Menon BK, Eesa M, Rempel JL, Thornton J, Roy D, Jovin TG, Willinsky RA, Sapkota BL, et al. Randomized assessment of rapid endovascular treatment of ischemic stroke. N Engl J Med. 2015;372(11): 1019–30.
112. Saver JL, Goyal M, Bonafe A, Diener HC, Levy EI, Pereira VM, Albers GW, Cognard C, Cohen DJ, Hacke W, et al. Stent-retriever thrombectomy after intravenous t-PA vs. t-PA alone in stroke. N Engl J Med. 2015;372(24):2285–95.
113. Jovin TG, Chamorro A, Cobo E, de Miquel MA, Molina CA, Rovira A, San Roman L, Serena J, Abilleira S, Ribo M, et al. Thrombectomy within 8 hours after symptom onset in ischemic stroke. N Engl J Med. 2015;372(24):2296–306.
114. Berkhemer OA, Majoie CB, Dippel DW. Endovascular therapy for ischemic stroke. N Engl J Med. 2015;372(24):2363.
115. Goyal M, Yu AY, Menon BK, Dippel DW, Hacke W, Davis SM, Fisher M, Yavagal DR, Turjman F, Ross J, et al. Endovascular therapy in acute ischemic stroke: challenges and transition from trials to bedside. Stroke. 2016;47(2): 548–53.
116. Albers GW, Goyal M, Jahan R, Bonafe A, Diener HC, Levy EI, Pereira VM, Cognard C, Cohen DJ, Hacke W, et al. Ischemic core and hypoperfusion volumes predict infarct size in SWIFT PRIME. Ann Neurol. 2016;79(1):76–89.
117. Goyal M, Menon BK, van Zwam WH, Dippel DW, Mitchell PJ, Demchuk AM, Davalos A, Majoie CB, van der Lugt A, de Miquel MA, et al. Endovascular thrombectomy after large-vessel ischaemic stroke: a meta-analysis of individual patient data from five randomised trials. Lancet. 2016;387(10029): 1723–31.
118. Saver JL, Goyal M, van der Lugt A, et al. Time to treatment with endovascular thrombectomy and outcomes from ischemic stroke: a meta-analysis. JAMA. 2016;316(12):1279–89.
119. Nogueira RG, Jadhav AP, Haussen DC, Bonafe A, Budzik RF, Bhuva P, Yavagal DR, Ribo M, Cognard C, Hanel RA et al. Thrombectomy 6 to 24 hours after stroke with a mismatch between deficit and infarct. N Engl J Med. 2018; 378(1):11–21.
120. Kidwell CS, Jahan R, Gornbein J, Alger JR, Nenov V, Ajani Z, Feng L, Meyer BC, Olson S, Schwamm LH, et al. A trial of imaging selection and endovascular treatment for ischemic stroke. N Engl J Med. 2013;368(10):914–23.
121. Broderick JP, Palesch YY, Demchuk AM, Yeatts SD, Khatri P, Hill MD, Jauch EC, Jovin TG, Yan B, Silver FL, et al. Endovascular therapy after intravenous t-PA versus t-PA alone for stroke. N Engl J Med. 2013;368(10):893–903.
122. Mokin M, Khalessi AA, Mocco J, Lanzino G, Dumont TM, Hanel RA, Lopes DK, Fessler RD 2nd, Ringer AJ, Bendok BR, et al. Endovascular treatment of acute ischemic stroke: the end or just the beginning? Neurosurg Focus. 2014;36(1):E5.
123. Mocco J, O'Kelly C, Arthur A, Meyers PM, Hirsch JA, Woo HH, Rasmussen PA, Albuquerque FC, Turk A, Tarr R, et al. Randomized clinical trials: the double edged sword. J Neurointerv Surg. 2013;5(5):387–90.
124. Goyal M, Shamy M, Menon BK, Saver JL, Diener HC, Mocco J, Pereira VM, Jovin TG, Zaidat O, Levy EI, et al. Endovascular stroke trials: why we must enroll all eligible patients. Stroke. 2013;44(12):3591–5.
125. Campbell BC, Hill MD, Rubiera M, Menon BK, Demchuk A, Donnan GA, Roy D, Thornton J, Dorado L, Bonafe A, et al. Safety and efficacy of solitaire stent Thrombectomy: individual patient data meta-analysis of randomized trials. Stroke. 2016;47(3):798–806.
126. Saver JL, Jahan R, Levy EI, Jovin TG, Baxter B, Nogueira RG, Clark W, Budzik R, Zaidat OO. Solitaire flow restoration device versus the merci retriever in patients with acute ischaemic stroke (SWIFT): a randomised, parallel-group, non-inferiority trial. Lancet. 2012;380(9849):1241–9.
127. Bracard S, Ducrocq X, Mas JL, Soudant M, Oppenheim C, Moulin T. Guillemin F, investigators T: mechanical thrombectomy after intravenous alteplase versus alteplase alone after stroke (THRACE): a randomised controlled trial. Lancet Neurol. 2016;15(11):1138–47.
128. Mocco J, Kuo S, Khatri P, Zaidat OO. 186 the THERAPY trial: a prospective, randomized, concurrent controlled trial to evaluate the role of mechanical Embolectomy as adjunctive treatment to IV rtPA for acute ischemic stroke. Neurosurgery. 2013;60(Suppl 1);181–2.
129. Smith WS, Sung G, Saver J, Budzik R, Duckwiler G, Liebeskind DS, Lutsep HL, Rymer MM, Higashida RT, Starkman S, et al. Mechanical thrombectomy for acute ischemic stroke: final results of the multi MERCI trial. Stroke. 2008; 39(4):1205–12.
130. Berlis A, Lutsep H, Barnwell S, Norbash A, Wechsler L, Jungreis CA, Woolfenden A, Redekop G, Hartmann M, Schumacher M. Mechanical thrombolysis in acute ischemic stroke with endovascular photoacoustic recanalization. Stroke. 2004;35(5):1112–6.
131. Meurer WJ, Barth BE, Gaddis G, Vilke GM, Lam SH. Rapid systematic review: intra-arterial Thrombectomy ("clot retrieval") for selected patients with acute ischemic stroke. J Emerg Med. 2017;52(2):255–61.
132. Investigators PPST. The penumbra pivotal stroke trial: safety and effectiveness of a new generation of mechanical devices for clot removal in intracranial large vessel occlusive disease. Stroke. 2009;40(8):2761–8.
133. Alshekhlee A, Pandya DJ, English J, Zaidat OO, Mueller N, Gupta R, Nogueira RG. Merci mechanical thrombectomy retriever for acute ischemic stroke therapy: literature review. Neurology. 2012;79(13 Suppl 1):S126–34.
134. Lee W, Sitoh YY, Lim CC, Lim WE, Hui FK. The MERCI retrieval system for the management of acute ischaemic stroke–the NNI Singapore experience. Ann Acad Med Singap. 2009;38(9):749–55.
135. Nogueira RG, Schwamm LH, Hirsch JA. Endovascular approaches to acute stroke, part 1: drugs, devices, and data. AJNR Am J Neuroradiol. 2009;30(4): 649–61.
136. Yeo LL, Paliwal P, Teoh HL, Seet RC, Chan BP, Wakerley B, Liang S, Rathakrishnan R, Chong VF, Ting EY, et al. Early and continuous neurologic improvements after intravenous thrombolysis are strong predictors of favorable long-term outcomes in acute ischemic stroke. J Stroke Cerebrovasc Dis. 2013;22(8):e590–6.
137. Sekoranja L, Loulidi J, Yilmaz H, Lovblad K, Temperli P, Comelli M, Sztajzel RF. Intravenous versus combined (intravenous and intra-arterial) thrombolysis in acute ischemic stroke: a transcranial color-coded duplex sonography–guided pilot study. Stroke. 2006;37(7):1805–9.
138. Rubiera M, Ribo M, Pagola J, Coscojuela P, Rodriguez-Luna D, Maisterra O, Ibarra B, Pineiro S, Meler P, Romero FJ, et al. Bridging intravenous-intra-arterial rescue strategy increases recanalization and the likelihood of a good outcome in nonresponder intravenous tissue plasminogen activator-treated patients: a case-control study. Stroke. 2011;42(4):993–7.
139. Ribo M, Molina CA, Alvarez B, Rubiera M, Alvarez-Sabin J, Matas M. Intra-arterial administration of microbubbles and continuous 2-MHz ultrasound insonation to enhance intra-arterial thrombolysis. J Neuroimaging. 2010; 20(3):224–7.
140. Lewandowski CA, Frankel M, Tomsick TA, Broderick J, Frey J, Clark W, Starkman S, Grotta J, Spilker J, Khoury J, et al. Combined intravenous and intra-arterial r-TPA versus intra-arterial therapy of acute ischemic stroke: emergency Management of Stroke (EMS) bridging trial. Stroke. 1999;30(12):2598–605.

141. Kass-Hout T, Kass-Hout O, Mokin M, Thesier DM, Yashar P, Orion D, Jahshan S, Hopkins LN, Siddiqui AH, Snyder KV, et al. Is bridging with intravenous thrombolysis of any benefit in endovascular therapy for acute ischemic stroke? World Neurosurg. 2014;82(3–4):e453–8.
142. Wechsler LR, Jovin TG. Intravenous recombinant tissue-type plasminogen activator in the extended time window and the US Food and Drug Administration: confused about the time. Stroke. 2012;43(9):2517–9.
143. IMS Study Investigators. Combined intravenous and intra-arterial recanalization for acute ischemic stroke: the Interventional Management of Stroke Study. Stroke. 2004;35(4):904–11.
144. IMS II Trial Investigators. The Interventional Management of Stroke (IMS) II Study. Stroke. 2007;38(7):2127–35.
145. Zaidat OO, Lazzaro MA, Gupta R, Yavagal DR, Rasmussen PA, Hirsch JA, Castonguay AC, Tarr RW: Interventional Management of Stroke III trial: establishing the foundation. J Neurointerv Surg 2012, 4(4):235-237.
146. Rha JH, Saver JL. The impact of recanalization on ischemic stroke outcome: a meta-analysis. Stroke. 2007;38(3):967–73.
147. Levy EI, Rahman M, Khalessi AA, Beyer PT, Natarajan SK, Hartney ML, Fiorella DJ, Hopkins LN, Siddiqui AH, Mocco J. Midterm clinical and angiographic follow-up for the first Food and Drug Administration-approved prospective, single-arm trial of primary stenting for stroke: SARIS (stent-assisted Recanalization for acute ischemic stroke). Neurosurgery. 2011;69(4):915–20. discussion 920
148. Levy EI, Siddiqui AH, Crumlish A, Snyder KV, Hauck EF, Fiorella DJ, Hopkins LN, Mocco J. First Food and Drug Administration-approved prospective trial of primary intracranial stenting for acute stroke: SARIS (stent-assisted recanalization in acute ischemic stroke). Stroke. 2009;40(11):3552–6.
149. Zaidat OO, Suarez JI, Santillan C, Sunshine JL, Tarr RW, Paras VH, Selman WR, Landis DM. Response to intra-arterial and combined intravenous and intra-arterial thrombolytic therapy in patients with distal internal carotid artery occlusion. Stroke. 2002;33(7):1821–6.
150. Nogueira RG, Yoo AJ, Masrur S, Batista LM, Hakimelahi R, Hirsch JA, Schwamm LH. Safety of full-dose intravenous recombinant tissue plasminogen activator followed by multimodal endovascular therapy for acute ischemic stroke. J Neurointerv Surg. 2013;5(4):298–301.
151. Gupta R, Vora NA, Horowitz MB, Tayal AH, Hammer MD, Uchino K, Levy EI, Wechsler LR, Jovin TG. Multimodal reperfusion therapy for acute ischemic stroke: factors predicting vessel recanalization. Stroke. 2006;37(4):986–90.
152. Lin DD, Gailloud P, Beauchamp NJ, Aldrich EM, Wityk RJ, Murphy KJ. Combined stent placement and thrombolysis in acute vertebrobasilar ischemic stroke. AJNR Am J Neuroradiol. 2003;24(9):1827–33.
153. Gupta R, Tayal AH, Levy EI, Cheng-Ching E, Rai A, Liebeskind DS, Yoo AJ, Hsu DP, Rymer MM, Zaidat OO, et al. Intra-arterial thrombolysis or stent placement during endovascular treatment for acute ischemic stroke leads to the highest recanalization rate: results of a multicenter retrospective study. Neurosurgery. 2011;68(6):1618–22. discussion 1622-1613
154. Ghobrial GM, Chalouhi N, Rivers L, Witte S, Davanzo J, Dalyai R, Gardecki ML, Jabbour P, Gonzalez F, Dumont AS, et al. Multimodal endovascular management of acute ischemic stroke in patients over 75 years old is safe and effective. J Neurointerv Surg. 2013;5(Suppl 1):i33–7.
155. Egashira Y, Yoshimura S, Enomoto Y, Ishiguro M, Yamada K, Tanaka Y, Iwama T. Efficacy and limitations of multimodal endovascular revascularization other than clot retrieval for acute stroke caused by large-vessel occlusion. J Stroke Cerebrovasc Dis. 2013;22(6):851–6.
156. Yoon W, Park MS, Cho KH. Low-dose intra-arterial urokinase and aggressive mechanical clot disruption for acute ischemic stroke after failure of intravenous thrombolysis. AJNR Am J Neuroradiol. 2010;31(1):161–4.
157. Nogueira RG, Schwamm LH, Buonanno FS, Koroshetz WJ, Yoo AJ, Rabinov JD, Pryor JC, Hirsch JA. Low-pressure balloon angioplasty with adjuvant pharmacological therapy in patients with acute ischemic stroke caused by intracranial arterial occlusions. Neuroradiology. 2008;50(4):331–40.
158. Lin R, Vora N, Zaidi S, Aleu A, Jankowitz B, Thomas A, Gupta R, Horowitz M, Kim S, Reddy V, et al. Mechanical approaches combined with intra-arterial pharmacological therapy are associated with higher recanalization rates than either intervention alone in revascularization of acute carotid terminus occlusion. Stroke. 2009;40(6):2092–7.
159. Leker RR, Grigoriadis S, Cohen JE. Endovascular reperfusion therapy for acute ischemic stroke: a meta-analysis. Neurol Res. 2010;32(8):787–91.
160. Cohen JE, Itshayek E, Moskovici S, Gomori JM, Fraifeld S, Eichel R, Leker RR. State-of-the-art reperfusion strategies for acute ischemic stroke. J Clin Neurosci. 2011;18(3):319–23.
161. Bhatia R, Hill MD, Shobha N, Menon B, Bal S, Kochar P, Watson T, Goyal M, Demchuk AM. Low rates of acute recanalization with intravenous recombinant tissue plasminogen activator in ischemic stroke: real-world experience and a call for action. Stroke. 2010;41(10):2254–8.
162. Demchuk AM, Goyal M, Yeatts SD, Carrozzella J, Foster LD, Qazi E, Hill MD, Jovin TG, Ribo M, Yan B, et al. Recanalization and clinical outcome of occlusion sites at baseline CT angiography in the interventional Management of Stroke III trial. Radiology. 2014;273(1):202–10.
163. Koga M, Arihiro S, Miyashita F, Yamamoto H, Yamada N, Nagatsuka K, Minematsu K, Toyoda K. Factors associated with early recanalization failure following intravenous rt-PA therapy for ischemic stroke. Cerebrovasc Dis. 2013;36(4):299–305.
164. Neumann-Haefelin T, du Mesnil de Rochemont R, Fiebach JB, Gass A, Nolte C, Kucinski T, Rother J, Siebler M, Singer OC, Szabo K, et al. Effect of incomplete (spontaneous and postthrombolytic) recanalization after middle cerebral artery occlusion: a magnetic resonance imaging study. Stroke. 2004; 35(1):109–14.
165. Wunderlich MT, Goertler M, Postert T, Schmitt E, Seidel G, Gahn G, Samii C, Stolz E. Recanalization after intravenous thrombolysis: does a recanalization time window exist? Neurology. 2007;68(17):1364–8.
166. Mazighi M, Meseguer E, Labreuche J, Serfaty JM, Laissy JP, Lavallee PC, Cabrejo L, Guidoux C, Lapergue B, Klein IF, et al. Dramatic recovery in acute ischemic stroke is associated with arterial recanalization grade and speed. Stroke. 2012;43(11):2998–3002.
167. Alexandrov AV, Hall CE, Labiche LA, Wojner AW, Grotta JC. Ischemic stunning of the brain: early recanalization without immediate clinical improvement in acute ischemic stroke. Stroke. 2004;35(2):449–52.
168. Baron JC. Perfusion thresholds in human cerebral ischemia: historical perspective and therapeutic implications. Cerebrovasc Dis. 2001;11(Suppl 1): 2–8.
169. Bardutzky J, Shen Q, Henninger N, Schwab S, Duong TQ, Fisher M. Characterizing tissue fate after transient cerebral ischemia of varying duration using quantitative diffusion and perfusion imaging. Stroke. 2007; 38(4):1336–44.
170. Shen Q, Fisher M, Sotak CH, Duong TQ. Effects of reperfusion on ADC and CBF pixel-by-pixel dynamics in stroke: characterizing tissue fates using quantitative diffusion and perfusion imaging. J Cereb Blood Flow Metab. 2004;24(3):280–90.
171. Markus R, Reutens DC, Kazui S, Read S, Wright P, Pearce DC, Tochon-Danguy HJ, Sachinidis JI, Donnan GA. Hypoxic tissue in ischaemic stroke: persistence and clinical consequences of spontaneous survival. Brain. 2004;127(Pt 6): 1427–36.
172. Darby DG, Barber PA, Gerraty RP, Desmond PM, Yang Q, Parsons M, Li T, Tress BM, Davis SM. Pathophysiological topography of acute ischemia by combined diffusion-weighted and perfusion MRI. Stroke. 1999;30(10): 2043–52.
173. Baron JC. Mapping the ischaemic penumbra with PET: implications for acute stroke treatment. Cerebrovasc Dis. 1999;9(4):193–201.
174. Choi JH, Bateman BT, Mangla S, Marshall RS, Prabhakaran S, Chong J, Mohr JP, Mast H, Pile-Spellman J. Endovascular recanalization therapy in acute ischemic stroke. Stroke. 2006;37(2):419–24.
175. Bang OY, Saver JL, Buck BH, Alger JR, Starkman S, Ovbiagele B, Kim D, Jahan R, Duckwiler GR, Yoon SR, et al. Impact of collateral flow on tissue fate in acute ischaemic stroke. J Neurol Neurosurg Psychiatry. 2008;79(6):625–9.
176. Leng X, Fang H, Leung TW, Mao C, Miao Z, Liu L, Wong KS, Liebeskind DS. Impact of collaterals on the efficacy and safety of endovascular treatment in acute ischaemic stroke: a systematic review and meta-analysis. J Neurol Neurosurg Psychiatry. 2016;87(5):537–44.
177. Mazighi M, Chaudhry SA, Ribo M, Khatri P, Skoloudik D, Mokin M, Labreuche J, Meseguer E, Yeatts SD, Siddiqui AH, et al. Impact of onset-to-reperfusion time on stroke mortality: a collaborative pooled analysis. Circulation. 2013; 127(19):1980–5.
178. Leker RR, Eichel R, Keigler G, Gomori JM, Cohen JE. Occlusion site does not impact outcome in patients with carotid stroke undergoing endovascular reperfusion. Int J Stroke. 2015;10(4):560–4.
179. Leslie-Mazwi TM, Hirsch JA, Falcone GJ, Schaefer PW, Lev MH, Rabinov JD, Rost NS, Schwamm L, Gonzalez RG. Endovascular stroke treatment outcomes after patient selection based on magnetic resonance imaging and clinical criteria. JAMA neurol. 2016;73(1):43–9.
180. Leigh R, Zaidat OO, Suri MF, Lynch G, Sundararajan S, Sunshine JL, Tarr R, Selman W, Landis DM, Suarez JI. Predictors of hyperacute clinical worsening

in ischemic stroke patients receiving thrombolytic therapy. Stroke. 2004; 35(8):1903–7.
181. Alvarez-Sabin J, Molina CA, Ribo M, Arenillas JF, Montaner J, Huertas R, Santamarina E, Rubiera M. Impact of admission hyperglycemia on stroke outcome after thrombolysis: risk stratification in relation to time to reperfusion. Stroke. 2004;35(11):2493–8.
182. Arnold M, Mattle S, Galimanis A, Kappeler L, Fischer U, Jung S, De Marchis GM, Gralla J, Mono ML, Brekenfeld C, et al. Impact of admission glucose and diabetes on recanalization and outcome after intra-arterial thrombolysis for ischaemic stroke. Int J Stroke. 2014;9(8):985–91.
183. Koga M, Reutens DC, Wright P, Phan T, Markus R, Pedreira B, Fitt G, Lim I, Donnan GA. The existence and evolution of diffusion-perfusion mismatched tissue in white and gray matter after acute stroke. Stroke. 2005;36(10):2132–7.
184. Kucinski T, Koch C, Eckert B, Becker V, Kromer H, Heesen C, Grzyska U, Freitag HJ, Rother J, Zeumer H. Collateral circulation is an independent radiological predictor of outcome after thrombolysis in acute ischaemic stroke. Neuroradiology. 2003;45(1):11–8.
185. Bhaskar S, Bivard A, Stanwell P, Parsons M, Attia JR, Nilsson M, Levi C. Baseline collateral status and infarct topography in post-ischaemic perilesional hyperperfusion: an arterial spin labelling study. J Cereb Blood Flow Metab. 2017;37(3):1148–62.
186. Lima FO, Furie KL, Silva GS, Lev MH, Camargo EC, Singhal AB, Harris GJ, Halpern EF, Koroshetz WJ, Smith WS, et al. The pattern of leptomeningeal collaterals on CT angiography is a strong predictor of long-term functional outcome in stroke patients with large vessel intracranial occlusion. Stroke. 2010;41(10):2316–22.
187. Liebeskind DS, Tomsick TA, Foster LD, Yeatts SD, Carrozzella J, Demchuk AM, Jovin TG, Khatri P, von Kummer R, Sugg RM, et al. Collaterals at angiography and outcomes in the interventional Management of Stroke (IMS) III trial. Stroke. 2014;45(3):759–64.
188. Sheth SA, Sanossian N, Hao Q, Starkman S, Ali LK, Kim D, Gonzalez NR, Tateshima S, Jahan R, Duckwiler GR, et al. Collateral flow as causative of good outcomes in endovascular stroke therapy. J Neurointerv Surg. 2016; 8(1):2–7.
189. Miteff F, Levi CR, Bateman GA, Spratt N, McElduff P, Parsons MW. The independent predictive utility of computed tomography angiographic collateral status in acute ischaemic stroke. Brain. 2009;132(Pt 8):2231–8.
190. Seyman E, Shaim H, Shenhar-Tsarfaty S, Jonash-Kimchi T, Bornstein NM, Hallevi H. The collateral circulation determines cortical infarct volume in anterior circulation ischemic stroke. BMC Neurol. 2016;16(1):206.
191. Marks MP, Lansberg MG, Mlynash M, Olivot JM, Straka M, Kemp S, McTaggart R, Inoue M, Zaharchuk G, Bammer R, et al. Effect of collateral blood flow on patients undergoing endovascular therapy for acute ischemic stroke. Stroke. 2014;45(4):1035–9.
192. Bang OY, Saver JL, Kim SJ, Kim GM, Chung CS, Ovbiagele B, Lee KH, Liebeskind DS. Collateral flow predicts response to endovascular therapy for acute ischemic stroke. Stroke. 2011;42(3):693–9.
193. Liebeskind DS, Kim D, Starkman S, Changizi K, Ohanian AG, Jahan R, Vinuela F. Collateral failure? Late mechanical thrombectomy after failed intravenous thrombolysis. J Neuroimaging. 2010;20(1):78–82.
194. Tsivgoulis G, Safouris A, Katsanos AH, Arthur AS, Alexandrov AV. Mechanical thrombectomy for emergent large vessel occlusion: a critical appraisal of recent randomized controlled clinical trials. Brain Behav. 2016;6(2):e00418.
195. Mokin M, Fargen KM, Primiani CT, Ren Z, Dumont TM, Brasiliense LBC, Dabus G, Linfante I, Kan P, Srinivasan VM, et al. Vessel perforation during stent retriever thrombectomy for acute ischemic stroke: technical details and clinical outcomes. J Neurointerv Surg. 2017;9(10):922–28.
196. Schumacher HC, Meyers PM, Yavagal DR, Harel NY, Elkind MS, Mohr JP, Pile-Spellman J. Endovascular mechanical thrombectomy of an occluded superior division branch of the left MCA for acute cardioembolic stroke. Cardiovasc Intervent Radiol. 2003;26(3):305–8.
197. Kwolek CJ, Crawford RS. Training the next generation of vascular specialists: current status and future perspectives. J Endovasc Ther. 2009;16(1_suppl): 42–52.
198. Endovascular Therapy Following Imaging Evaluation for Ischemic Stroke 3 (DEFUSE 3). [https://clinicaltrials.gov/ct2/show/NCT02586415].
199. POSITIVE Stroke Clinical Trial [https://clinicaltrials.gov/ct2/show/NCT01852201].
200. Trevo and Medical Management Versus Medical Management Alone in Wake Up and Late Presenting Strokes [https://clinicaltrials.gov/ct2/show/NCT02142283].
201. Griessenauer CJ, Schirmer CM. Dawn of an even newer era: mechanical Thrombectomy for acute ischemic stroke beyond 6 to 8 hours. World Neurosurg. 2017;104:968–9.
202. Hacke W. A new DAWN for imaging-based selection in the treatment of acute stroke. N Engl J Med. 2018;378(1):81–3.
203. Brinjikji W, Murad MH, Rabinstein AA, Cloft HJ, Lanzino G, Kallmes DF. Conscious sedation versus general anesthesia during endovascular acute ischemic stroke treatment: a systematic review and meta-analysis. AJNR Am J Neuroradiol. 2015;36(3):525–9.
204. Abou-Chebl A, Lin R, Hussain MS, Jovin TG, Levy EI, Liebeskind DS, Yoo AJ, Hsu DP, Rymer MM, Tayal AH, et al. Conscious sedation versus general anesthesia during endovascular therapy for acute anterior circulation stroke: preliminary results from a retrospective, multicenter study. Stroke. 2010; 41(6):1175–9.
205. John S, Thebo U, Gomes J, Saqqur M, Farag E, Xu J, Wisco D, Uchino K, Hussain MS. Intra-arterial therapy for acute ischemic stroke under general anesthesia versus monitored anesthesia care. Cerebrovasc Dis. 2014;38(4):262–7.
206. van den Berg LA, Koelman DL, Berkhemer OA, Rozeman AD, Fransen PS, Beumer D, Dippel DW, van der Lugt A, van Oostenbrugge RJ, van Zwam WH, et al. Type of anesthesia and differences in clinical outcome after intra-arterial treatment for ischemic stroke. Stroke. 2015;46(5):1257–62.
207. Sedation vs. Intubation for Endovascular Stroke TreAtment (SIESTA). [https://clinicaltrials.gov/ct2/show/NCT02126085].
208. General Or Local Anaestesia in Intra Arterial THerapy (GOLIATH) [https://clinicaltrials.gov/ct2/show/NCT02317237].
209. Sedation Versus General Anesthesia for Endovascular Therapy in Acute Stroke - Impact on Neurological Outcome (ANSTROKE). [https://clinicaltrials.gov/ct2/show/NCT01872884].
210. Mokin M, Rojas H, Levy EI. Randomized trials of endovascular therapy for stroke [mdash] impact on stroke care. Nat Rev Neurol. 2016;12(2):86–94.
211. Lowhagen Henden P, Rentzos A, Karlsson JE, Rosengren L, Leiram B, Sundeman H, Dunker D, Schnabel K, Wikholm G, Hellstrom M, et al. General anesthesia versus conscious sedation for endovascular treatment of acute ischemic stroke: the AnStroke trial (anesthesia during stroke). Stroke. 2017; 48(6):1601–7.
212. Schonenberger S, Pfaff J, Uhlmann L, Klose C, Nagel S, Ringleb PA, Hacke W, Kieser M, Bendszus M, Mohlenbruch MA, et al. The impact of conscious sedation versus general anesthesia for stroke Thrombectomy on the predictive value of collateral status: a post hoc analysis of the SIESTA trial. AJNR Am J Neuroradiol. 2017;38(8):1580–85.
213. Schonenberger S, Uhlmann L, Hacke W, Schieber S, Mundiyanapurath S, Purrucker JC, Nagel S, Klose C, Pfaff J, Bendszus M, et al. Effect of conscious sedation vs general anesthesia on early neurological improvement among patients with ischemic stroke undergoing endovascular Thrombectomy: a randomized clinical trial. JAMA. 2016;316(19):1986–96.
214. Schonewille WJ, Algra A, Serena J, Molina CA, Kappelle LJ. Outcome in patients with basilar artery occlusion treated conventionally. J Neurol Neurosurg Psychiatry. 2005;76(9):1238–41.
215. Tountopoulou A, Ahl B, Weissenborn K, Becker H, Goetz F. Intra-arterial thrombolysis using rt-PA in patients with acute stroke due to vessel occlusion of anterior and/or posterior cerebral circulation. Neuroradiology. 2008;50(1):75–83.
216. Lindsberg PJ, Mattle HP. Therapy of basilar artery occlusion: a systematic analysis comparing intra-arterial and intravenous thrombolysis. Stroke. 2006; 37(3):922–8.
217. Schonewille WJ, Wijman CA, Michel P, Rueckert CM, Weimar C, Mattle HP, Engelter ST, Tanne D, Muir KW, Molina CA et al: Treatment and outcomes of acute basilar artery occlusion in the basilar artery international cooperation study (BASICS): a prospective registry study. Lancet Neurol 2009, 8(8):724-730.
218. Nagel S, Kellert L, Mohlenbruch M, Bosel J, Rohde S, Ringleb P. Improved clinical outcome after acute basilar artery occlusion since the introduction of endovascular thrombectomy devices. Cerebrovasc Dis. 2013;36(5–6):394–400.
219. Nagel S, Schellinger PD, Hartmann M, Juettler E, Huttner HB, Ringleb P, Schwab S, Kohrmann M. Therapy of acute basilar artery occlusion: intraarterial thrombolysis alone vs bridging therapy. Stroke. 2009;40(1):140–6.
220. Pfefferkorn T, Mayer TE, Opherk C, Peters N, Straube A, Pfister HW, Holtmannspotter M, Muller-Schunk S, Wiesmann M, Dichgans M. Staged escalation therapy in acute basilar artery occlusion: intravenous thrombolysis and on-demand consecutive endovascular mechanical thrombectomy: preliminary experience in 16 patients. Stroke. 2008;39(5): 1496–500.

221. Basilar Artery International Cooperation Study (BASICS) [https://clinicaltrials.gov/ct2/show/NCT01717755].
222. van der Hoeven EJ, Schonewille WJ, Vos JA, Algra A, Audebert HJ, Berge E, Ciccone A, Mazighi M, Michel P, Muir KW, et al. The basilar artery international cooperation study (BASICS): study protocol for a randomised controlled trial. Trials. 2013;14:200.
223. Huo X, Gao F, Sun X, Ma N, Song L, Mo D, Liu L, Wang B, Zhang X, Miao Z. Endovascular mechanical Thrombectomy with the solitaire device for the treatment of acute basilar artery occlusion. World neurosurg. 2016;89:301–8.
224. Mourand I, Machi P, Milhaud D, Picot MC, Lobotesis K, Arquizan C, Costalat V, Heroum C, Sablot D, Bouly S, et al. Mechanical thrombectomy with the solitaire device in acute basilar artery occlusion. J Neurointerv Surg. 2014; 6(3):200–4.
225. Direct Transfer to an Endovascular Center Compared to Transfer to the Closest Stroke Center in Acute Stroke Patients With Suspected Large Vessel Occlusion. [https://clinicaltrials.gov/ct2/show/NCT02795962].
226. Statistical Plan for the MOST trial [http://www.berryconsultants.com/wp-content/uploads/2015/08/MOST.pdf].
227. Alberts MJ, Latchaw RE, Jagoda A, Wechsler LR, Crocco T, George MG, Connolly ES, Mancini B, Prudhomme S, Gress D, et al. Revised and updated recommendations for the establishment of primary stroke centers: a summary statement from the brain attack coalition. Stroke. 2011;42(9):2651–65.
228. Latchaw RE, Alberts MJ, Lev MH, Connors JJ, Harbaugh RE, Higashida RT, Hobson R, Kidwell CS, Koroshetz WJ, Mathews V, et al. Recommendations for imaging of acute ischemic stroke: a scientific statement from the American Heart Association. Stroke. 2009;40(11):3646–78.
229. Pereira VM, Krings T. Comeback victory. Am J Neuroradiol. 2015;36(5):821–4.
230. Malhotra K, Liebeskind DS. Imaging in endovascular stroke trials. J Neuroimaging. 2015;25(4):517–27.
231. Marler JR, Tilley BC, Lu M, Brott TG, Lyden PC, Grotta JC, Broderick JP, Levine SR, Frankel MP, Horowitz SH, et al. Early stroke treatment associated with better outcome: the NINDS rt-PA stroke study. Neurology. 2000;55(11):1649–55.
232. Wahlgren N, Ahmed N, Davalos A, Ford GA, Grond M, Hacke W, Hennerici MG, Kaste M, Kuelkens S, Larrue V, et al. Thrombolysis with alteplase for acute ischaemic stroke in the safe implementation of Thrombolysis in stroke-monitoring study (SITS-MOST): an observational study. Lancet. 2007; 369(9558):275–82.
233. Toni D, Lorenzano S, Agnelli G, Guidetti D, Orlandi G, Semplicini A, Toso V, Caso V, Malferrari G, Fanucchi S, et al. Intravenous thrombolysis with rt-PA in acute ischemic stroke patients aged older than 80 years in Italy. Cerebrovasc Dis. 2008;25(1–2):129–35.
234. Rha JH, Shrivastava VP, Wang Y, Lee KE, Ahmed N, Bluhmki E, Hermansson K, Wahlgren N. Thrombolysis for acute ischaemic stroke with alteplase in an Asian population: results of the multicenter, multinational safe implementation of Thrombolysis in stroke-non-European Union world (SITS-NEW). Int J Stroke. 2014;9(Suppl A100):93–101.
235. Grunwald IQ, Walter S, Papanagiotou P, Krick C, Hartmann K, Dautermann A, Fassbender K, Haass A, Bolar LJ, Reith W, et al. Revascularization in acute ischaemic stroke using the penumbra system: the first single center experience. Eur J Neurol. 2009;16(11):1210–6.
236. Hui FK, Narayanan S, Cawley CM. Posterior-to-anterior circulation access using the penumbra stroke system for mechanical thrombectomy of a right middle cerebral artery thrombus. World neurosurg. 2010;73(1):17–21.
237. Kalia JS, Zaidat OO. Using a distal access catheter in acute stroke intervention with penumbra, merci and gateway. A technical case report. Interv Neuroradiol. 2009;15(4):421–4.
238. Chow K, Gobin YP, Saver J, Kidwell C, Dong P, Vinuela F. Endovascular treatment of dural sinus thrombosis with rheolytic thrombectomy and intra-arterial thrombolysis. Stroke. 2000;31(6):1420–5.
239. Curtin KR, Shaibani A, Resnick SA, Russell EJ, Simuni T. Rheolytic catheter thrombectomy, balloon angioplasty, and direct recombinant tissue plasminogen activator thrombolysis of dural sinus thrombosis with preexisting hemorrhagic infarctions. AJNR Am J Neuroradiol. 2004;25(10):1807–11.
240. Dashti SR, Hu YC, Yao T, Fiorella D, Mitha AP, Albuquerque FC, McDougall CG. Mechanical thrombectomy as first-line treatment for venous sinus thrombosis: technical considerations and preliminary results using the AngioJet device. J Neurointerv Surg. 2013;5(1):49–53.
241. Iskander A, Nayak A, Chauhan MS. Submassive pulmonary embolism and paradoxical embolic stroke treated with percutaneous rheolytic thrombectomy and closure of the patent foramen ovale. Catheter Cardiovasc Interv. 2005;64(3):356–60.
242. Tomsick T, Broderick J, Carrozella J, Khatri P, Hill M, Palesch Y, Khoury J. Revascularization results in the interventional Management of Stroke II trial. AJNR Am J Neuroradiol. 2008;29(3):582–7.
243. Kim SM, Lee DH, Kwon SU, Choi CG, Kim SJ, Suh DC. Treatment of acute ischemic stroke: feasibility of primary or secondary use of a self-expanding stent (Neuroform) during local intra-arterial thrombolysis. Neuroradiology. 2012;54(1):35–41.
244. Mitra D, Herwadkar A, Gholkar A. Use of neuroform stent in a patient with acute stroke caused by spontaneous petrous segment internal carotid artery dissection: a case report. Interv Neuroradiol. 2004;10(2):155–60.
245. Dumont TM, Natarajan SK, Eller JL, Mocco J, Kelly WH Jr, Snyder KV, Hopkins LN, Siddiqui AH, Levy EI. Primary stenting for acute ischemic stroke using the Enterprise vascular reconstruction device: early results. J Neurointerv Surg. 2014;6(5):363–72.
246. Lee KY, Chen DY, Hsu HL, Chen CJ, Tseng YC. Undersized angioplasty and stenting of symptomatic intracranial tight stenosis with Enterprise: evaluation of clinical and vascular outcome. Interv Neuroradiol. 2016;22(2):187–95.
247. Natarajan SK, Sonig A, Mocco J, Dumont TM, Thind H, Hartney ML, Snyder KV, Hopkins LN, Siddiqui AH, Levy EI. Primary stenting for acute ischemic stroke using the Enterprise intracranial stent: 2-year results of a phase-I trial. J Vasc Interv Neurol. 2015;8(3):62–7.
248. Coutinho JM, Liebeskind DS, Slater LA, Nogueira RG, Baxter BW, Levy EI, Siddiqui AH, Goyal M, Zaidat OO, Davalos A, et al. Mechanical Thrombectomy for isolated M2 occlusions: a post hoc analysis of the STAR, SWIFT, and SWIFT PRIME studies. AJNR Am J Neuroradiol. 2016;37(4):667–72.
249. Coutinho JM, Liebeskind DS, Slater LA, Nogueira RG, Clark W, Davalos A, Bonafe A, Jahan R, Fischer U, Gralla J, et al. Combined intravenous Thrombolysis and Thrombectomy vs Thrombectomy alone for acute ischemic stroke: a pooled analysis of the SWIFT and STAR studies. JAMA Neurol. 2017;74(3):268–74.
250. Lopez-Cancio E, Jovin TG, Cobo E, Cerda N, Jimenez M, Gomis M, Hernandez-Perez M, Caceres C, Cardona P, Lara B, et al. Endovascular treatment improves cognition after stroke: a secondary analysis of REVASCAT trial. Neurology. 2017;88(3):245–51.
251. Mokin M, Levy EI, Siddiqui AH, Goyal M, Nogueira RG, Yavagal DR. V MP, Saver JL. Association of clot burden score with radiographic and clinical outcomes following solitaire stent retriever thrombectomy: analysis of the SWIFT PRIME trial. J Neurointerv Surg. 2016;9(10):929–32.
252. Shireman TI, Wang K, Saver JL, Goyal M, Bonafe A, Diener HC, Levy EI, Pereira VM, Albers GW, Cognard C, et al. Cost-effectiveness of solitaire stent retriever Thrombectomy for acute ischemic stroke: results from the SWIFT-PRIME trial (solitaire with the intention for Thrombectomy as primary endovascular treatment for acute ischemic stroke). Stroke. 2017;48(2):379–87.
253. Broussalis E, Trinka E, Hitzl W, Wallner A, Chroust V, Killer-Oberpfalzer M. Comparison of stent-retriever devices versus the merci retriever for endovascular treatment of acute stroke. AJNR Am J Neuroradiol. 2013;34(2):366–72.
254. Davalos A, Pereira VM, Chapot R, Bonafe A, Andersson T, Gralla J. Retrospective multicenter study of solitaire FR for revascularization in the treatment of acute ischemic stroke. Stroke. 2012;43(10):2699–705.
255. Dippel DW, Majoie CB, Roos YB, van der Lugt A, van Oostenbrugge RJ, van Zwam WH, Lingsma HF, Koudstaal PJ, Treurniet KM, van den Berg LA, et al. Influence of device choice on the effect of intra-arterial treatment for acute ischemic stroke in MR CLEAN (multicenter randomized clinical trial of endovascular treatment for acute ischemic stroke in the Netherlands). Stroke. 2016;47(10):2574–81.
256. Haussen DC, Lima A, Nogueira RG. The Trevo XP 3x20 mm retriever ('Baby Trevo') for the treatment of distal intracranial occlusions. J Neurointerv Surg. 2016;8(3):295–9.
257. Hentschel KA, Daou B, Chalouhi N, Starke RM, Clark S, Gandhe A, Jabbour P, Rosenwasser R, Tjoumakaris S. Comparison of non-stent retriever and stent retriever mechanical thrombectomy devices for the endovascular treatment of acute ischemic stroke. J Neurosurg. 2016;126(4):1123–30.
258. Imahori T, Tanaka K, Koyama J, Arai A, Shiomi R, Iwahashi H, Yokote A, Matsushima K, Matsui D, Kobayashi M, et al. Mechanical Thrombectomy using the Trevo ProVue in 50 consecutive patients with anterior circulation stroke: a single-center experience after approval of the stent retriever in Japan. Neurol Med Chir (Tokyo). 2017;57(3):128–35.
259. Kim SK, Baek BH, Heo TW, Yoon W. Successful cross-circulation stent-retriever Embolectomy through posterior communicating artery for acute MCA occlusion by using Trevo XP ProVue. Neurointervention. 2016;11(1):55–8.

260. Rohde S, Haehnel S, Herweh C, Pham M, Stampfl S, Ringleb PA, Bendszus M. Mechanical thrombectomy in acute embolic stroke: preliminary results with the revive device. Stroke. 2011;42(10):2954–6.
261. Saleh M, Spence JN, Nayak S, Pearce G, Tennuci C, Roffe C. Safety and efficacy of the Aperio thrombectomy device when compared to the solitaire AB/FR and the revive devices in a pulsatile flow system. Am J Cardiovasc Dis. 2012;2(4):301–8.
262. Kallenberg K, Solymosi L, Taschner CA, Berkefeld J, Schlamann M, Jansen O, Arnold S, Tomandl B, Knauth M, Turowski B: Endovascular stroke therapy with the Aperio thrombectomy device. J Neurointerv Surg 2016, 8(8):834-839.
263. Roth C, Junk D, Papanagiotou P, Keuler A, Korner H, Schumacher M, Reith W. A comparison of 2 stroke devices: the new Aperio clot-removal device and the solitaire AB/FR. AJNR Am J Neuroradiol. 2012;33(7):1317–20.
264. Kabbasch C, Mpotsaris A, Liebig T, Soderman M, Holtmannspotter M, Cronqvist M, Thornton J, Mendes Pereira V, Andersson T. First-in-man procedural experience with the novel EmboTrap(R) revascularization device for the treatment of ischemic stroke-a European multicenter series. Clin Neuroradiol. 2016;26(2):221–8.
265. Prothmann S, Schwaiger BJ, Gersing AS, Reith W, Niederstadt T, Felber A, Kurre W. Acute Recanalization of Thrombo-embolic ischemic stroke with pREset (ARTESp): the impact of occlusion time on clinical outcome of directly admitted and transferred patients. J Neurointerv Surg. 2017;9(9): 817–22.
266. Cerejo R, John S, Bauer A, Hussain MS, Bain M, Rasmussen P, Hui F, Masaryk T, Toth G. Emergent mechanical thrombectomy for acute stroke using the Mindframe capture LP system: initial single-center experience. J Neurointerv Surg. 2016;8(11):1178–80.
267. Protto S, Pienimaki JP, Seppanen J, Matkaselka I, Ollikainen J, Numminen H, Sillanpaa N. TREVO and capture LP have equal technical success rates in mechanical thrombectomy of proximal and distal anterior circulation occlusions. J Neurointerv Surg. 2017;9(7):644–9.
268. Raoult H, Redjem H, Bourcier R, Gaultier-Lintia A, Daumas-Duport B, Ferre JC, Eugene F, Fahed R, Bartolini B, Piotin M, et al. Mechanical thrombectomy with the ERIC retrieval device: initial experience. J Neurointerv Surg. 2017; 9(6):574–77.
269. Mohlenbruch MA, Kabbasch C, Kowoll A, Broussalis E, Sonnberger M, Muller M, Wiesmann M, Trenkler J, Killer-Oberpfalzer M, Weber W, et al. Multicenter experience with the new SOFIA plus catheter as a primary local aspiration catheter for acute stroke thrombectomy. J Neurointerv Surg. 2017;9(12): 1223–27.
270. Stampfl S, Kabbasch C, Muller M, Mpotsaris A, Brockmann M, Liebig T, Wiesmann M, Bendszus M, Mohlenbruch MA. Initial experience with a new distal intermediate and aspiration catheter in the treatment of acute ischemic stroke: clinical safety and efficacy. J Neurointerv Surg. 2016;8(7):714–8.
271. Wong JH, Do HM, Telischak NA, Moraff AM, Dodd RL, Marks MP, Ingle SM, Heit JJ. Initial experience with SOFIA as an intermediate catheter in mechanical thrombectomy for acute ischemic stroke. J Neurointerv Surg. 2016;
272. Kowoll A, Weber A, Mpotsaris A, Behme D, Weber W. Direct aspiration first pass technique for the treatment of acute ischemic stroke: initial experience at a European stroke center. J Neurointerv Surg. 2016;8(3):230–4.
273. Kim YS, Kwak HS, Chung GH, Hwang SB. Manual aspiration thrombectomy using the penumbra catheter in patients with acute M1 occlusion: a single-center study. Interv Neuroradiol. 2015;21(6):694–9.
274. Park JS, Kwak HS. Manual aspiration Thrombectomy using penumbra catheter in patients with acute M2 occlusion : a single-center analysis. J Korean Neurosurg Soc. 2016;59(4):352–6.
275. Schumacher HC, Gupta R, Higashida RT, Meyers PM. Advances in revascularization for acute ischemic stroke treatment. Expert Rev Neurother. 2005;5(2):189–201.
276. Mahon BR, Nesbit GM, Barnwell SL, Clark W, Marotta TR, Weill A, Teal PA, Qureshi AI. North American clinical experience with the EKOS MicroLysUS infusion catheter for the treatment of embolic stroke. AJNR Am J Neuroradiol. 2003;24(3):534–8.
277. Jiang WJ, Yu W, Du B, Gao F, Cui LY. Outcome of patients with >/=70% symptomatic intracranial stenosis after wingspan stenting. Stroke. 2011; 42(7):1971–5.
278. Li TX, Gao BL, Cai DY, Wang ZL, Zhu LF, Xue JY, Bai WX, He YK, Li L. Wingspan stenting for severe symptomatic intracranial atherosclerotic Stenosis in 433 patients treated at a single medical center. PLoS One. 2015; 10(9):e0139377.
279. Murias Quintana E, Vega Valdes P, Morales Deza E, Gil Garcia A, Cuellar Saenz H, Salgado Bernal AL, Cadenas Rodriguez M, Benavente Fernandez L, Delgado MG, Riesco Perez N, et al. Endovascular reconstruction of internal carotid artery dissection in patients with acute ischemic stroke using the wingspan stent. Interv Neuroradiol. 2016;22(6):700–4.
280. Qureshi AI, Al-Senani FM, Husain S, Janjua NA, Lanzino G, Lavados PM, Nguyen T, Raymond J, Shah QA, Suarez JI, et al. Intracranial angioplasty and stent placement after stenting and aggressive medical management for preventing recurrent stroke in intracranial stenosis (SAMMPRIS) trial: present state and future considerations. J Neuroimaging. 2012;22(1):1–13.
281. Sung SM, Lee TH, Cho HJ, Sol YL, Park KH, Jung DS, Kim CW. Recanalization with wingspan stent for acute middle cerebral artery occlusion in failure or contraindication to intravenous thrombolysis: a feasibility study. AJNR Am J Neuroradiol. 2012;33(6):1156–61.
282. Wang ZL, Gao BL, Li TX, Cai DY, Zhu LF, Xue JY, Bai WX, Li ZS. Outcomes of middle cerebral artery angioplasty and stenting with wingspan at a high-volume center. Neuroradiology. 2016;58(2):161–9.
283. Xavier AR, Tiwari A, Purai N, Rayes M, Pandey P, Kansara A, Narayanan S, Chaturvedi S. Safety and efficacy of intracranial stenting for acute ischemic stroke beyond 8 h of symptom onset. J Neurointerv Surg. 2012;4(2):94–100.
284. Zhao T, Zhu WY, Xiong XY, Li J, Wang L, Ding HY, Wei F, Zhou Y, Gong ZL, Cheng SY, et al. Safety and efficacy of wingspan stenting for severe symptomatic atherosclerotic Stenosis of the middle cerebral artery: analysis of 278 continuous cases. J Stroke Cerebrovasc Dis. 2016;25(10):2368–72.
285. Lee MS, Singh V, Wilentz JR, Makkar RR. AngioJet thrombectomy. J Invasive Cardiol. 2004;16(10):587–91.
286. Lee JS, Demchuk AM. Choosing a Hyperacute stroke imaging protocol for proper patient selection and time efficient endovascular treatment: lessons from recent trials. J Stroke. 2015;17(3):221–8.
287. International Multicenter Registry for Mechanical Recanalization Procedures in Acute Stroke [https://clinicaltrials.gov/ct2/show/NCT01399762].
288. Imaging Guided Patient Selection for Interventional Revascularization Therapy (START) [https://clinicaltrials.gov/ct2/show/NCT00963989].
289. Endovascular Acute Stroke Intervention Trial - the EASI Trial [https://clinicaltrials.gov/ct2/show/NCT02157532].

Association of fibrinogen level with early neurological deterioration among acute ischemic stroke patients with diabetes

Seong-Joon Lee[1], Ji Man Hong[1], Sung Eun Lee[1], Dae Ryong Kang[2], Bruce Ovbiagele[3], Andrew M. Demchuk[4] and Jin Soo Lee[1*]

Abstract

Background: Diabetes mellitus (DM) is a risk factor for early neurological deterioration (END) in acute ischemic stroke. The prothrombotic protein fibrinogen is frequently elevated in patients with diabetes, and may be associated with poorer prognoses. We evaluated whether fibrinogen is associated with END in patients with diabetes after acute ischemic stroke.

Methods: We included 3814 patients from a single hospital database admitted within 72 h of onset of ischemic stroke. END was defined as an increase in the National Institutes of Health Stroke Scale (NIHSS) ≥2 within 7 days post-admission. In the total population (END, $n = 661$; non-END, $n = 3153$), univariate and multivariate analyses were performed to assess fibrinogen as an independent predictor for END. We then performed propensity score matching and univariate analyses for DM (END, $n = 261$; non-END, $n = 522$) and non-DM populations (END, $n = 399$; non-END, $n = 798$). Multiple logistic analyses were performed after matching for fibrinogen as a risk factor in each subgroup.

Results: Fibrinogen levels were higher in the END group than in the non-END group (367 ± 156 mg/dL vs. 347 ± 122 mg/dL, $p = 0.002$), though they were not associated with END in logistic regression analyses. Fibrinogen levels were found to be an independent predictor for END, but only in the DM population (fibrinogen levels 300–599 mg/dL, odds ratio: 1.618, 95% confidence interval: 1.037–2.525, $p = 0.034$, fibrinogen levels ≥600 mg/dL, 2.575, 1.018–6.514, $p = 0.046$; non-DM population, $p = 0.393$). The diabetes-fibrinogen interaction for the entire cohort was $p = 0.101$.

Conclusions: Elevated fibrinogen is dose-dependently associated with END in patients with diabetes following acute ischemic stroke.

Keywords: Cerebral infarction, Disease progression, Diabetes mellitus, Fibrinogen, Intracranial thrombosis

Background

Diabetes mellitus (DM) and hyperglycemia negatively affect the outcome and pathophysiology of acute ischemic stroke. The associations between DM and early neurological deterioration (END) [1, 2], more comorbidities [3], severe handicap and disability [4, 5], and increased mortality [3], have been repeatedly reported in both case-control [6] and cohort studies [7]. When the effects of hyperglycemia are included, these patients also present with more severe lesion size [8], more symptomatic intracranial hemorrhages [9, 10], edema [11], and mortality [12]. Although END is more frequently encountered in diabetic patients, the specific mechanisms underlying how DM promotes END are among the least clear. In clinical practice, being able to anticipate END would allow for more timely intervention; thus, gaining further insight into the mechanisms of END specific to patients with DM would improve the ability to identify and intervene in END in a population seemingly more susceptible

* Correspondence: jinsoo22@gmail.com
[1]Department of Neurology, Ajou University School of Medicine, Ajou University Medical Center, San 5, Woncheon-dong, Yeongtong-gu, Suwon, Kyungki-do 443–721, South Korea
Full list of author information is available at the end of the article

to it. One possible mechanism linking DM with adverse outcomes of stroke involves fibrinogen, a prothrombotic protein, and acute phase reactant that is consistently elevated in patients with diabetes [13, 14]. In fact, a large body of evidence identifies fibrinogen as a mediator in the development of coronary artery thrombi and future cardiac events [15, 16]. However, the association of hyperfibrinogenemia and END in acute ischemic stroke has not yet been demonstrated. In this study, we evaluated whether elevated fibrinogen levels in patients with diabetes and acute ischemic stroke are associated with END in a large, single-center population.

Methods

Study population

We performed a retrospective study that was approved by the Institutional Review Board, and performed in accordance with the ethical standards of the 1964 Declaration of Helsinki and its later amendments, incorporating consecutive patients enrolled in a hospital stroke database. From this database, we reviewed consecutive patients from Jan. 2000 to Dec. 2015. Among them, we included 3814 patients with acute ischemic stroke within 72 h of onset, and with available National Institutes of Health Stroke Scale (NIHSS) data.

Data acquisition

For this study, the diagnosis of DM was defined as either a prior diagnosis of diabetes, or glycated hemoglobin (HbA1c) levels >6.1% at admission, according to a previous study which showed that prediabetic levels of hba1c >6.1% were associated with increased stroke recurrence [17]. Lab data concerning the hemostatic profiles such as fibrinogen, fibrin degradation products (FDP), D-dimer, and classic stroke risk factors were obtained on the day of admission, before initiation of intravenous tissue plasminogen activators for those who were applicable. Acute inflammatory markers, erythrocyte sedimentation rate (ESR), and standard C-reactive protein (CRP) levels were included in the analysis, to compare with fibrinogen. Components of metabolic syndrome were also analyzed. Lab data routinely taken to evaluate diabetic status, such as fasting glucose levels, urine glucose, urine protein, and HbA1c levels were also included in the analysis. Trial of Org 10,172 in Acute Stroke Treatment (TOAST) classification, and NIHSS scores on admission and at discharge were also collected from the database.

Propensity score matching and statistical analysis

END was defined as a NIHSS score increase of 2 or more within 7 days after admission. A number of studies have, for the definition of END, used an increase of ≥2 points in the total NIHSS score within 7 days [18], as modified from a previous study. We have incorporated such sensitive criteria to define END for such subtle changes call for action in clinical practice. Because END in patients with acute ischemic stroke can be influenced by a greater initial NIHSS and TOAST classification, we used propensity score matching to adjust for well-known confounding factors. First, among the 3814 patients with acute stroke, we performed univariate and multivariate analyses to document the effects of fibrinogen and other predictive factors of END. Multivariate analysis was performed, adjusting for age, sex, presence of hypertension, diabetes mellitus, initial NIHSS score, and TOAST classification. The p value for the diabetes status x fibrinogen level interaction was also calculated in the logistic regression model. For subgroup analysis, the patients were divided into DM (n = 1360) and non-DM (n = 2454) populations. In each subgroup, a 1:2 propensity score matching of END patients and non-END patients was performed, adjusting for age, sex, initial NIHSS score, and TOAST classification (Additional file 1: Figure S1A-B). Differences between the two groups were analyzed before and after propensity score matching, using a χ^2 test for categorical variables and Student's t-test for continuous variables. Multiple logistic regression analysis was performed, adjusting for baseline clinical variables known to be associated with END such as age, sex, hypertension, initial NIHSS, and TOAST classification, as well as with potentially significant factors determined in the univariate analysis ($p < 0.005$), to verify the significance of fibrinogen levels on END. All statistical analyses were performed using IBM SPSS Statistics 20 software (Chicago, IL).

Results

Among 3814 patients with acute stroke, 661 cases (17.3%) experienced early neurological deterioration. Patients in the END group were significantly older (65.3 ± 12.6 vs. 63.5 ± 13.5, p = 0.001), and more frequently had a history of DM (39.6% vs. 34.8%, p = 0.019), a history of hypertension (70.0% vs. 65.8%, p = 0.039), a higher initial NIHSS (8.2 ± 6.7 vs. 5.6 ± 6.3, $p < 0.001$), higher fasting glucose (151 ± 66 vs. 144 ± 63 mg/dL, p = 0.005), higher urine protein positivity (22.7% vs. 14.6%, $p < 0.001$), and higher fibrinogen levels (367 ± 156 vs. 347 ± 122 mg/dL, p = 0.002) (Table 1). In the multiple regression analysis of the total population, higher fibrinogen levels were not significantly associated with END after adjusting for confounders (p = 0.195) (Table 2). The interaction between diabetes status and fibrinogen levels regarding END was not statistically significant in the entire cohort (p = 0.101).

There were 1360 diabetic and 2454 non-diabetic patients. In the DM population (END = 262, non-END = 1098), a diagnosis of hypertension (81.6% vs. 74.6%, p = 0.017), initial NIHSS (10.4 ± 10.6 vs. 3.6 ± 5.7,

Table 1 Comparison of baseline data in patients with acute ischemic stroke admitted within 72 h

	END (n = 661)	Non-END (n = 3153)	P
Age	65.3 ± 12.6	63.5 ± 13.5	0.001
Male sex	409 (61.9%)	2017 (64.0%)	0.309
Hypertension	462 (70.0%)	2052 (65.8%)	0.039
Diabetes mellitus	262 (39.6%)	1098 (34.8%)	0.019
Initial NIHSS	8.2 ± 6.7	5.6 ± 6.3	<0.001
Discharge NIHSS	10.5 ± 10.3	3.2 ± 5.4	<0.001
TOAST			<0.001
Cardioembolism	160 (24.2%)	718 (22.8%)	
Atherosclerosis	201 (30.4%)	818 (25.9%)	
Small artery disease	159 (24.1%)	614 (19.5%)	
Others	141 (21.3%)	1003 (31.8%)	
Fasting glucose (mg/dL)	151 ± 66	144 ± 63	0.005
Glycated hemoglobin (%)	6.65 ± 1.57	6.46 ± 1.36	0.051
Urine protein positivity	100/441 (22.7%)	276/1896 (14.6%)	<0.001
Fibrinogen (mg/dL)	367 ± 156	347 ± 122	0.002
ESR (mm)	18.15 ± 17.09	17.57 ± 17.01	0.439
CRP (mg/dL)	0.81 ± 2.00	0.73 ± 2.33	0.459
BMI	23.8 ± 3.2	24.0 ± 3.4	0.163
Metabolic syndrome	288 (43.6%)	1295 (41.1%)	0.236
Lipid panel			
T.chol (mg/dL)	179.54 ± 42.07	179.15 ± 51.46	0.857
LDL (mg/dL)	107.42 ± 37.48	105.68 ± 35.45	0.262
HDL (mg/dL)	45.65 ± 12.87	45.94 ± 13.40	0.616
TG (mg/dL)	139.77 ± 122.26	142.83 ± 117.81	0.552

END early neurological deterioration, *NIHSS* National Institutes of Health Stroke Scale, *TOAST* trial of Org 10,172 in acute stroke treatment, *ESR* erythrocyte sedimentation rate, *CRP* c-reactive protein, *BMI* body mass index, *T.chol* total cholesterol, *LDL* low density lipoprotein, *HDL* high density lipoprotein, *TG* triglyceride

$p < 0.001$), urine protein positivity (35.1% vs. 21.2%, $p < 0.001$), and fibrinogen levels (392.9 ± 204.2 mg/dL, $p = 0.012$) were significantly higher in the END population versus the non-END population (Table 3). Propensity score matching was performed for age, sex, initial NIHSS, and TOAST classification, with a relative multivariate imbalance measure L1 of 0.621 before matching, and 0.609 after matching. No covariate exhibited a large imbalance. After matching, proteinuria (34.7% vs. 23.4%, $p = 0.007$, and hyperfibrinogenemia (392.8 ± 204.6 vs. 361 ± 123.1 mg/dL, $p = 0.009$) were still significantly associated with END (Table 3). In the propensity score-matched population, further logistic regression analysis adjusting for age, sex, hypertension, TOAST classification, and positive proteinuria was done, and fibrinogen was significantly associated with END in the DM population (fibrinogen <300 mg/dL as reference; fibrinogen levels 300 ~ 599 mg/dL, odds ratio: 1.618, 95% confidence interval: 1.037–2.525, $p = 0.034$, fibrinogen levels ≥600 mg/dL, 2.575, 1.018–6.514, $p = 0.046$) (Table 4).

In the non-DM population (END = 399, Non-END = 2055), age (65.3 ± 13.2 vs. 62.7 ± 14.3, $p < 0.001$), initial NIHSS (8.4 ± 6.8 vs. 5.6 ± 6.3, $p < 0.001$), and fasting glucose levels (125.6 ± 30.9 vs. 122.1 ± 29.7 mg/dL, $p = 0.036$) were significantly higher in the END group, as were differences in TOAST classification ($p < 0.001$) (Additional file 2: Table S1). Propensity score matching was performed for age, sex, initial NIHSS, and TOAST classification, with a relative multivariate imbalance measure L1 of 0.581 before matching, and 0.525 after matching. No covariate exhibited a large imbalance. After matching, TOAST classification ($p = 0.003$), elevated total cholesterol (179.5 ± 41.3 vs. 173.6 ± 38.4 mg/dL, $p = 0.015$), and elevated low density lipoprotein (108.2 ± 37.4 vs. 102.8 ± 34.3 mg/dL, $p = 0.015$) were significantly associated with END (Additional file 2: Table S1). In further regression analysis in the matched population, including age, male sex, presence of hypertension, initial NIHSS, TOAST classification, and total cholesterol levels as covariables, fibrinogen did

Table 2 A logistic regression model including potential factors associated with early neurologic deterioration in patients with acute ischemic stroke admitted within 72 h

	Odds ratio (95% confidence interval)	P
Age	1.00 (1.00–1.01)	0.605
Male sex	0.94 (0.78–1.14)	0.551
Hypertension	1.14 (0.93–1.40)	0.194
Diabetes mellitus	1.11 (0.92–1.33)	0.268
Initial NIHSS	1.07 (1.05–1.08)	<0.001
TOAST		<0.001
Cardioembolism	Reference	
Atherosclerosis	1.38 (1.07–1.78)	0.013
Small artery disease	1.97 (1.48–2.63)	<0.001
Others	0.94 (0.71–1.24)	0.652
Fibrinogen (mg/dL)		0.195
0–300 mg/dL	Reference	
300–600 mg/dL	1.20 (0.97–1.49)	0.091
> 600 mg/dL	1.36 (0.78–2.37)	0.195

NIHSS National Institutes of Health Stroke Scale, *TOAST* trial of Org 10,172 in acute stroke treatment

not prove to be associated with END (p = 0.393) (Additional file 2: Table S2).

Discussion

The results of this study suggest that hyperfibrinogenemia in patients with acute stroke and DM is associated with END, using both propensity score matching and multiple logistic regression analysis. Whereas the influence of hyperfibrinogenemia on END was consistently seen in the DM subgroup, it disappeared in the non-DM subgroup.

Hyperfibrinogenemia itself may directly induce a higher frequency of END in diabetic individuals through activation of the coagulation cascade. Fibrinogen forms fibrin clots as part of the final common stages of both the extrinsic and intrinsic pathways of the coagulation cascade [19]. Atherogenesis and the growth of atheromatous lesions are also initiated in part by fibrin deposition [20, 21]. Fibrinogen also facilitates platelet aggregation by binding to the glycoprotein IIb/IIIa receptor, increasing its reactivity [22].

Hyperfibrinogenemia may also indirectly reflect a prothrombotic condition induced by hyperinsulinemia and prolonged glycation. Levels of fibrinogen in diabetic patients correlate with insulin resistance and metabolic syndrome [13]. Prolonged glycation also induces a prothrombotic condition. Studies on fibrin clot structure under diabetic conditions have shown fibrinogen to be glycated in vivo [23], causing a change in the fibrin clot structure that reduces permeability [24], decreases fibrinolysis [25], and decreases α-chain crosslinking [26]. Thus, the effects of insulin resistance and prolonged glycation increase the risk of thrombosis, which underpins the development of vascular disease [27]. These studies lead us to assume that fibrinogen levels may represent a marker of platelet aggregation or progression to a prothrombotic phenotype in patients with diabetes [27].

This is the first study to link diabetic hyperfibrinogenemia to a higher frequency of END after ischemic stroke. Epidemiological studies have established that elevated fibrinogen levels are strongly and independently correlated with the risks of coronary arterial disease (CAD), stroke, and peripheral arterial disease [16, 28–31]. In stroke, carotid artery stenosis is significantly associated with elevated fibrinogen levels [32], and placebo data analysis in the Stroke Treatment with Ancrod Trial (STAT) and European Stroke Treatment with Ancrod Trial (ESTAT) has shown that plasma fibrinogen levels at stroke onset are independently associated with a poor functional outcome [33]. However, it has not been reported that hyperfibrinogenemia in patients with diabetes is associated with END in the acute stroke period.

It is conceivable that stronger antiplatelet treatments might be needed for patients with diabetes and hyperfibrinogenemia following acute ischemic stroke. Of note, elevated fibrinogen levels in our group of patients with diabetes may be linked to antiplatelet resistance, which may in turn result in END. Previous large scale trials, such as the Japanese Primary Prevention of Atherosclerosis with Aspirin for Diabetes (JPAD) trial [34], and the Prevention of Progression of Arterial Disease and Diabetes (POPAPAD) trial [35], have shown low efficacy of aspirin monotherapy for prevention of cardiovascular events in patients with diabetes. In addition, recent data show that responses to clopidogrel in patients with diabetes are suboptimal [36]. Such data suggest that diabetes is associated with considerable resistance to aspirin and clopidogrel therapy, and such insufficient antiplatelet responses could be an underlying causal factor for the frequent END observed in this population. In accordance with the elevated fibrinogen levels in our data, a recent study evaluating platelet aggregation characteristics in acute coronary syndrome found antiplatelet drug resistance to be significantly associated with metabolic syndrome, and fibrinogen levels and high sensitivity-CRP were higher in this population [37]. Serum fibrinogen levels appeared to be strongly associated with drug resistance [37]. In this case, elevated fibrinogen levels may call for more radical choices for antiplatelet therapy in such a population.

Apart from the antiplatelet issue, the idea that reduced fibrin, which is formed by fibrinogen in blood, may reduce blood viscosity, improve blood flow, and help remove the blood clot blocking the artery and re-establish

Table 3 Comparison before and after propensity score matching[a] in patients with diabetes and acute ischemic stroke admitted within 72 h

	Before matching			After matching		
	END (*n* = 262)	Non-END (*n* = 1098)	P	END (*n* = 261)	Non-END (*n* = 522)	P
Age	65.3 ± 11.8	65.1 ± 11.7	0.771	65.3 ± 11.8	64.8 ± 11.8	0.593
Male sex	160 (61.1%)	700 (63.8%)	0.418	159 (60.9%)	315 (60.3%)	0.877
Hypertension	213 (81.6%)	812(74.6%)	0.017	213 (81.6%)	431 (82.6%)	0.741
Initial NIHSS	8.0 ± 6.6	5.7 ± 6.4	<0.001	7.9 ± 6.6	7.6 ± 6.8	0.562
Discharge NIHSS	10.4 ± 10.6	3.6 ± 5.7	<0.001	10.4 ± 10.5	4.8 ± 6.5	<0.001
TOAST			0.167	76 (23.4%)		0.169
Cardioembolism	52 (19.8%)	221 (20.1%)		52 (19.9%)	111 (21.3%)	
Atherosclerosis	88 (33.6%)	328 (29.8%)		88 (33.7%)	163 (31.2%)	
Small artery disease	64 (24.4%)	235 (21.4%)		64 (24.5%)	102 (19.5%)	
Others	58 (22.1%)	314 (28.6%)		57 (21.8%)	146 (28.0%)	
Fasting glucose (mg/dL)	190.9 ± 84.1	184.0 ± 85.5	0.238	190.7 ± 84.2	189.5 ± 87.8	0.852
Glycated hemoglobin (%)	7.5 ± 1.7	7.3 ± 1.5	0.119	7.5 ± 1.7	7.4 ± 1.6	0.392
Urine protein positivity	59 (35.1%)	143 (21.2%)	<0.001	58 (34.7%)	76 (23.4%)	0.007
Fibrinogen (mg/dL)	392.9 ± 204.2	359.0 ± 119.1	0.012	392.8 ± 204.6	361.1 ± 123.1	0.009
ESR (mm)	22.0 ± 20.5	21.2 ± 20.1	0.547	22.0 ± 20.5	21.3 ± 18.9	0.643
CRP (mg/dL)	0.9 ± 2.3	0.9 ± 2.8	0.931	0.9 ± 2.3	1.1 ± 3.2	0.528
BMI				24.2 ± 3.3	24.5 ± 3.2	0.317
Metabolic syndrome	149 (56.9%)	609 (55.5%)	0.681	149 (57.1%)	305 (58.4%)	0.720
Lipid panel						
T.chol (mg/dL)	179.6 ± 43.2	181.7 ± 69.0	0.629	179.3 ± 43.0	182.2 ± 47.4	0.396
LDL (mg/dL)	106.3 ± 37.7	106.1 ± 37.4	0.919	106.0 ± 37.4	107.5 ± 38.1	0.604
HDL (mg/dL)	43.7 ± 11.7	43.9 ± 15.0	0.825	43.7 ± 11.7	44.0 ± 12.1	0.775
TG (mg/dL)	158.6 ± 113.5	163.4 ± 133.4	0.600	158.7 ± 113.7	165.6 ± 153.3	0.521

END early neurological deterioration, *NIHSS* National Institutes of Health Stroke Scale, *TOAST* trial of Org 10,172 in acute stroke treatment, *ESR* erythrocyte sedimentation rate, *CRP* c-reactive protein, *BMI* body mass index, *T.chol* total cholesterol, *LDL* low density lipoprotein, *HDL* high density lipoprotein, *TG* triglyceride
[a] Age, sex, initial NIHSS and TOAST were adjusted

blood flow has inspired clinical trials testing the therapeutic effects of the fibrin-depleting agents ancrod and defibrase [38]. In eight trials involving 5701 patients, fibrin-depleting agents marginally reduced the proportion of patients who were dead or disabled at the end of follow-up, and there were fewer stroke recurrences in the treatment group than in the control group. However, symptomatic intracranial hemorrhage was about twice as common in the treatment group compared with the control group [38]. The use of fibrin-depleting agents to reduce blood viscosity in patients with DM and elevated fibrinogen at risk for END holds similar problems. Plasma fibrinogen levels are associated with silent cerebrovascular lesions [39], and although this relationship may be evidence that increased viscosity by fibrinogen is a risk factor for stroke, deep white matter hyperintensities, on the other hand, are a known risk factor for intracerebral hemorrhage [40]. Accordingly, the use of fibrin-depleting agents in patients with DM may confer a higher risk of hemorrhagic complications. Thus, while the selective use of fibrin-depleting agents in patients with DM and END may be considered, further clinical studies to address the risks are needed prior to making such treatment a recommendation.

We acknowledge that our study has limitations. First, due to the retrospective nature of the study, there may be selection bias. We tried to minimize this issue by maximizing the number of patients included in the study and including adequate propensity score matching. Second, our somewhat long temporal definition of END (<7 days) incorporates a range of heterogeneous underlying mechanisms, and different definitions are used in other reports. Due to the retrospective nature and large number of enrolled patients in the study, the heterogeneity of END could not be addressed in this study. Third, because of the focus on lab data in this study, medication factors and imaging variables such as intracranial occlusion, stenosis, or diffusion weighted image volume were not included for analysis. However, variables that may have similar implications such as TOAST classification, and NIHSS

Table 4 A logistic regression model for END after propensity score matching[a] in patients with diabetes mellitus admitted within 72 h of acute ischemic stroke

	Odds ratio (95% confidence interval)	P
Age	1.01 (0.99–1.03)	0.397
Male sex	1.22 (0.80–1.87)	0.352
Hypertension	1.01 (0.584–1.74)	0.982
Initial NIHSS	1.01 (0.98–1.05)	0.434
TOAST		0.098
Cardioembolism	Reference	
Atherosclerosis	1.24 (0.71–2.16)	0.445
Small artery disease	2.01 (1.00–4.02)	0.049
Others	0.95 (0.51–1.75)	0.858
Positive urine proteins	1.40 (0.90–2.17)	0.140
Fibrinogen per 300 mg/dl		0.044
0–300 mg/dL	Reference	
300–600 mg/dL	1.62 (1.04–2.53)	0.034
> 600 mg/dL	2.60 (1.02–6.51)	0.046

END early neurological deterioration, *NIHSS* National Institutes of Health Stroke Scale, *TOAST* trial of Org 10,172 in acute stroke treatment
[a] Age, sex, initial NIHSS and TOAST were adjusted

scores were included, and the large patient numbers included may supplement such limitations. We hope to address these issues in later prospective studies.

Conclusion

In conclusion, hyperfibrinogenemia at admission in patients with acute ischemic stroke and DM is independently associated with END. This finding suggests that an elevated fibrinogen level is a marker of a prothrombotic or antiplatelet-resistant condition related to DM that could affect the patient's prognosis. On the other hand, these results also reveal a category of patients wherein fibrin-depleting therapy could be significantly more effective.

Abbreviations

CAD: Coronary arterial disease; CRP: C-reactive protein; DM: Diabetes mellitus; END: Early neurological deterioration; ESR: Erythrocyte sedimentation rate; FDP: Fibrin degradation products; HbA1c: Glycated hemoglobin; NIHSS: National Institute of Health Stroke Scale; TOAST: Trial of Org 10,172 in acute stroke treatment

Acknowledgements

None.

Funding

This work was supported by Basic Science Research Program through the National Research Foundation of Korea funded by the Ministry of Education (NRF-2014R1A1A1008249, J.S.L.). The funding body had no role in the design of the study, collection, analysis, and interpretation of the data, and in writing of the manuscript.

Authors' contributions

SJL contributed to analysis and interpretation of data, preparation and review of the manuscript. JMH contributed to patient data acquisition and review of the manuscript. SEL contributed to patient data acquisition of the manuscript. DRK contributed to statistical analysis of the data. BO contributed to analysis and interpretation of data and review of the manuscript. AMD contributed to analysis and interpretation of data and review of the manuscript. JSL contributed to analysis and interpretation of data, preparation and review of the manuscript. All the authors have read and approved the final version of the manuscript.

Competing interests

The authors declare that they have no competing interests.

Author details

[1]Department of Neurology, Ajou University School of Medicine, Ajou University Medical Center, San 5, Woncheon-dong, Yeongtong-gu, Suwon, Kyungki-do 443-721, South Korea. [2]Center of Biomedical Data Science/ Institute of Genomic Cohort, Yonsei University Wonju College of Medicine, Wonju, South Korea. [3]Department of Neurology, Medical University of South Carolina, Charleston, SC, USA. [4]Calgary Stroke Program, Departments of Clinical Neurosciences and Radiology, Hotchkiss Brain Institute, University of Calgary, Calgary, AB, Canada.

References

1. Davalos A, Toni D, Iweins F, Lesaffre E, Bastianello S, Castillo J. Neurological deterioration in acute ischemic stroke: potential predictors and associated factors in the European cooperative acute stroke study (ECASS) I. Stroke. 1999;30(12):2631–6.
2. Kim BJ, Park J-M, Kang K, Lee SJ, Ko Y, Kim JG, Cha J-K, Kim D-H, Nah H-W, Han M-K, et al. Case Characteristics, Hyperacute Treatment, and Outcome Information from the Clinical Research Center for Stroke-Fifth Division Registry in South Korea. J Stroke. 2015;17(1):38–53.
3. Kamalesh M, Shen J, Eckert GJ. Long term postischemic stroke mortality in diabetes: a veteran cohort analysis. Stroke. 2008;39(10):2727–31.
4. Megherbi SE, Milan C, Minier D, Couvreur G, Osseby GV, Tilling K, Di Carlo A, Inzitari D, Wolfe CD, Moreau T, et al. Association between diabetes and stroke subtype on survival and functional outcome 3 months after stroke: data from the European BIOMED Stroke Project. Stroke. 2003;34(3):688–94.
5. Lee S-J, Hong JM, Lee M, Huh K, Choi JW, Lee JS. Cerebral Arterial Calcification Is an Imaging Prognostic Marker for Revascularization Treatment of Acute Middle Cerebral Arterial Occlusion. J Stroke. 2015;17(1): 67–75.
6. Barber M, Wright F, Stott DJ, Langhorne P. Predictors of early neurological deterioration after ischaemic stroke: a case-control study. Gerontology. 2004; 50(2):102–9.
7. Weimar C, Mieck T, Buchthal J, Ehrenfeld CE, Schmid E, Diener HC. Neurologic worsening during the acute phase of ischemic stroke. Arch Neurol. 2005;62(3):393–7.
8. Els T, Klisch J, Orszagh M, Hetzel A, Schulte-Monting J, Schumacher M, Lucking CH. Hyperglycemia in patients with focal cerebral ischemia after intravenous thrombolysis: influence on clinical outcome and infarct size. Cerebrovasc Dis. 2002;13(2):89–94.
9. Lansberg MG, Albers GW, Wijman CA. Symptomatic intracerebral hemorrhage following thrombolytic therapy for acute ischemic stroke: a review of the risk factors. Cerebrovasc Dis. 2007;24(1):1–10.
10. Demchuk AM, Morgenstern LB, Krieger DW, Linda Chi T, Hu W, Wein TH, Hardy RJ, Grotta JC, Buchan AM. Serum glucose level and diabetes predict tissue plasminogen activator-related intracerebral hemorrhage in acute ischemic stroke. Stroke. 1999;30(1):34–9.
11. Berger L, Hakim AM. The association of hyperglycemia with cerebral edema in stroke. Stroke. 1986;17(5):865–71.
12. Candelise L, Landi G, Orazio EN, Boccardi E. Prognostic significance of hyperglycemia in acute stroke. Arch Neurol. 1985;42(7):661–3.
13. Meigs JB, Mittleman MA, Nathan DM, Tofler GH, Singer DE, Murphy-Sheehy PM, Lipinska I, D'Agostino RB, Wilson PW. Hyperinsulinemia, hyperglycemia,

and impaired hemostasis: the Framingham Offspring Study. JAMA. 2000; 283(2):221–8.
14. Dunn EJ, Ariens RA. Fibrinogen and fibrin clot structure in diabetes. Herz. 2004;29(5):470–9.
15. Koenig W. Fibrin(ogen) in cardiovascular disease: an update. Thromb Haemost. 2003;89(4):601–9.
16. Ernst E. Fibrinogen as a cardiovascular risk factor–interrelationship with infections and inflammation. Eur Heart J. 1993;14 Suppl K:82–7.
17. Wu S, Shi Y, Wang C, Jia Q, Zhang N, Zhao X, Liu G, Wang Y, Liu L, Wang Y, et al. Glycated hemoglobin independently predicts stroke recurrence within one year after acute first-ever non-cardioembolic strokes onset in A Chinese cohort study. PLoS One. 2013;8(11):e80690.
18. Kanamaru T, Suda S, Muraga K, Okubo S, Watanabe Y, Tsuruoka S, Kimura K. Albuminuria predicts early neurological deterioration in patients with acute ischemic stroke. J Neurol Sci. 2017;372:417–20.
19. Herrick S, Blanc-Brude O, Gray A, Laurent G. Fibrinogen. Int J Biochem Cell Biol. 1999;31(7):741–6.
20. Forsyth CB, Solovjov DA, Ugarova TP, Plow EF. Integrin alpha(M)beta(2)-mediated cell migration to fibrinogen and its recognition peptides. J Exp Med. 2001;193(10):1123–33.
21. Tousoulis D, Papageorgiou N, Androulakis E, Briasoulis A, Antoniades C, Stefanadis C. Fibrinogen and cardiovascular disease: genetics and biomarkers. Blood Rev. 2011;25(6):239–45.
22. Schneider DJ, Taatjes DJ, Howard DB, Sobel BE. Increased reactivity of platelets induced by fibrinogen independent of its binding to the IIb-IIIa surface glycoprotein: a potential contributor to cardiovascular risk. J Am Coll Cardiol. 1999;33(1):261–6.
23. Hammer MR, John PN, Flynn MD, Bellingham AJ, Leslie RD. Glycated fibrinogen: a new index of short-term diabetic control. Ann Clin Biochem. 1989;26(Pt 1):58–62.
24. Brownlee M, Vlassara H, Cerami A. Nonenzymatic glycosylation reduces the susceptibility of fibrin to degradation by plasmin. Diabetes. 1983;32(7):680–4.
25. Bobbink IW, Tekelenburg WL, Sixma JJ, de Boer HC, Banga JD, de Groot PG. Glycated proteins modulate tissue-plasminogen activator-catalyzed plasminogen activation. Biochem Biophys Res Commun. 1997;240(3):595–601.
26. Lutjens A, Jonkhoff-Slok TW, Sandkuijl C, vd Veen EA, vd Meer J. Polymerisation and crosslinking of fibrin monomers in diabetes mellitus. Diabetologia. 1988; 31(11):825–30.
27. Grant PJ. Diabetes mellitus as a prothrombotic condition. J Intern Med. 2007;262(2):157–72.
28. Lee AJ, Lowe GD, Woodward M, Tunstall-Pedoe H. Fibrinogen in relation to personal history of prevalent hypertension, diabetes, stroke, intermittent claudication, coronary heart disease, and family history: the Scottish Heart Health Study. Br Heart J. 1993;69(4):338–42.
29. Qizilbash N, Jones L, Warlow C, Mann J. Fibrinogen and lipid concentrations as risk factors for transient ischaemic attacks and minor ischaemic strokes. BMJ. 1991;303(6803):605–9.
30. Wilhelmsen L, Svardsudd K, Korsan-Bengtsen K, Larsson B, Welin L, Tibblin G. Fibrinogen as a risk factor for stroke and myocardial infarction. N Engl J Med. 1984;311(8):501–5.
31. Danesh J, Lewington S, Thompson SG, Lowe GD, Collins R, Kostis JB, Wilson AC, Folsom AR, Wu K, Benderly M, et al. Plasma fibrinogen level and the risk of major cardiovascular diseases and nonvascular mortality: an individual participant meta-analysis. JAMA. 2005;294(14):1799–809.
32. Kofoed SC, Wittrup HH, Sillesen H, Nordestgaard BG. Fibrinogen predicts ischaemic stroke and advanced atherosclerosis but not echolucent, rupture-prone carotid plaques: the Copenhagen City Heart Study. Eur Heart J. 2003; 24(6):567–76.
33. del Zoppo GJ, Levy DE, Wasiewski WW, Pancioli AM, Demchuk AM, Trammel J, Demaerschalk BM, Kaste M, Albers GW, Ringelstein EB. Hyperfibrinogenemia and functional outcome from acute ischemic stroke. Stroke. 2009;40(5):1687–91.
34. Ogawa H, Nakayama M, Morimoto T, Uemura S, Kanauchi M, Doi N, Jinnouchi H, Sugiyama S, Saito Y, Japanese Primary Prevention of Atherosclerosis With Aspirin for Diabetes Trial I. Low-dose aspirin for primary prevention of atherosclerotic events in patients with type 2 diabetes: a randomized controlled trial. JAMA. 2008;300(18):2134–41.
35. Belch J, MacCuish A, Campbell I, Cobbe S, Taylor R, Prescott R, Lee R, Bancroft J, MacEwan S, Shepherd J, et al. The prevention of progression of arterial disease and diabetes (POPADAD) trial: factorial randomised placebo controlled trial of aspirin and antioxidants in patients with diabetes and asymptomatic peripheral arterial disease. BMJ. 2008;337:a1840.
36. Hall HM, Banerjee S, McGuire DK. Variability of clopidogrel response in patients with type 2 diabetes mellitus. Diab Vasc Dis Res. 2011;8(4):245–53.
37. Paul R, Banerjee AK, Guha S, Chaudhuri U, Ghosh S, Mondal J, Bandyopadhyay R. Study of platelet aggregation in acute coronary syndrome with special reference to metabolic syndrome. Int J Appl Basic Med Res. 2013;3(2):117–21.
38. Hao Z, Liu M, Counsell C, Wardlaw JM, Lin S, Zhao X. Fibrinogen depleting agents for acute ischaemic stroke. Cochrane Database Syst Rev. 2012;3: CD000091.
39. Aono Y, Ohkubo T, Kikuya M, Hara A, Kondo T, Obara T, Metoki H, Inoue R, Asayama K, Shintani Y, et al. Plasma fibrinogen, ambulatory blood pressure, and silent cerebrovascular lesions: the Ohasama study. Arterioscler Thromb Vasc Biol. 2007;27(4):963–8.
40. Neumann-Haefelin T, Hoelig S, Berkefeld J, Fiehler J, Gass A, Humpich M, Kastrup A, Kucinski T, Lecei O, Liebeskind DS, et al. Leukoaraiosis is a risk factor for symptomatic intracerebral hemorrhage after thrombolysis for acute stroke. Stroke. 2006;37(10):2463–6.

7

Prognostic models for complete recovery in ischemic stroke

Nampet Jampathong, Malinee Laopaiboon*, Siwanon Rattanakanokchai and Porjai Pattanittum

Abstract

Background: Prognostic models have been increasingly developed to predict complete recovery in ischemic stroke. However, questions arise about the performance characteristics of these models. The aim of this study was to systematically review and synthesize performance of existing prognostic models for complete recovery in ischemic stroke.

Methods: We searched journal publications indexed in PUBMED, SCOPUS, CENTRAL, ISI Web of Science and OVID MEDLINE from inception until 4 December, 2017, for studies designed to develop and/or validate prognostic models for predicting complete recovery in ischemic stroke patients. Two reviewers independently examined titles and abstracts, and assessed whether each study met the pre-defined inclusion criteria and also independently extracted information about model development and performance. We evaluated validation of the models by medians of the area under the receiver operating characteristic curve (AUC) or c-statistic and calibration performance. We used a random-effects meta-analysis to pool AUC values.

Results: We included 10 studies with 23 models developed from elderly patients with a moderately severe ischemic stroke, mainly in three high income countries. Sample sizes for each study ranged from 75 to 4441. Logistic regression was the only analytical strategy used to develop the models. The number of various predictors varied from one to 11. Internal validation was performed in 12 models with a median AUC of 0.80 (95% CI 0.73 to 0.84). One model reported good calibration. Nine models reported external validation with a median AUC of 0.80 (95% CI 0.76 to 0.82). Four models showed good discrimination and calibration on external validation. The pooled AUC of the two validation models of the same developed model was 0.78 (95% CI 0.71 to 0.85).

Conclusions: The performance of the 23 models found in the systematic review varied from fair to good in terms of internal and external validation. Further models should be developed with internal and external validation in low and middle income countries.

Keywords: Stroke, Cerebral ischemia, Prognosis, Ischemic stroke, Prognostic model, Systematic review

Background

Globally, stroke is the second leading cause of death following ischemic heart disease and the third leading cause of disability [1, 2]. In 2013, 6.5 million deaths from stroke (51% died from ischemic stroke), 113 million disability-adjusted life years were lost because of stroke (58% due to ischemic stroke) and 10.3 million of people with new strokes (67% were ischemic stroke) [1]. In 2015, prevalence of stroke was 42.4 million people, which included ischemic stroke for 24.9 million. There were 6.3 million stroke deaths worldwide, and 3.0 million individuals died of ischemic stroke [2].

Minimizing the time to treatment for stroke is the important key to improving chances of an excellent outcome (time lost is brain lost) [3]. It is also important to be able to predict the outcomes of diseases or treatments. Most physicians use their own clinical experience in predicting their patients' outcomes for making decisions in patient care management. The accuracy of these informal predictions is unclear. Care management might

* Correspondence: malinee@kku.ac.th; laopaiboonmalinee@yahoo.co.uk
Department of Epidemiology and Biostatistics, Faculty of Public Health, Khon Kaen University, 123 Mittraphap Road, Nai-Muang, Muang District, Khon Kaen 40002, Thailand

be improved if the physicians combined their clinical forecasts with the formal predictions provided by statistical models. This may be more accurate than relying simply on clinical experience. Prognostic models are statistical tools to assist physicians in making decisions which may affect their patients' outcomes [4].

Accurate prognostic models of the functional outcome of a complete recovery in patients after ischemic stroke could be beneficial to neurological care practices for a number of reasons. Firstly, the information of developed prognostic model could be used to select appropriate treatments and action plans in individual patient management, including patient counseling. Secondly, they could be used to improve rehabilitation and discharge planning. Lastly, in light of a weakening economy, prognostic models could be used to make the best clinical choices for patients with regard to specific clinical scenarios which may reduce health care costs [5].

To date, several studies have developed prognostic models to predict functional outcomes after ischemic stroke, and each model has different strengths and weaknesses. Since models do not always work well in practice, it is recommended that, before a prognostic model is used in clinical practice, the performance of the model should be properly evaluated. This process is known as model validation and involves an assessment of calibration (the agreement between the observed and predicted outcomes) and discrimination (the model's ability to discriminate between those patients who are likely or unlikely to experience a particular prognostic event). A poor calibration usually reflects over-fitting of the model in the development sample. At least the models should be determined the internal validity (for example, using 'bootstrap sampling') to assess validity for the setting where the development data originated from. Another aspect is the external validity (using patient data not used for the development model) to assess generalizability [6, 7].

There may be danger in moving too quickly to use these models without appropriate validation and understanding of their limitations. The purpose of this study was to systematically review and synthesize performance of existing prognostic models which have been used to predict the probability of complete recovery in ischemic stroke and to investigate their quality.

Methods

Selection criteria

We included studies predicting the outcome of complete recovery after ischemic stroke and in which complete recovery was assessed by scores on at least one of the following instruments: the Barthel Index (BI) ≥ 95/100 or 19/20, the Glasgow Outcome Scale (GOS) score = 1, the Oxford Handicap Scale (OHS) score ≤ 2, and the Modified Rankin Scale (mRS) score ≤ 1. A further criterion was that the studies reported model performance by the use of the concordance statistic, area under the receiver operating characteristic curve (AUC) or calibration performance. There were no restrictions on timing of the outcome evaluation, age of the patients, or type/severity of ischemic stroke.

Search strategy

We searched PUBMED, SCOPUS, CENTRAL, ISI Web of Science and OVID MEDLINE for prognostic models published from inception until 4 December, 2017, using the search terms listed in the Additional file 1 without restrictions on publication language. We also reviewed the reference lists of relevant studies.

Study selection and data extraction

Study titles and abstracts were independently screened and selected by two reviewers (NJ and SR) using the specified criteria. If a decision could not be made based on the abstracts, we then considered their full texts. Disagreement was resolved through discussion with a third reviewer (ML). We extracted the performance measures (concordance statistics, AUCs and performance calibrations) of both types of prediction model: development models and validation models. We also extracted study characteristics: author(s), publication year, setting, study design, definition of outcome, number of subjects, number of outcome events, age, ischemic stroke severity and duration of follow-up.

Quality assessment

We assessed the study quality based on an adaptation of the tool developed by D'Amico et al. [8]. We showed how each study performed according to each of various major methodological requirements for prognosis research studies. The assessment items were as follows:

- Did the prognostic study use a cohort design?
- Were the predictors clearly defined and details provided of how they were measured?
- Were the missing data handled appropriately with statistical imputation?
- Was some form of stepwise analysis used for selecting predictors in a multivariable analysis?
- Was the sample size adequate as defined by an events-per-variable ratio of 10 or more?
- Was the final model validated on the patients who were used to generate the model (internal validation)?
- Was the final model validated on the patients who were not used to generate the model (external validation)?

Statistical analysis

We qualitatively synthesized model performances because each separate model had a different combination of predictor variables. We used frequencies and medians with 95% confidence intervals to describe the model performance which included its calibration (how closely predicted values agree with the observed values) and discrimination (the model's ability to discriminate between patients developing and not developing an outcome event, e.g., complete recovery cases and non-complete recovery cases among ischemic patients). The assessment of calibration was performed using either the Hosmer-Lemshow chi-square test or a calibration curve. The assessment of discrimination was conducted using either the AUC or the concordance statistic (C-statistic) along with a 95% CI. The discrimination of each model was evaluated in accordance with the suggestions by Hosmer and Lemeshow: excellent (AUC $\geq$ 0.90), good (AUC $\geq$ 0.80 and $<$ 0.90), fair (AUC $\geq$ 0.70 and $<$ 0.80), and poor (AUC $<$ 0.70). Calibration was judged as good when a calibration curve closely resembled the line representing perfect calibration (the pre-specified acceptable absolute mean error for the calibration curve was $<$ 0.4) or when the Hosmer-Lemshow chi-square test was non-significant [9, 10]. We estimated the 95% CIs for AUCs using Hanley's method for a study which presented only AUCs. The estimation required three quantities: total sample size, number of events and an AUC [11]. If two or more models assessed discrimination performance in terms of validation, we performed a random-effects inverse-variance meta-analysis using Stata version 10.1 [12].

Results

A total of 896 articles were found by searching the electronic databases, and 10 studies were eligible [13–22]. Seven studies were development studies; while three were validation studies (see Fig. 1). Twenty three different models were identified.

Patient characteristics of included models

All included models were developed from elderly patients in high income countries: five studies from the United States of America [13–16, 22], three from Germany [17–19] and one from the Netherlands [21]. One study [20] did not report study setting but used data from the Virtual International Stroke Trials

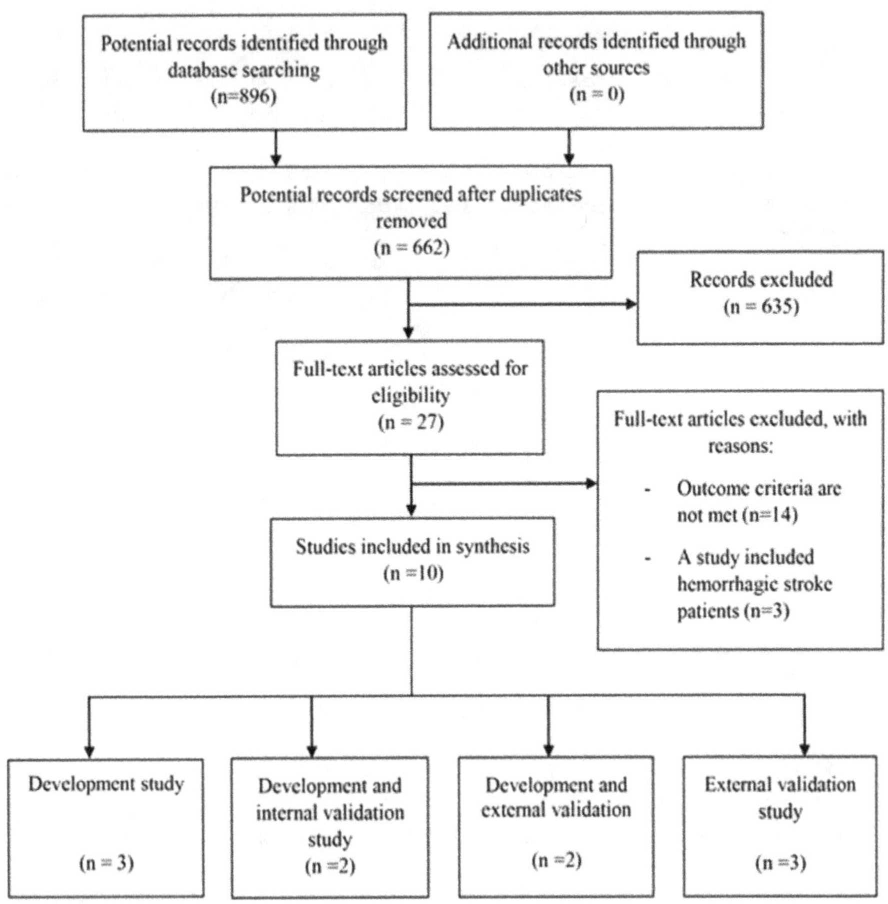

Fig. 1 Study flow diagram

Archive (VISTA) which included patients from many different countries.

Twenty models were developed from patients with a moderately severe ischemic stroke based on the NIHSS score [23], but for three models ischemic stroke severity was not reported. The sample sizes from which the models were developed ranged from 75 to 4441, the complete recovery cases ranged from 33 to 1970 and were measured at around 90 days after ischemic stroke diagnosed in six studies [13–16, 20, 22], at 100 days in three studies [17–19], and at 365 days in one study [21]. Table 1 presents the characteristics of the models.

Table 1 Characteristics of prognostic models

First author (year)	Setting	Study period	Study design	Model No.	Type of model	Definition of outcome	Participants				No. of complete recovery	Events per variable	Duration of follow-up
							n	Age	Male	NIHSS score			
Johnston (2000)	America	May 1993 - Dec 1994	Cohort	1	Internal	BI ≥ 95	222	68.7[b]	–	10 (5, 15)[a]	125	125	90 days
				2								21	
				3								18	
				4		GOS = 1	222	68.7[b]	–	10 (5, 15)[a]	108	108	
				5								18	
				6								16	
Johnston (2003)	America	–	Cohort	3	External	BI ≥ 95	199	67 (59,74)[a]	59%	15(10, 20)[a]	78	12	90 days
				6		GOS = 1					62	9	
Johnston (2002)	America	May 1993 - Dec 1994	Cohort	7	Internal	BI ≥ 95	206	69 (12)[b]	–	10 (5, 16)[a]	92	92	90 days
				8								92	
				9								46	
				10		GOS = 1	206	69 (12)[b]	–	10 (5, 16)[a]	99	99	
				11								99	
				12								50	
Johnston (2007)	America	–	Cohort	13	Development	BI ≥ 95	382	69 (58, 77)[a]	53.9%	14 (10, 18)[a]	123	25	90 days
		May 2000 & Aug 2005			External		266	70 (58, 78)[a]	53.0%	5 (3, 10)[a]	167	34	
		–		14	Development		382	69 (58, 77)[a]	53.9%	14 (10, 18)[a]	123	16	
		May 2000 & Aug 2005			External		266	70 (58, 78)[a]	53.0%	5 (3, 10)[a]	167	21	
		–		15	Development	mRS ≤ 1	382	69 (58, 77)[a]	53.9%	14 (10, 18)[a]	75	15	
		May 2000 & Aug 2005			External		266	70 (58, 78)[a]	53.0%	5 (3, 10)[a]	148	30	
		–		16	Development		382	69(58, 77)[a]	53.9%	14 (10, 18)[a]	75	10	
		May 2000 & Aug 2005		16	External	mRS ≤ 1	266	70 (58, 78)[a]	53.0%	5 (3, 10)[a]	148	19	90 days
Weimar (2002)	Germany	1998 - 1999	Cohort	17	Development	BI ≥ 95	1743	68.1 (12.7)[b]	59.2%	6.9 (6.2)[b]	1021	102	100 days
German Stroke Study Collaboration (2004)	Germany	Feb 2001 - Mar 2002	Cohort		External	BI ≥ 95	1470	67.9 (12.4)[b]	57.3%	6.4 (6.0)[b]	831	76	100 days
Weimar (2004)	Germany	–	Cohort	18	Development	BI ≥ 95	1079	67.0 (12.3)[b]	60.5%	–	644	322	100 days
		Feb 2001 - Mar 2002	Cohort		External	BI ≥ 95	1307	68.2 (12.5)[b]	56.5%	7.6 (6.9)[b]	722	361	100 days
Konig (2008)	–	–	Cohort		External	BI ≥ 95	4441	68.8 (12.3)[b]	55.8%	13.4 (6.5)[b]	1970	985	90 days
Schiemanck (2006)	Netherland	1999 - 2001	Cohort	19	Development	BI ≥ 19	75	63 (15)[b]	47%	11 (6)[b]	33	17	365 days
				20								7	
Patti (2016)	America	2013 - 2014	Cohort	21	Development	mRS ≤ 1	414	70 (50, 69)[a]	50%	5 (2, 13)[a]	230	77	90 days
				22			204	–	–	–	–	–	
				23			210	–	–	–	–	–	

[a]Median (25th–75th percentile); [b] Mean (SD); – indicates not stated

Model predictors

A total of 24 different variables were included in the 23 models. The number of variables included in each model ranged from 1 to 11. The National Institutes of Health Stroke Scale (NIHSS) was the most common predictor (70.8%) followed by age (62.5%) and infarct volume (50.0%). Table 2 presents details of predictor variables.

Quality of prognostic models

All 10 studies used a cohort design. Details about the measurement of predictors were presented for 13 of the 23 models (56.5%). All of the 10 studies handled missing data by excluding subjects from the analyses. The full model approach (all the candidate predictors included in the multivariable analysis) was the most common method used (69.6%) for selection of predictors by multivariable modeling [13, 14, 16]. Two studies [13, 14] reported 12 development models (model No.1-12) but provided no information on their discrimination performances. However, they did report their discrimination performances on internal validation, but for only one model (model No. 9) was calibration performance reported in the internal validation. Five studies [15, 16, 18–20] reported external validation in nine models (model No.3, 6 and 13-18). Calibration performances were reported for six of these nine models, and four of them (model No. 3, 6, 13 and 15) showed good calibration. There was only one study which provided a 95% confidence interval for the AUC [21]; those of the other nine studies [13–20, 22] were estimated using Hanley's method (see Table 4). There were only two models (model No.3 and No.6) which were validated both internally and externally. Table 3 presents details of quality of prognostic models.

Table 2 Predictors included in final model

No. of model	1	2	3	4	5	6	7	8	9	10	11	12	13	14	15	16	17	18	19	20	21	22	23	Total (%)
Predictors included																								
NIHSS score		*	*		*	*	*		*	*		*	*	*	*	*	*	*			*	*	*	17 (70.8)
Age		*	*		*	*							*	*	*	*	*	*	*	*	*	*	*	15 (62.5)
Infarct volume	*		*	*		*		*	*		*	*								*				12 (50.0)
Infarct volume < 29.5 mL																					*			
Infarct volume < 31.2 mL																						*		
Infarct volume < 25.5 mL																							*	
History of diabetes mellitus		*	*		*	*							*	*	*	*	*							9 (37.5)
History of stroke		*	*		*	*											*				*	*	*	8 (33.3)
Prestroke disability		*	*		*	*							*	*	*	*								8 (33.3)
Small-vessel stroke		*	*		*	*																		4 (16.7)
Tissue-type plasminogen activator (t-PA use)													*	*	*	*								4 (16.7)
Preadmission modified Rankin scale																	*				*	*	*	4 (16.7)
Sex																	*				*	*	*	4 (16.7)
Atrial fibrillation																					*	*	*	3 (12.5)
Congestive heart failure																					*	*	*	3 (12.5)
Antiplatelet use																					*	*	*	3 (12.5)
Diffusion-weighted imaging lesion volume (DWI)														*		*								2 (8.3)
Time to DWI scan														*		*								2 (8.3)
Time by DWI interaction														*		*								2 (8.3)
Barthel index																			*	*				2 (8.3)
Neurological complications																	*							1 (4.2)
Fever > 38 °C																	*							1 (4.2)
Lenticulostriate arteries infarction																	*							1 (4.2)
Right arm weakness																	*							1 (4.2)
Left arm weakness																	*							1 (4.2)
Days to poststroke MRI scan																				*				1 (4.2)
Hemisphere (left/right)																				*				1 (4.2)
Total	1	6	7	1	6	7	1	1	2	1	1	2	5	8	5	8	11	2	2	5	9	9	9	

*indicates the predictor included in the final model

Table 3 Quality assessment of prognostic models

Assessment items	All models ($n = 23$)
Study design	
Cohort study	23 (100%)
Variables	
Description of measurement of predictors	
Yes	13 (56.5%)
No	10 (43.5%)
Loss to follow-up	
< 10%	10 (43.5%)
≥ 10%	13 (56.5%)
Analysis	
More than 10 events per variable	
Yes	22 (95.7%)
No	1 (4.3%)
Method for selection of predictors during multivariable modeling	
Forward Selection	2 (8.7%)
Backward Elimination	3 (13.0%)
Stepwise selection	0
Full model approach	16 (69.6%)
Unknown	2 (8.7%)
Handling of missing data	
Estimated statistically	0
Excluded	23 (100%)
Model performance	
Internal validity	
Performance reported AUC (Discrimination)	
Yes	12 (52.2%)
95% CI presented	0
No	11 (47.8%)
Calibration	
Yes	1 (4.3)
No	22 (95.7%)
External validity	
Performance reported AUC (Discrimination)	
Yes	8 (34.9%)
95% CI presented	2 out of 8 (25.0%)
No	15 (65.1%)
Calibration	
Yes	6 (26.1%)
No	17 (73.9%)

Model performances

There were 11 development models which reported AUC values. The median AUC was 0.80 (95% CI 0.77 to 0.85) (see Table 4 and Fig. 2).

Internal validation

Model performance was evaluated using internal validation by bootstrapping methods in 12 models (model No.1-12). The models were validated in samples of 222 [13] and 206 [14] elderly patients with a moderately severe ischemic stroke. The number of events ranged from 92 to 125 (see Table 1). The median AUC for discrimination performance on internal validation was 0.82 (95% CI 0.73 to 0.87); there was only model No. 9 which was reported to have good calibration (see Table 4 and Fig. 3).

External validation

Two studies [16, 19] reported external validation in their five developed models (model No.13-16 and 18). Model No.18 was validated in two different samples in two studies [19, 20]; one study included patients from Germany [19] and another study included patients from many countries [20]. Three other studies [15, 18, 20] reported external validation of four pre-existing models (model No 3, 6, 17 and 18).

On external validation discrimination and calibration performance were reported in six models (model No. 3, 6 and 13-16). Four of the six models had good discrimination with a median AUC of 0.81 (95% CI 0.80 to 0.83), and good calibration (model No. 3, 6, 13 and 15). Three other models (model No.17, model No.18 reported in two external populations) reported only discrimination performance. The pooled AUC value for model No. 18 was 0.78 (95% CI 0.71 to 0.85; two studies) (see Fig. 4). The median AUC of these nine validation models was 0.80 (95% CI 0.76 to 0.82) (see Table 4 and Fig. 5).

Discussion

This systematic review identified 23 prognostic models from ten studies for complete recovery in ischemic stroke. None of these models provided complete information about the model performance which included both internal and external validation. While most prognostic models (18/23) were validated and half of the models (12/23) reported fair to good discrimination on internal validation, only one model showed good calibration. Nearly one third of the models (9/23) were externally validated, and reported fair to good discrimination performance, but only a quarter of the models (6/23) reported nearly perfect calibration. Only two models were validated both internally and externally but not in complete process of the model performance. There was only one model in which a meta-analysis could be performed, and the pooled AUC was fair.

The models were developed and validated in elderly patients mainly with a moderately severe stroke and mainly from high income countries. In addition, most of the developed models were not externally validated. These factors are likely to limit the application of the models to other populations and settings.

Table 4 Model performances

No. of model	Calibration		Discrimination; AUC (95%CI)		
	Internal validation	External validation	Development model	Internal validation	External validation
1	–	–	–	0.73 (0.66 to 0.80)	–
2	–	–	–	0.80 (0.74 to 0.86)	–
3	–	closely resembling perfect calibration	–	0.84 (0.79 to 0.89)	0.83 (0.77 to 0.89)
4	–	–	–	0.74 (0.67 to 0.81)	–
5	–	–	–	0.79 (0.73 to 0.85)	–
6	–	closely resembling perfect calibration	–	0.84 (0.79 to 0.89)	0.81 (0.75 to 0.87)
7	–	–	–	0.87 (0.82 to 0.92)	–
8	–	–	–	0.70 (0.63 to 0.77)	–
9	closely resembling perfect calibration, mean absolute error = 0.01	–	–	0.87 (0.82 to 0.92)	–
10	–	–	–	0.89 (0.84 to 0.94)	–
11	–	–	–	0.72 (0.65 to 0.79)	–
12	–	–	–	0.89 (0.84 to 0.94)	–
13	–	closely resembling perfect calibration, mean absolute error = 0.33	0.80 (0.75 to 0.85)	–	0.82 (0.76 to 0.88)
14	–	mean absolute errors = 0.4, less well calibrated	0.79 (0.74 to 0.84)	–	0.80 (0.73 to 0.87)
15	–	closely resembling perfect calibration, mean absolute error = 0.37	0.79 (0.73 to 0.85)	–	0.80 (0.74 to 0.86)
16	–	mean absolute errors = 0.4, less well calibrated	0.78 (0.71 to 0.85)	–	0.76 (0.69 to 0.83)
17	–	–	0.80 (0.78 to 0.82)	–	0.78 (0.75 to 0.81)
18	–	–	0.86 (0.84 to 0.88)	–	0.74 (0.71 to 0.77) 0.81 (0.80 to 0.82)
19	–	–	0.84 (0.75 to 0.94)	–	–
20	–	–	0.87 (0.79 to 0.95)	–	–
21	–	–	0.74 (0.69 to 0.79)	–	–
22	–	–	0.82	–	–
23	–	–	0.70	–	–
Median AUC (95% CI)			0.80 (0.77 to 0.85)	0.82 (0.73 to 0.87)	0.80 (0.76 to 0.82)

In our review, we conducted a systematic search of several electronic databases. All of the included studies used a cohort design. For half of all the identified models more than 10% of their subjects' data was missing. The model performance analyses were handled by excluding the subjects with missing data. This strategy could lead to biased conclusions if the reasons for missing data were related to the important prognostic indicators or outcomes.

There are some issues related to the assessed quality of the prognostic models. Firstly, our search was performed up to 4 December, 2017. No attempt was made to search unpublished studies. Studies were selected and extracted independently by two reviewers. We did not assess publication bias by any statistical tests or funnel plot asymmetry due to insufficient data. However, we assessed and presented the quality of all the 10 selected studies for each important quality features listed in our methods section.

No. of Model	Discriminant ability	AUC (95% CI)
1		-
2		-
3		-
4		-
5		-
6		-
7		-
8		-
9		-
10		-
11		-
12		-
13	Good	0.80 (0.75 to 0.85)
14	Fair	0.79 (0.74 to 0.84)
15	Fair	0.79 (0.73 to 0.85)
16	Fair	0.78 (0.71 to 0.85)
17	Good	0.80 (0.78 to 0.82)
18	Good	0.86 (0.84 to 0.88)
19	Good	0.84 (0.75 to 0.94)
20	Good	0.87 (0.79 to 0.95)
21	Fair	0.74 (0.69 to 0.79)
22	Good	0.82
23	Fair	0.70

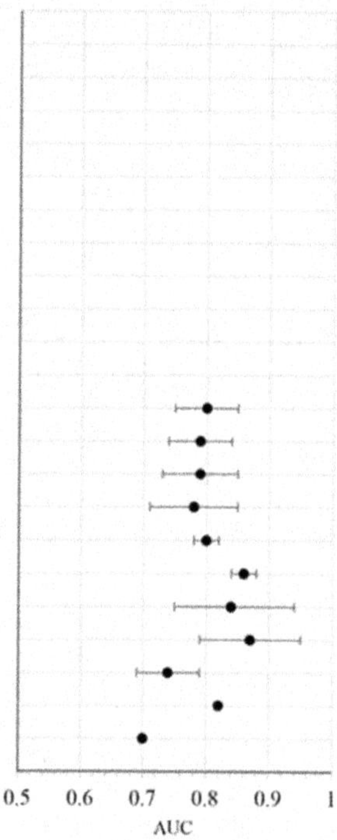

Fig. 2 Discrimination performance in development models

No. of Model	Discriminant ability	AUC (95% CI)
1	Fair	0.73 (0.66 to 0.80)
2	Good	0.80 (0.74 to 0.86)
3	Good	0.84 (0.79 to 0.89)
4	Fair	0.74 (0.67 to 0.81)
5	Fair	0.79 (0.73 to 0.85)
6	Good	0.84 (0.79 to 0.89)
7	Good	0.87 (0.82 to 0.92)
8	Fair	0.70 (0.63 to 0.77)
9	Good	0.87 (0.82 to 0.92)
10	Good	0.89 (0.84 to 0.94)
11	Fair	0.72 (0.65 to 0.79)
12	Good	0.89 (0.84 to 0.94)

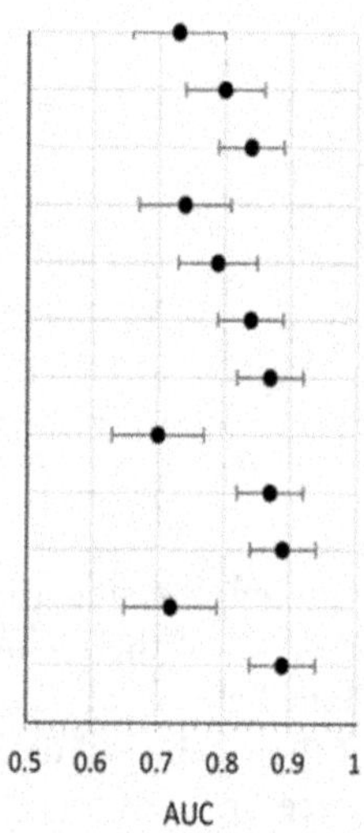

Fig. 3 Discrimination performance in internal validation models

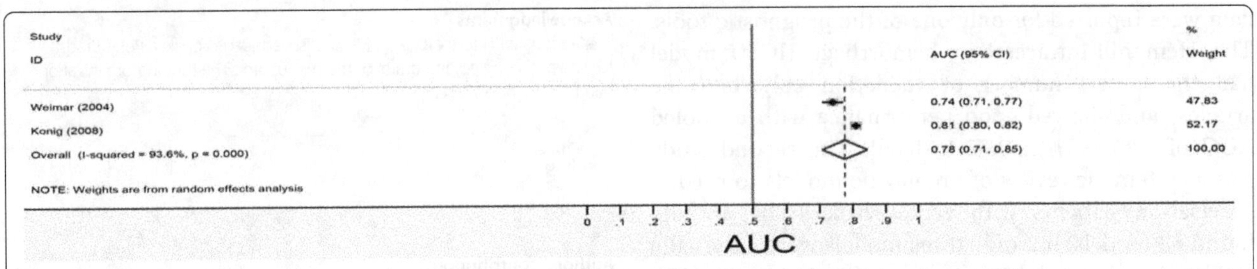

Fig. 4 Meta-analysis of the areas under the receiver operating characteristic curve (AUC) for previous prognostic models

Secondly, about 70% (16/23) of the models used the full model approach in predictor selection (all the candidate predictors included in the multivariable analysis) [13, 14, 16]. This approach could reduce the risk of predictor selection bias and over-fitting. However, this technique is difficult to apply if the number of events is limited [6]. In our review, all of the models with the full model approach to predictor selection had fulfilled the requirement of more than 10 patients with complete recovery per predictor. Finally, incomplete measures of the prognostic model performances were reported in all included models. The 95% confidence intervals of the estimated performance indices were rarely reported. The 95% confidence intervals for AUCs which we estimated using Hanley's method may be slightly inaccurate, but this approach has been accepted in estimating the precision of AUCs when their standard errors are not reported. In addition, calibration performance was often ignored. Calibration is the important performance measure for application of the model in practice. A poor calibration reflects over-fitting of a model and can also be interpreted as reflecting a need for shrinkage of regression coefficients in a prognostic model [10].

To our knowledge, there are three previous systematic reviews of prognostic models in stroke, but their outcomes of interest were different from ours: for example, mortality in hemorrhagic stroke, recurrent stroke and survival outcome of stroke patients. Therefore, our results were not able to be compared directly to the results of previous reviews. However, while the discrimination performance of their prognostic models varied from poor to good, calibration performance was not considered. The first study was a systematic review of prognostic tools for early mortality in hemorrhagic stroke [24]. The authors selected 11 articles (12 prognostic tools), but validation

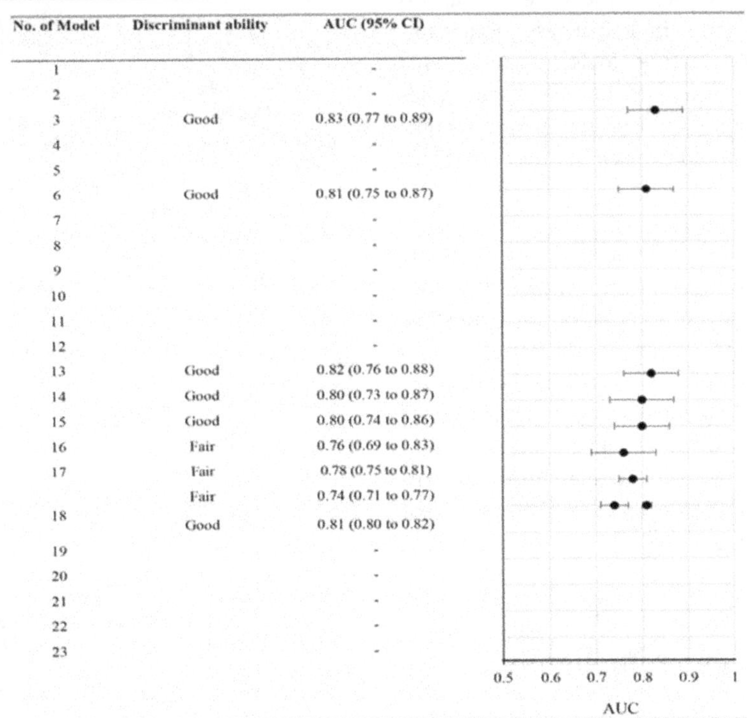

Fig. 5 Discrimination performance in external validation models

data were reported for only one of the prognostic tools. The Hemphill-intracerebral hemorrhage (ICH) model had the largest number of validation cohorts (nine articles) and showed good performance with a pooled AUC of 0.80 (95%CI 0.77 to 0.85). The second study was a systematic review of prognostic models to predict survival in patients with acute stroke. The authors found 83 models, but only three models were externally validated and showed fair to good discrimination [25]. The final study was a systematic review of prediction models for recurrent stroke and myocardial infarction after stroke. The authors showed that the models for recurrent stroke discriminate poorly between patients with and without a recurrent stroke with the pooled AUCs of 0.60 (95% CI 0.59 to 0.62) for the Essen Stroke Risk Score (ESRS) and 0.62 (95% CI 0.60 to 0.64) for the Stroke Prognosis Instrument II (SPI-II) [26].

Our findings suggest that some of the current prognostic models for predicting complete recovery from ischemic stroke may be clinically useful when applied to patients from high income countries who have experienced moderately severe ischemic stroke. Model No. 9 which was developed by Johnston et al. [14] suggests that the model was not over-fitted to the data set and is likely to be useful in predicting complete recovery from ischemic stroke in a similar population. Models No.3, 6, 13 and 15 involving eight predictors, including NIHSS score, age, infarct volume, history of diabetes mellitus and stroke, prestroke disability, small-vessel stroke and tissue-type plasminogen activator (t-PA use). Some were overlapped among the models as shown in Table 2. These models fulfilled the majority of the methodological requirements and showed acceptable performances in the external validation for both discrimination and calibration. We recommend that these models should be used in other settings.

Conclusions

This systematic review has shown that, while many prognostic models have been published, they are rarely validated in external populations, and most of the models were developed from elderly patients with moderately severe ischemic stroke, mainly in high income countries. There is a need for the development of models in other settings, especially in low and middle income populations. All models should be validated, and performance measures should be reported which address the two key issues of discrimination and calibration.

Abbreviations

AUC: Area under a receiver operating characteristic (ROC) curve; BI: Barthel Index; C-statistics: Concordance statistics; CT: Computerized tomography; ESRS: Essen Stroke Risk Score; GOS: Glasgow Outcome Scale; MRI: Magnetic resonance imaging; mRS: Modified Rankin Scale; NIHSS: National Institutes of Health Stroke Scale; OHS: Oxford Handicap Scale; SPI-II: Stroke Prognosis Instrument II

Acknowledgments

The authors wish to thank a native English language speaker, Peter Bradshaw, for line and copy editing drafts of the manuscript. The funding organization had no role in this research.

Funding

Not applicable.

Authors' contributions

NJ, ML and PP developed the protocol. NJ conducted the systematic review. NJ and SR conducted the literature search and the data extraction. NJ and ML drafted the manuscript. All authors read and approved the final manuscript.

Competing interests

The authors declare that they have no competing interests.

References

1. Feigin VL, Norrving B, Mensah GA. Global burden of stroke. Circ Res. 2017;120:439–48.
2. Benjamin EJ, Virani SS, Callaway CW, Chang AR, Cheng S, Chiuve SE, et al. Heart disease and stroke statistics-2018 update: a report from the American Heart Association. Circulation. 2018;137:1–442.
3. Moser DK, Kimble LP, Alberts MJ, Alonzo A, Croft JB, Dracup K, Evenson KR, Go AS, Hand MM, Kothari RU, Mensah GA. Reducing delay in seeking treatment by patients with acute coronary syndrome and stroke: a scientific statement from the American Heart Association Council on cardiovascular nursing and stroke council. J Cardiovasc Nurs. 2007;22:326–43.
4. Steyerberg E, Moons KGM, van der Windt D, Hayden J, Perel P, Schroter S, et al. Prognosis research strategy (PROGRESS) series 3: prognostic model research. PLoS Med. 2013;10:e1001381.
5. Vogenberg FR. Predictive and prognostic Models: implications for healthcare decision-making in a modern recession. American health & drug benefits. 2009;2:218.
6. Pavlou M, Ambler G, Seaman SR, Guttmann O, Elliott P, King M, et al. How to develop a more accurate risk prediction model when there are few events relative to the number of predictors. BMJ (Clinical research ed). 2015;351:h3868.
7. Justice AC, Covinsky KE, Berlin JA. Assessing the generalizability of prognostic information. Ann Intern Med. 1999;130:515–24.
8. D'Amico G, Malizia G, D'Amico M. Prognosis research and risk of bias. Intern Emerg Med. 2016;11:251–60.
9. Kleinbaum D, Klein M. Logistic regression: a self- learning text. 3rd ed. New York: Springer; 2010.
10. Steyerberg EW, Vickers AJ, Cook NR, Gerds T, Gonen M, Obuchowski N, Pencina MJ, Kattan MW. Assessing the performance of prediction models: a framework for some traditional and novel measures. Epidemiology (Cambridge, Mass). 2010;21:128.
11. Hanley A, Mcneil J, Hanley JA, BJ MN. The meaning and use of the area under a receiver operating characteristic (ROC) curve. Radiology. 1982;143:29–36.
12. StataCorp. Stata statistical software,Release 10. College Station: StataCorp LP; 2007.
13. Johnston KC, Connors AF, Wagner DP, Knaus WA, Wang X, Haley EC. A predictive risk model for outcomes of ischemic stroke. Stroke. 2000;31:448–55.
14. Johnston KC, Wagner DP, Haley EC, Connors AF. Combined clinical and imaging information as an early stroke outcome measure. Stroke. 2002;33:466–72.
15. Johnston KC, Connors AF Jr, Wagner DP, Haley EC Jr. Predicting outcome in ischemic stroke: external validation of predictive risk models. 2003;34:200–2.
16. Johnston KC, Wagner DP, Wang X-Q, Newman GC, Thijs V, Sen S, et al. Validation of an acute ischemic stroke model: does diffusion-weighted imaging lesion volume offer a clinically significant improvement in prediction of outcome? Stroke. 2007;38:1820–5.
17. Weimar C, Ziegler A, König IR, Diener HC. Predicting functional outcome and survival after acute ischemic stroke. J Neurol. 2002;249:888–95.
18. German Stroke Study Collaboration. Predicting outcome after acute ischemic stroke: an external validation of prognostic models. Neurology. 2004;62:581–5.

19. Weimar C, König IR, Kraywinkel K, Ziegler A, Diener HC. Age and National Institutes of Health stroke scale score within 6 hours after onset are accurate predictors of outcome after cerebral ischemia. Stroke. 2004;35:158–62.
20. König IR, Ziegler A, Bluhmki E, Hacke W, Bath PM, Sacco RL, Diener HC, Weimar C. Predicting long-term outcome after acute ischemic stroke. Stroke. 2008;39:1821–6.
21. Schiemanck SK, Kwakkel G, Post MW, Kappelle LJ, Prevo AJ. Predicting long-term independency in activities of daily living after middle cerebral artery stroke. Stroke. 2006;37:1050–4.
22. Patti J, Helenius J, Puri AS, Henninger N. White matter Hyperintensity–adjusted critical infarct thresholds to predict a favorable 90-day outcome. Stroke. 2016;47:2526–33.
23. Hage V. The NIH stroke scale: a window into neurological status. NurseCom Nursing Spectrum (Greater Chicago). 2011;24:44–9.
24. Mattishent K, Kwok CS, Ashkir L, Pelpola K, Myint PK, Loke YK. Prognostic tools for early mortality in hemorrhagic stroke: systematic review and meta-analysis. J Clin Neurol. 2015;11:339–48.
25. Counsell C, Dennis M. Systematic review of prognostic models in patients with acute stroke. Cerebrovasc Dis. 2001;12:159–70.
26. Thompson DD, Murray GD, Dennis M, Sudlow CL, Whiteley WN. Formal and informal prediction of recurrent stroke and myocardial infarction after stroke: a systematic review and evaluation of clinical prediction models in a new cohort. BMC Med. 2014;12:58.

8

Atrial fibrillation is not uncommon among patients with ischemic stroke and transient ischemic stroke in China

Xiaomeng Yang[1], Shuya Li[2], Xingquan Zhao[1,3], Liping Liu[4,5], Yong Jiang[2,3], Zixiao Li[1,6], Yilong Wang[2,6*] and Yongjun Wang[1,5,6*]

Abstract

Background: Atrial fibrillation (AF) is reported to be a less frequent cause of ischemic stroke in China than in Europe and North America, but it is not clear whether this is due to underestimation. Our aim was to define the true frequency of AF-associated stroke, to determine the yield of 6-day Holter ECG to detect AF in Chinese stroke patients, and to elucidate predictors of newly detected AF.

Methods: Patients with acute ischemic stroke or transient ischemic attack (TIA) were enrolled in a prospective, multicenter cohort study of 6-day Holter monitoring within 7 days after stroke onset at 20 sites in China between 2013 and 2015. Independent predictors of newly-detected AF were determined by multivariate analysis.

Results: Among 1511 patients with ischemic stroke and TIA (mean age 63 years, 33.1% women), 305 (20.2%) had either previously known (196, 13.0%) or AF newly-detected by electrocardiography (53, 3.5%) or by 6-day Holter monitoring (56/1262, 4.4%). A history of heart failure (OR = 4.70, 95%CI, 1.64–13.5), advanced age (OR = 1.06, 95%CI, 1.04–1.09), NIHSS at admission (OR = 1.06, 95%CI, 1.02–1.10), blood high density lipoprotein (HDL) (OR = 1.52, 95%CI, 1.09–2.13), together with blood triglycerides (OR = 0.64, 95%CI, 0.45–0.91) were independently associated with newly-detected AF.

Conclusions: Contrary to previous reports, AF-associated stroke is frequent (20%) in China if systemically sought. Prolonged noninvasive cardiac rhythm monitoring importantly increases AF detection in patients with recent ischemic stroke and TIA in China. Advanced age, history of heart failure, and higher admission NIHSS and higher level of HDL were independent indicators of newly-detected AF.

Keywords: Atrial fibrillation, Prolonged ECG monitoring, ischemic stroke, transient ischemic attack, China

Background

The fraction of strokes associated with atrial fibrillation has been reported to be lower in China than in European and North American stroke populations [1–3], but it is not clear whether this is due to its under-detection and hence leading to suboptimal secondary prevention. Recent studies have demonstrated that prolonged (> 24 h) of cardiac rhythm monitoring importantly increases detection of paroxysmal atrial fibrillation in post-stroke patients [4–6], but this has not previously been assessed in Chinese stroke patients, who are on average relatively young. We sought to determine the true frequency of AF-associated stroke and yield of prolonged cardiac rhythm monitoring to detect paroxysmal AF in Chinese patients with recent ischemic stroke and TIA.

* Correspondence: yilong528@gmail.com; yongjunwang1962@gmail.com
[2]Tiantan Clinical Trial and Research Center for Stroke, Department of Neurology, Beijing Tiantan Hospital, Capital Medical University, No.6 Tiantanxili, Dongcheng District, Beijing 100050, China
[1]Vascular Neurology, Department of Neurology, Beijing Tiantan Hospital, Capital Medical University, No. 6 Tiantan Xili, Dongcheng District, Beijing 100050, China
Full list of author information is available at the end of the article

Methods

Subjects

From October 2013 to June 2015, we recruited consecutive patients within 7 days of the index event of ischemic stroke or TIA from 20 Chinese hospitals. Clinical TIAs with an acute ischemic lesion visualized on computerized tomography (CT) or magnetic resonance imaging (MRI) were classified as strokes. The exclusionary criteria were 1) age < 18 years; 2) patients who were unable or unwilling to give informed consent; and 3)patients who were found not to have a stroke or TIA (stroke mimics). The study complied with the Declaration of Helsinki, and protocol was approved by the institutional review board (IRB) of Beijing Tiantan Hospital, Capital Medical University. All patients or their legal representatives provided written informed consent.

Data collection

Clinical data included demographic information, stroke risk factors, detailed medical history and treatments. Stroke severity was assessed using the National Institutes of Health Stroke Scale (NIHSS) [7] assessed by physicians. Patients received routine stroke care according to his/her condition including CT or MRI, 12-channel surface electrocardiography (ECG), transthoracic echocardiography, ultrasound of the cervical arteries, and routine blood analysis including, for example, lipid profile, blood glucose, liver enzymes and creatinine. Previously known AF was diagnosed according to the medical history reported by the patients and the prior medical records of the patients in our study.

Holter monitoring

The 6-day Holter monitoring initiated within 7 days after the index event using a commercially available 3-lead monitor device (iHolter, Yocaly Information Science & Technology Co., Ltd. Jinan, Shandong, China). It is an autotriggered device that uses an event detection algorithm to capture asymptomatic paroxysmal events, including paroxysmal AF. The event detection algorithm uses RR interval variability and QRS morphology analysis to detect all possible AF events that are then transmitted to a central core laboratory for manual review and confirmation based on standard diagnostic criteria (absence of p wave activity and irregular RR interval). ECG recordings were analyzed in a central core laboratory by two investigators who were independent of our study team and who were unaware of clinical and neuroimaging results using dedicated analysis software (DoctorClient, Software Version 1.5.0.16). All Holter ECG recordings with suspected AF were subsequently evaluated by another independent observer. Bursts of AF on ECG were reported by the number of beats of each occurrence. The first time and longest duration of bursts of AF for each patient were also recorded. The device defined AF as ≥ 1 period of > 30 s duration of an absolute arrhythmia without detectable P-waves and episodes < 30 s require manual review of all possible AF events [8, 9]. Atrial flutter and AF were not discriminated as both arrhythmias carry a similar stroke risk and often coincide [10].

Statistical analyses

Continuous data are given as median, range and categorical variables are given as absolute number and percentage. Mann–Whitney U test (continuous variables) and Pearson $\chi 2$ tests (categorical variables) were used to compare groups. Significance was assumed when the 2-sided probability value was <0.05. A multivariate analysis was performed using logistic regression, all factors that associated with detected AF in univariate analysis were included ($P< 0.05$). For calculation of 95% confidence interval (CI), binominal distribution was assumed. Statistical analysis was performed using SAS version 9.2 (SAS Institute Inc., Cary, NC).

Results

Patient population

During the study period, 1556 patients with stroke or TIA were admitted to the participating stroke units. Because of artifacts, interruptions for clinical procedures, and early detachment of the monitoring leads by patients, 1511 patients (1441 with ischemic stroke and 70with TIA) were included (Fig. 1). The mean age of the study cohort was 63 years, and 33.1% were women.

Detection of Atrial fibrillation

Among 1511 patients with ischemic stroke and TIA, 305 (20.2%) had previously known ((196, 13.0%) or newly detected AF on electrocardiography (53, 3.5%), and 4.4% of patients had unsuspected AF detected by 6-day Holter monitoring (56/1262). The median duration from index event (TIA/stroke) to initiation of monitoring was 4 days (range, 2–5 days). Prolonged Holter monitoring was well tolerated, yielding a median ECG recording duration of 5 days (range, 5–6 days). Cumulative overall detection rates of 56 unsuspected AF detected by 6-day Holter monitoring were shown in Fig. 2. Patients with TIA/stroke frequently revealed other significant dysrhythmias, including 1) premature atrial complexes (1099,72.7%); 2) premature ventricular complexes (1123, 74.3%); 3) atrial tachycardia (728, 48.2%);4) ventricular tachycardia (142, 9.4%).

Patient characteristics

Cohort characteristics, comparing patients with and without AF, are presented in Table 1. Older patients (median 72 vs. median 61; $P < 0.001$) and patients who are not current smokers (81.0% vs. 63.8%; $P < 0.001$) were more likely to have AF. Patients with AF were presented more frequently with previous ischemic stroke (27.2% vs. 21.1%; $P = 0.02$), coronary heart disease (17.7% vs. 8.3%; $P < 0.001$), heart failure (9.5% vs. 1.0%;

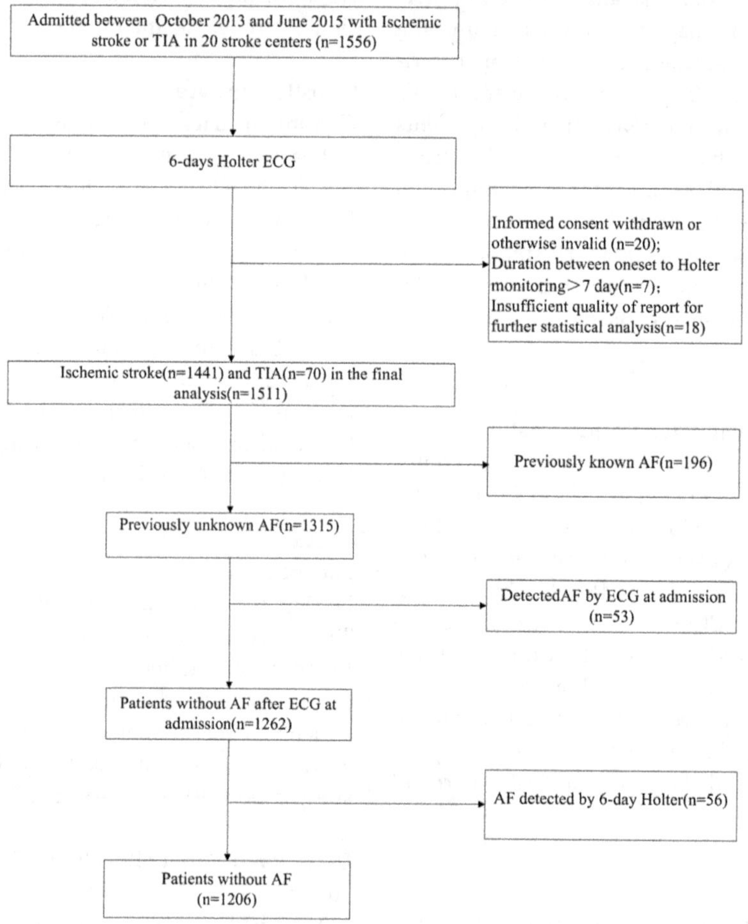

Fig. 1 Flow chart of the study

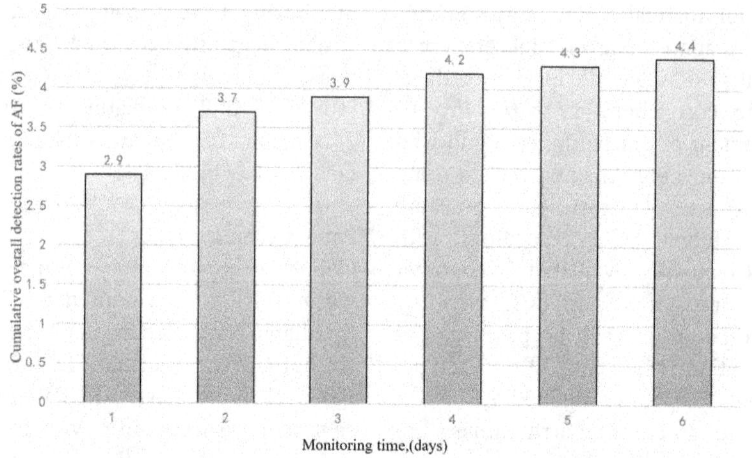

Fig. 2 Cumulative overall detection rates of 56 unsuspected AF detected by 6-day Holter monitoring

Table 1 Patient features associated with AF

Variables	All patients ($n = 1511$)	Without AF ($n = 1206$)	With AF ($n = 305$)	*P* Value
Age,yr. (median[IQR])	63(55–73)	61(53–71)	72(64–78)	< 0.001
Women, n(%)	500(33.1)	385 (31.9)	115(37.7)	0.06
BMI,Kg/m^2 (median[IQR])	24.2(22.0–26.4)	24.2(22.0–26.4)	24.2(21.5–26.3)	0.08
Current smoker,n(%)	494(32.7)	436(36.2)	58(19.0)	< 0.001
Medical history, (%)				
Hypertension	949(62.8)	750 (62.2)	199 (65.2)	0.32
Diabetes	326(21.6)	254 (21.1)	72 (23.6)	0.33
Hyperlipidemia	227(15.0)	192 (15.9)	35(11.5)	0.052
Ischemic stroke	337(22.3)	254 (21.1)	83 (27.2)	0.02
TIA	43(2.8)	36 (3.0)	7(2.3)	0.52
MI	45(3.0)	33 (2.7)	12 (3.9)	0.27
Coronary heart disease	154(10.2)	100(8.3)	54(17.7)	< 0.001
Peripheral arterial disease	32(2.1)	23(1.9)	9(3.0)	0.26
Heart failure	41(2.7)	12 (1.0)	29(9.5)	< 0.001
Blood analysis(mmol/L)				
Triglycerides	1.33(0.90–1.91)	1.40(0.96–2.00)	1.05(0.78–1.56)	< 0.001
LDL	2.70(2.20–3.31)	2.74(2.23–3.35)	2.57(2.05–3.22)	0.001
HDL	1.12(0.96–1.34)	1.12(0.96–1.34)	1.20(1.00–1.41)	0.002
Cholesterol	4.52 (3.90–5.24)	4.55(3.93–5.29)	4.35(3.76–5.06)	0.002
Fasting blood-glucose	5.49(4.92–6.81)	5.47(4.92–6.81)	5.60(4.94–6.83)	0.42
Clinical features(median[IQR])				
NIHSS at admission	3(1–6)	3(1–6)	4(2–9)	< 0.001

IQR indicates interquartile range, *TIA* transient ischemic attack, *MI* myocardial infarction, *NIHSS* the National Institutes of Health Stroke Scale, *LDL* low density lipoprotein, *HDL* high density lipoprotein

$P < 0.001$) and higher NIHSS score at admission (median 4 vs. 3; P < 0.001). Considering laboratory tests, patients with AF had, on average, lower levels of triglycerides (median 1.05 vs. 1.40; $P < 0.001$) and LDL (median 2.57 vs. median 2.74; $P = 0.001$) and cholesterol (median 4.35 vs. median 4.55; $P = 0.002$)) and had higher levels of HDL (median1.20 vs. 1.12; $P < 0.001$).

In multivariable analysis (Table 2), a history of coronary heart disease (OR = 1.65, 95%CI, 1.08–2.50) and heart failure (OR = 7.11,95%CI,3.22–15.72), advanced age (OR = 1.06, 95%CI, 1.05–1.08), admission NIHSS (OR = 1.06, 95%CI, 1.04–1.09), HDL (OR = 1.41, 95%CI, 1.02–1.94) together with current smoker (OR = 0.68, 95%CI, 0.48–0.97) and blood triglycerides (OR = 0.78, 95%CI, 0.65–0.94) were independently associated with AF in patients with ischemic stroke and TIA.

Table 2 Multivariate analysis of clinical features associated with AF

Variables	OR	95% CI	*P* value
Age	1.06	1.04–1.08	< 0.001
Previous coronary heart disease	2.00	1.31–3.05	0.001
Previous heart failure	7.36	3.38–16.05	< 0.001
NIHSS at admission	1.05	1.03–1.08	< 0.001
Current smoker	0.65	0.45–0.93	0.02
Triglycerides	0.76	0.63–0.91	0.004

NIHSS indicates the National Institutes of Health Stroke Scale

We also compared the characteristics of patients with previously known/ newly-detected AF and without AF (Table 3). Older patients (median 72 vs. median 61; $P < 0.001$) and patients who are not current smokers (77.1% vs. 63.8%; $P = 0.006$) were more likely to have newly-detected AF. Patients with newly-detected AF were presented more frequently with previous TIA (6.4% vs. 1.0%; $P < 0.001$), coronary heart disease (17.4% vs. 8.3%; $P = 0.001$), heart failure (6.4% vs. 1.0%; P < 0.001), higher NIHSS score at admission (median 4 vs. 3; $P < 0.001$) and less frequently with previous hyperlipidemia (8.3% vs. 15.9%; $P = 0.03$). Considering laboratory tests, patients with newly-detected AF had, on average, lower levels of triglycerides (median 1.03 vs. 1.40; $P < 0.001$) and cholesterol (median 4.38 vs. median 4.55; $P = 0.05$)) and had higher levels of HDL (median1.22 vs. 1.12; $P = 0.002$).

In multivariable analysis (Table 4), a history of heart failure (OR = 4.70, 95%CI, 3.22–15.72), advanced age

Table 3 Patient characteristics with previously known, newly detected AF or without AF

Variables	Without AF (*n* = 1206)	Previously known AF (*n* = 196)	Newly detected AF (*n* = 109)	*P* Value*	*P* Value†
Age, yr. (median[IQR])	61(53–71)	72(64–78)	72(64–78)	< 0.001	< 0.001
Women, n (%)	385(31.9)	75(38.3)	40 (36.7)	0.08	0.31
BMI, Kg/m^2 (median[IQR])	24.2(22.0–26.4)	24.2(21.3–26.4)	23.8(21.9–25.6)	0.27	0.11
Current smoker, n (%)	436(36.2)	33(16.8)	25(22.9)	< 0.001	0.006
Medical history, (%)					
Hypertension	750(62.2)	136(69.4)	63 (57.8)	0.053	0.37
Diabetes	254(21.1)	46(23.5)	26 (23.9)	0.45	0.50
Hyperlipidemia	192(15.9)	26(13.3)	9(8.3)	0.34	0.03
Ischemic stroke	254(21.1)	67(34.2)	16 (14.7)	< 0.001	0.11
TIA	12(1.0)	6(3.1)	7 (6.4)	0.95	< 0.001
MI	33(2.7)	7(3.6)	5(4.6)	0.52	0.42
Coronary heart disease	100(8.3)	35(17.9)	19 (17.4)	< 0.001	0.001
Peripheral arterial disease	23(1.9)	8(4.1)	1(0.9)	0.10	0.71
Heart failure	12(1.0)	22(11.2)	7(6.4)	< 0.001	< 0.001
Blood analysis (mmol/L)					
Triglycerides	1.40(0.96–2.00)	1.05(0.75–1.60)	1.03(0.81–1.48)	< 0.001	< 0.001
LDL	2.74(2.23–3.35)	2.49(2.03–3.25)	2.65(2.13–3.17)	0.003	0.07
HDL	1.12(0.96–1.34)	1.19(0.99–1.38)	1.22(1.02–1.45)	0.06	0.002
Cholesterol	4.55(3.93–5.29)	4.28(3.73–5.14)	4.38(3.77–4.94)	0.01	0.05
Fasting blood-glucose	5.47(4.92–6.81)	5.63(4.98–7.10)	5.50(4.87–6.51)	0.18	0.67
Clinical features (median[IQR])					
NIHSS at admission	3(1–6)	4(2–9)	4(2–10)	< 0.001	< 0.001

IQR indicates interquartile range, *TIA* transient ischemic attack, *MI* myocardial infarction, *NIHSS* the National Institutes of Health Stroke Scale, *LDL* low density lipoprotein, *HDL* high density lipoprotein
**P* values for comparation between patients with previously known AF and those without AF
†P values for comparation between patients with newly-detected AF and those without AF

(OR = 1.06, 95%CI, 1.04–1.09), admission NIHSS (OR = 1.06, 95%CI, 1.02–1.10), HDL (OR = 1.52, 95%CI, 1.09–2.13) together with blood triglycerides (OR = 0.64, 95%CI, 0.45–0.91) were independently associated with newly-detected AF.

Discussion

Contrary to previous reports, AF-associated brain ischemia is frequent (20.2%) in China. Identification of AF after ischemic stroke or TIA is crucial to optimize appropriate anticoagulation. This is the first study to demonstrate the yield of prolonged cardiac rhythm monitoring after ischemic stroke and TIA in Chinese patients with recent brain ischemia. This prospective multicenter study provides solid evidence that AF is considerably more common in patients with ischemic stroke and TIA than what has been reported in most previous population-based studies in China [2, 3, 11]. The underlying reasons are likely the increased duration of cardiac rhythm monitoring in comparison to prior studies and AF detection based upon a standardized automated arrhythmia detection algorithm and continuous review of monitoring data.

Table 4 Multivariate analysis of clinical features independently predictive of newly detected AF

Variables	OR	95% CI	*P* value
Age	1.06	1.04–1.09	< 0.001
Previous heart failure	4.70	1.64–13.5	0.004
NIHSS at admission	1.06	1.02–1.10	0.003
Triglycerides	0.64	0.45–0.91	0.01
HDL	1.52	1.09–2.13	0.02

NIHSS the National Institutes of Health Stroke Scale, *LDL* low density lipoprotein, *HDL* high density lipoprotein

However, when compared with the studies in western countries [12, 13], the overall detection rate of AF among stroke and TIA is still lower. In our study the detection rate of any new AF among patients without previously known AF were respectively 5.2% and 6.9% in the first 24 h and during the whole monitoring period while the rate were 6.2% and 14.1% in a recent review [14]. The discrepancy might be because the patients in our study are, on average younger (mean age, 63.0 years) than in studies reporting higher frequencies AF in which the mean ages was 68.4 years. When compared with studies with the similar monitoring duration, Stahrenberg et al. [12]and Jabaudon et al. [15] have reported higher detection rates of new AF using 7-day continuous Holter monitoring and 7-day event-loop recording (ELR) device (12.5% and 14.8% respectively). The early time point of monitoring after symptom onset (9.5 h) and relatively older patients in their studies may be the explanation for the difference.

In our study, we found that patients with history of previous coronary heart disease have a higher likelihood of AF which is consistent with previous study [16]. We suppose that the explanation might be that coronary heart disease shares similar risk factors such as aging and systemic vascular risk factors with AF which may cause an abnormal atrial tissue substrate or atrial cardiopathy, that can result in AF.

We also found that current smoker was less likely to have AF in our study which is in accordance with previous study [13]. However, this is inconsistent with recent study investigating the association between smoking and AF in community population which have shown smoking was associated with the incidence of AF [17]. We speculate that the inconsistency may lie in the different population. As we known smoking is an important and potent risk factor for atherosclerosis which may be the main reason for stroke in patients without AF, accordingly the percentage of current smoker is higher in stroke patients without AF. Prospective studies about the association between smoking and AF in stroke patients are needed in the future.

Several factors were significantly associated with an increased risk of new AF detection, namely older age, NIHSS at admission and previous heart failure and HDL. Our results are in line with previous studies in which advanced age was shown to be associated with a higher incidence of AF and paroxysmal atrial fibrillation (pAF) after stroke [16, 18, 19]. This argues for a structural abnormality of the atria with age which may lead to electrical instability thus causing pAF. As cardioembolic strokes are frequently larger and associated with an adverse outcome than those due to other sources [20], we also found that higher NIHSS score at admission is an independent predictor of detection of AF.

In addition, we found that patients with history of heart failure to have a higher likelihood of newly detected AF which is in accordance with previous studies [16, 21]. Previous study also showed preexisting heart disease is the major cause of AF that is first diagnosed after stroke [21], so more intensified screening for AF in these patients may be essential and meaningful.

We also observed independent association between blood triglycerides/HDL and detected AF. The association between blood lipids and AF risk has been reported by several previous publications which have offered inconsistent results [22]. Lack of adjustment for important confounders and inclusion of lipid-lowering medication users may affect the finding in our study which should be explained in caution.

There are limitations to our study: firstly, patients enrolled in our study had, on average, relatively mild strokes which enabled them to complete the study protocol. As cardioembolism is likely to cause large, severe strokes, the detection rate of AF may be underestimated in our study. Secondly, because our analysis focused on the usefulness of Holter monitoring on detection of AF, detailed diagnostic workup such as transesophageal echocardiography or additional biomarkers were only completed in some patients. This limited the predictive model regarding clinical indicators that be associated with decreased risk of AF. Thirdly, some of the brief occurrences of AF may represent stroke-induced arrhythmias rather than being the cause of the stroke. However, whether pAF occurred before or after the stroke will always be difficult to clarify because prestroke monitoring is not available.

Conclusion

In conclusion, we found that AF is more common among patients with ischemic stroke and TIA in China than those previously reported. For the first time in a Chinese population, we have demonstrated that AF can be detected in an important fraction of patients with ischemic stroke and TIA via prolonged monitoring evaluation. Clinicians should plan the best available combination of post-stroke atrial fibrillation screening methods to increase yield of AF detection in the shortest possible time after stroke or TIA in order to optimize secondary antithrombotic management.

Abbreviations

AF: Atrial fibrillation; CI: Confidence interval; CT: Computerized tomography; ELR: Event-loop recording; HDL: High density lipoprotein; IQR: Interquartile range; LDL: low density lipoprotein; MI: Myocardial infarction; MRI: Magnetic resonance imaging; NIHSS: National Institutes of Health Stroke Scale; OR: Odds-Ratio; pAF: Paroxysmal Atrial fibrillation; TIA: Transient ischemic attack

Acknowledgments

We thank all participating hospitals, their physicians and nurses.

Funding

This study was funded by grants from the Ministry of Science and Technology of the People's Republic of China (2011BAI08B02, 2012ZX09303, and 2013BAI09B03), Beijing Institute for Brain Disorders (BIBD-PXM2013_014226_07_000084).
This study was sponsored and funded by Bayer HealthCare Pharmaceuticals. Bayer HealthCare Pharmaceuticals took no part in the design of the study and collection, analysis, and interpretation of data and in writing the manuscript.

Authors' contributions

Dr. LPL, Dr. XQZ, Dr. WLW, Dr. YJW, contributed to the design of the study; Dr. XMY, Dr. SYL and Dr. ZXL contribute to acquisition of data and interpretation of data. Dr. YJ contributes to data cleansing and analysis. Dr. XMY contributes to Literature search and draft writing. All authors read and approved the final manuscript.

Competing interests

This study was sponsored and funded by Bayer HealthCare Pharmaceuticals.

Author details

[1]Vascular Neurology, Department of Neurology, Beijing Tiantan Hospital, Capital Medical University, No. 6 Tiantan Xili, Dongcheng District, Beijing 100050, China. [2]Tiantan Clinical Trial and Research Center for Stroke, Department of Neurology, Beijing Tiantan Hospital, Capital Medical University, No.6 Tiantanxili, Dongcheng District, Beijing 100050, China. [3]Center of Stroke, Beijing Institute for Brain Disorders, Beijing, China. [4]Neuro-intensive Care Unit, Department of Neurology, Beijing Tiantan Hospital, Capital Medical University, Beijing, China. [5]Beijing Key Laboratory of Translational Medicine for Cerebrovascular Disease, No. 6 Tiantan Xili, Dongcheng District, Beijing 100050, China. [6]China National Clinical Research Center for Neurological Diseases, No. 6 Tiantan Xili, Dongcheng District, Beijing 100050, China.

References

1. Wang C, Yang Z, Wang C, Wang Y, Zhao X, Liu L, et al. Significant underuse of warfarin in patients with nonvalvular atrial fibrillation: results from the china national stroke registry. J Stroke Cerebrovasc Dis. 2014;23:1157–63.
2. Gao Q, Fu X, Wei JW, Chen X, Huang Y, Wang J, et al. Use of oral anticoagulation among stroke patients with atrial fibrillation in china: the chinaquest (quality evaluation of stroke care and treatment) registry study. Int J Stroke. 2013;8:150–4.
3. Lin S, Wu B, Hao ZL, Kong FY, Tao WD, Wang DR, et al. Characteristics, treatment and outcome of ischemic stroke with atrial fibrillation in a chinese hospital-based stroke study. Cerebrovasc Dis. 2011;31:419–26.
4. Wachter R, Groschel K, Gelbrich G, Hamann GF, Kermer P, Liman J, et al. Holter-electrocardiogram-monitoring in patients with acute ischaemic stroke (find-afrandomised): an open-label randomised controlled trial. Lancet Neurol. 2017;16:282–90.
5. Sanna T, Diener HC, Passman RS, Di Lazzaro V, Bernstein RA, Morillo CA, et al. Cryptogenic stroke and underlying atrial fibrillation. N Engl J Med. 2014; 370:2478–86.
6. Gladstone DJ, Spring M, Dorian P, Panzov V, Thorpe KE, Hall J, et al. Atrial fibrillation in patients with cryptogenic stroke. N Engl J Med. 2014;370:2467–77.
7. Brott T, Adams HP Jr, Olinger CP, Marler JR, Barsan WG, Biller J, et al. Measurements of acute cerebral infarction: a clinical examination scale. Stroke. 1989;20:864–70.
8. Kirchhof P, Auricchio A, Bax J, Crijns H, Camm J, Diener HC, et al. Outcome parameters for trials in atrial fibrillation: recommendations from a consensus conference organized by the german atrial fibrillation competence network and the european heart rhythm association. Europace. 2007;9:1006–23.
9. Fuster V, Ryden LE, Cannom DS, Crijns HJ, Curtis AB, Ellenbogen KA, et al. 2011 accf/aha/hrs focused updates incorporated into the acc/aha/esc 2006 guidelines for the management of patients with atrial fibrillation: a report of the american college of cardiology foundation/american heart association task force on practice guidelines developed in partnership with the european society of cardiology and in collaboration with the european heart rhythm association and the heart rhythm society. J Am Coll Cardiol. 2011;57:e101–98.
10. Camm AJ, Lip GY, De Caterina R, Savelieva I, Atar D, Hohnloser SH, et al. 2012 focused update of the esc guidelines for the management of atrial fibrillation: an update of the 2010 esc guidelines for the management of atrial fibrillation. Developed with the special contribution of the european heart rhythm association. Eur Heart J. 2012;33:2719–47.
11. Li SY, Zhao XQ, Wang CX, Liu LP, Liu GF, Wang YL, et al. One-year clinical prediction in chinese ischemic stroke patients using the chads2 and cha2ds2-vasc scores: the china national stroke registry. CNS Neurosci Ther. 2012;18:988–93.
12. Stahrenberg R, Weber-Kruger M, Seegers J, Edelmann F, Lahno R, Haase B, et al. Enhanced detection of paroxysmal atrial fibrillation by early and prolonged continuous holter monitoring in patients with cerebral ischemia presenting in sinus rhythm. Stroke. 2010;41:2884–8.
13. Friberg L, Rosenqvist M, Lindgren A, Terent A, Norrving B, Asplund K. High prevalence of atrial fibrillation among patients with ischemic stroke. Stroke. 2014;45:2599–605.
14. Kishore A, Vail A, Majid A, Dawson J, Lees KR, Tyrrell PJ, et al. Detection of atrial fibrillation after ischemic stroke or transient ischemic attack: a systematic review and meta-analysis. Stroke. 2014;45:520–6.
15. Jabaudon D, Sztajzel J, Sievert K, Landis T, Sztajzel R. Usefulness of ambulatory 7-day ecg monitoring for the detection of atrial fibrillation and flutter after acute stroke and transient ischemic attack. Stroke. 2004;35:1647–51.
16. Wohlfahrt J, Stahrenberg R, Weber-Kruger M, Groschel S, Wasser K, Edelmann F, et al. Clinical predictors to identify paroxysmal atrial fibrillation after ischaemic stroke. Eur J Neurol. 2014;21:21–7.
17. Chamberlain AM, Agarwal SK, Folsom AR, Duval S, Soliman EZ, Ambrose M, et al. Smoking and incidence of atrial fibrillation: results from the atherosclerosis risk in communities (ARIC) study. Heart Rhythm. 2011;8(8):1160–6.
18. Doliwa Sobocinski P, Anggardh Rooth E, Frykman Kull V, von Arbin M, Wallen H, Rosenqvist M. Improved screening for silent atrial fibrillation after ischaemic stroke. Europace. 2012;14:1112–6.
19. Alhadramy O, Jeerakathil TJ, Majumdar SR, Najjar E, Choy J, Saqqur M. Prevalence and predictors of paroxysmal atrial fibrillation on holter monitor in patients with stroke or transient ischemic attack. Stroke. 2010;41:2596–600.
20. Grau AJ, Weimar C, Buggle F, Heinrich A, Goertler M, Neumaier S, et al. Risk factors, outcome, and treatment in subtypes of ischemic stroke: the german stroke data bank. Stroke. 2001;32:2559–66.
21. Rizos T, Horstmann S, Dittgen F, Tager T, Jenetzky E, Heuschmann P, et al. Preexisting heart disease underlies newly diagnosed atrial fibrillation after acute ischemic stroke. Stroke. 2016;47:336–41.
22. Alonso A, Yin X, Roetker NS, Magnani JW, Kronmal RA, Ellinor PT, et al. Blood lipids and the incidence of atrial fibrillation: the multi-ethnic study of atherosclerosis and the framingham heart study. J Am Heart Assoc. 2014;3:e001211.

9

Clinical and radiological factors associated with unfavorable outcome after intravenous thrombolysis in patients with mild ischemic stroke

Dae-Hyun Kim[1,2*], Deok-Soo Lee[2], Hyun-Wook Nah[1,2] and Jae-Kwan Cha[1,2]

Abstract

Background: A significant proportion of patients with mild ischemic stroke become disabled despite receiving intravenous thrombolytic therapy. The purpose of this study was to assess the clinical and radiological factors associated with unfavorable outcomes in patients with minor ischemic stroke that received intravenous recombinant tissue plasminogen activator (rt-PA) therapy.

Methods: We identified anterior circulation stroke patients with initial National Institutes of Health Stroke Scale (NIHSS) scores ≤5 who received intravenous thrombolysis within 4.5 h of stroke onset and had pretreatment magnetic resonance (MR)/MR angiography using our prospective stroke database. We analyzed baseline characteristics, infarction patterns on diffusion-weighted imaging (DWI), and steno-occlusive lesions on MR angiography. Unfavorable outcome was defined as a modified Rankin Scale (mRS) score ≥ 2 at 90 days. Logistic regression was used to determine independent predictors of unfavorable outcomes.

Results: Among 121 patients (85 men; mean age, 63.4 ± 11.3 years) included in this study, 46 (38%) had unfavorable outcomes at 90 days and DWI lesion patterns showing infarction in the deep middle cerebral artery (MCA) territory involving the perforating artery area was observed in 47 (38.8%) patients. On multivariable analysis, unfavorable outcomes at 90 days were associated with diabetes [odds ratio (OR), 3.41; 95% confidence interval (CI), 1.06–10.9; $P = 0.039$), NIHSS score on admission (OR, 2.11; 95% CI, 1.35–3.30; $P = 0.001$), and infarction in the deep MCA territory on DWI (OR, 4.19; 95% CI, 1.63–10.8; $P = 0.003$). Lesions in the deep MCA territory was independently associated with early neurological deterioration ($P = 0.032$). The patients without deep MCA territory infarction had a higher prevalence of cardiac embolism ($P = 0.009$).

Conclusions: Higher NIHSS scores, diabetes, and deep MCA territory infarction may be useful for predicting unfavorable outcomes in patients with minor stroke treated with intravenous rt-PA therapy.

Keywords: Mild ischemic stroke, Recombinant tissue plasminogen activator, Diffusion-weighted imaging

* Correspondence: kdh6542@hanmail.net

[1]Busan-Ulsan Regional Cardiocerebrovascular Center, Dong-A University Hospital, Busan, Republic of Korea

[2]Department of Neurology, College of Medicine, Dong-A University, 1, 3-ga Dongdaesin-dong, Seo-gu, Busan 602-715, Republic of Korea

Background

More than half of all ischemic stroke patients exhibit a clinical syndrome with mild neurological deficit [1, 2]. Intravenous thrombolysis with recombinant tissue plasminogen activator (rt-PA) within 4.5 h has been proven to be an effective treatment for acute ischemic stroke, but its benefits and risks in mild strokes are still unclear [3]. When patients with a mild stroke received intravenous thrombolytic therapy, approximately 30% of them had an unfavorable outcome [3–5]. Thus, it is of great importance to identify the patients at risk of unfavorable outcomes in the acute phase to prevent neurological deterioration and to predict outcomes in minor ischemic strokes treated with intravenous thrombolysis.

Magnetic resonance imaging (MRI) with diffusion-weighted imaging (DWI) is superior to computed tomography (CT) for early detection of hyperacute and small ischemic lesions. Pretreatment DWI lesion patterns may be helpful in predicting clinical outcome in patients with acute ischemic stroke [6, 7]. Steno-occlusive lesions of the cerebral artery are associated with unfavorable outcomes in patients with minor strokes [8, 9]. However, it is unclear whether the pretreatment lesions pattern on DWI and the presence of steno-occlusive lesions in relevant arteries can predict outcome following rt-PA thrombolysis in patients with minor stroke.

The aim of our study was to elucidate the clinical and pretreatment radiological factors associated with an unfavorable outcome after intravenous thrombolysis in patients with minor stroke.

Methods

We identified 682 consecutive patients in our prospectively collected institutional stroke database treated with intravenous rt-PA therapy within 4.5 h after symptom onset, independent of performance of emergent endovascular treatment between January 2010 and December 2016. During this period, MRI was systematically adopted at our center as the first-line imaging modality [DWI, fluid-attenuated inversion recovery, gradient echo sequences, and time of flight magnetic resonance angiography (MRA)] in the absence of contraindications to MRI. Eligible patients were treated with intravenous rt-PA according to clinical guidelines. No upper or lower National Institutes of Health Stroke Scale (NIHSS) threshold was applied. Follow up MRI or CT were performed 24 h after intravenous rt-PA thrombolysis in all patients.

Patients were included in our study if they had an anterior circulation stroke with an initial NIHSS score of 1 to 5 and pretreatment MRI including DWI and MRA. We excluded patients who; (1) had a pre-stroke modified Rankin scale core (mRS) > 1, (2) received subsequent endovascular treatment combined with intravenous thrombolysis, (3) had no definitive evidence of focal hyperintensities in clinically relevant areas on initial or follow up DWI, or (4) had no follow-up data.

Demographic, clinical and laboratory data were collected from the prospectively collected stroke registry. Baseline data included initial NIHSS scores and onset-to-rt-PA treatment times. Mild stroke was defined as a baseline NIHSS score 1–5 [5]. The etiologic stroke subtype was defined according to the Trial of Org 10,172 in Acute Stroke Treatment (TOAST) criteria [10].

This study was approved by the Institutional Review Board of Dong-A University Hospital.

Imaging analysis

Two investigators (D.-H. K and D.-S. L) who were blinded to the patients' clinical characteristics reviewed the pretreatment DWI and MRA images and follow up DWI at 24 h after intravenous thrombolysis. Discrepancies were resolved by consensus. DWI lesion pattern were classified as perforating artery infarcts (PAI), pial infarcts, border-zone infarcts, territorial infarcts and PAI plus additional infarcts outside the perforating artery territory, by modification of previous studies (Fig. 1) [11].

These findings were also divided into two different groups according to the presence of infarcts in the territory of the perforating arteries involving the internal capsule, corona radiata, and basal ganglia. Deep middle cerebral artery (MCA) infarction with or without infarctions outside the perforating artery territory were classified as Group A while the other 3 lesion patterns were classified as Group B.

Stenosis or occlusion of the arteries related to ischemia were determined via analysis of the initial MRA, which included the entire internal carotid artery, MCA (M1 proximal, M1 distal, and M2 segment), and anterior cerebral artery (ACA; A1 segment). Arterial occlusion was defined as a complete loss of distal flow signal. Moderate to severe arterial stenosis was defined as a 50% narrowing of the lumen and focal signal loss in the presence of a distal flow signal.

Clinical outcomes

Early neurological deterioration (END) was defined as an increase of 2 or more points in the NIHSS scores between hospital days 0 and 5. Outcome was assessed using the mRS score at 3 months from stroke onset and was dichotomized into favorable (mRS 0–1) and unfavorable (mRS 2–6). Symptomatic intracerebral hemorrhage was defined as blood at any site in the brain associated with clinical deterioration resulting in an NIHSS score increase of ≥4 points [12].

Statistical analysis

The results are expressed as mean (standard deviation) or median (range), as appropriate, throughout the text

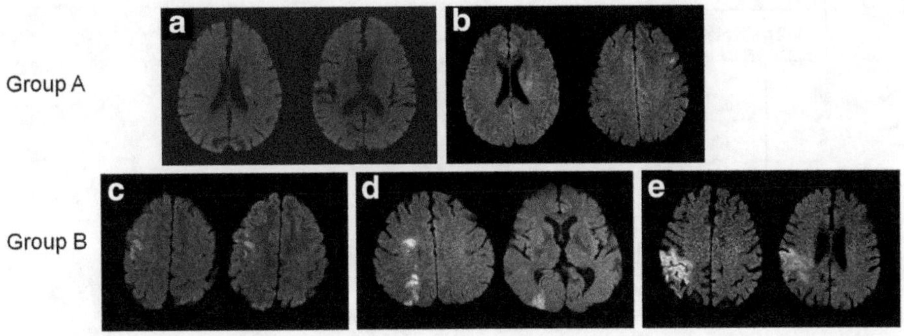

Fig. 1 Examples of the five different diffusion-weighted imaging patterns analyzed and the classification into two groups. Lesion patterns were classified as perforating artery infarcts (**a**), perforating artery infarcts with additional infarcts outside the perforating artery territory (**b**), pial infarcts (**c**), border-zone infarcts (**d**) and territorial infarcts (**e**)

and tables. The differences in patients' characteristics and their relation to 90-day outcomes (mRS ≤ 1 vs. mRS ≥ 2) were analyzed. For dichotomous outcomes, the chi-squared or Fisher's exact test are reported where appropriate. For outcomes with continuous data, comparisons were performed using Student's t test or the Mann-Whitney U test, depending on the normality of data distribution. Multivariate logistic regression analysis was performed to determine factors that could be considered to be independent predictors of unfavorable outcome after intravenous rt-PA thrombolysis. Variables showing a value of $P < 0.2$ in univariate analysis were included in the multivariate model. A probability value < 0.05 was considered statistically significant.

Results

A total of 202 patients with baseline NIHSS ≤5 were treated with intravenous thrombolysis. We excluded 42 patients with posterior circulation strokes, 18 patients without hyperintensity lesions on pretreatment and follow-up DWI, 5 patients who received endovascular treatment, 5 patients with an initial NIHSS of 0, 5 patients with unavailable or insufficient quality DWI, 3 patients with mRS 2–6 prior to the stroke, and 3 patients without an mRS assessment at 3 months Finally, 121 patients (85 men and 36 women; mean age, 63.4 ± 11.3 years) were included in the study (Fig. 2). The median baseline NIHSS score was 4 (interquartile range, 3–5). Among 121 patients, 46 (38%) had unfavorable outcomes (mRS score 2–6) at 90 days. Symptomatic intracerebral hemorrhages were rare (1.7%).

Table 1 presents the general characteristics and radiologic features of patients with and without unfavorable outcomes. In univariate analysis, diabetes ($P = 0.007$), non-cardiac embolism ($P = 0.04$), higher NIHSS scores ($P = 0.003$), and deep MCA territory infarction ($P < 0.001$) were more frequently observed in patients with an unfavorable outcome. The onset-to-rt-PA time was 141.6 ± 58 and 145.6 ± 67 min in the favorable and unfavorable groups, respectively, and did not differ significantly ($P = 0.728$). Visible arterial occlusion before rtPA was observed in 33% of patients. They were comprised of ICA occlusion ($N = 8$), M1 proximal occlusion ($N = 10$), M1 distal occlusion ($N = 11$), M2 occlusion ($N = 9$), and ACA occlusion ($N = 2$) on MRA. There was no difference in favorable outcome following intravenous thrombolysis between mild stroke patients with and without large artery occlusion.

After univariate analysis, hyperlipidemia ($P = 0.058$), age, sex, previous stroke, and steno-occlusive disease ($P = 0.181$) were also included in the multivariate logistic regression. Multivariate logistic regression analysis showed that diabetes [odds ratio (OR), 3.41; 95% confidence interval (CI), 1.06–10.9; $P = 0.039$], higher NIHSS scores on admission (OR, 2.11; 95% CI, 1.35–3.30; $P = 0.001$), and infarction in the deep MCA territory (OR, 4.19; 95% CI, 1.63–10.8; $P = 0.003$) were independently associated with unfavorable outcome (Table 2).

A DWI lesion pattern with infarction in the deep MCA territory (Group A) was observed in 47 (38.8%) patients. Group A was independently associated with END ($P = 0.032$) and moderate to severe (> 50%) stenosis in the relevant artery ($P = 0.019$). The patients without lesions in the deep MCA territory (Group B) had a higher prevalence of cardiac embolism ($P = 0.009$) (Additional file 1: Table S1, Fig. 3).

Discussion

This study showed that a large proportion (38%) of patients receiving intravenous thrombolysis for minor strokes will have an unfavorable outcome at 90 days. Symptomatic intracerebral hemorrhages were rare. Baseline NIHSS score, diabetes mellitus, and deep MCA infarction with lesions in the perforating artery territory were independently associated with unfavorable outcomes.

According to recent reports, age [5, 13], diabetes mellitus [5, 8, 9, 14], previous stroke [14], intra-or extracranial vascular occlusive lesions [8, 9] and NIHSS score [5, 15]

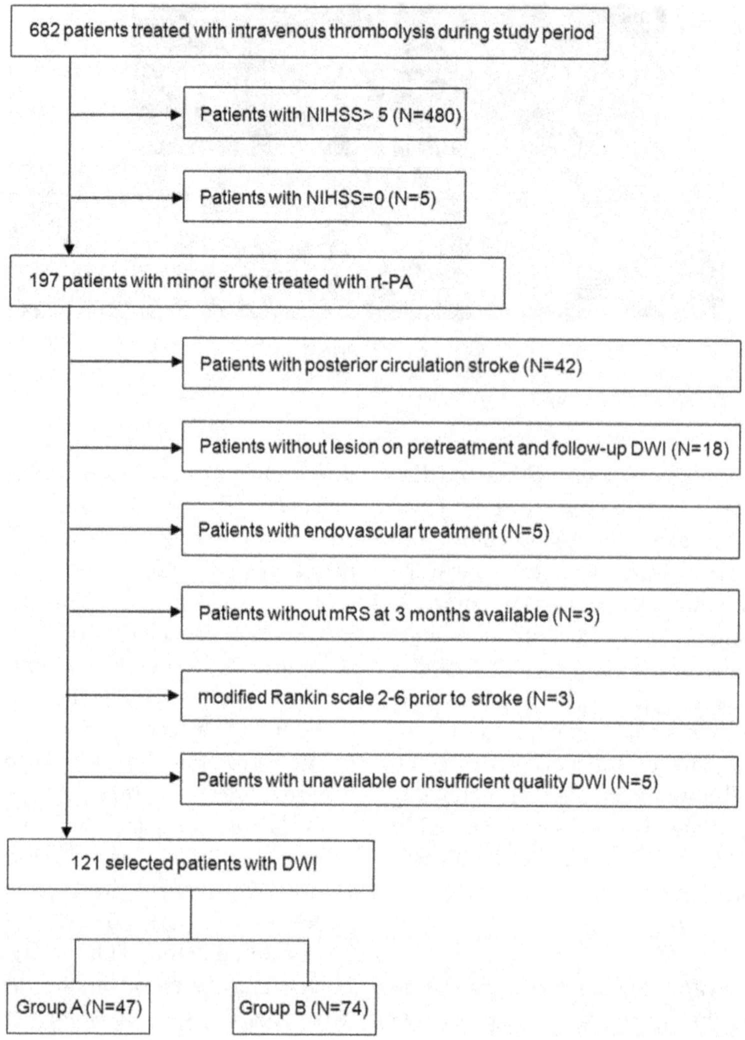

Fig. 2 Schematic description of the patient selection process

were associated with unfavorable outcomes in patients with minor strokes. However, these studies explored the factors associated with disability at 90 days in mild stroke patients not treated with thrombolytic therapy.

It remains to be determined whether the presence of steno-occlusive lesions leads to unfavorable outcomes in mild stroke patients following intravenous rt-PA treatment. As opposed to previous reports on non-thrombolytic therapy [8, 9], we did not find an association between large artery occlusion and unfavorable outcome following intravenous rt-PA therapy. This is in line with previous reports that also found no differences in outcome following intravenous thrombolysis between mild stroke patients with and without large artery occlusion [16, 17]. Mild stroke patients tend to have more distal artery occlusion, lower thrombus burden, and higher recanalization rates or have central occlusions with good collaterals [18–20]. This might be the reason why even patients with large artery occlusion do not have different outcome following intravenous rt-PA therapy compared to those without.

Previous studies have shown that acute lesion patterns may predict prognosis or stroke recurrence after ischemic stroke [11, 21] but it remains unclear whether such imaging factors are related to patient outcome after intravenous thrombolysis in mild ischemic stroke. Patients with perforating artery infarcts in the basal ganglia and corona radiata were more likely to have unfavorable outcomes in this study. These finding may be explained by several hypothesis.

First, Strambo et al. [15] reported that among all NIHSS items, only impairment of motor items is significantly associated with poor outcome in mild stroke. Since the deep MCA territory is crossed by the corticospinal tract [22] and is prone to damage by poor collateral flow [23], this area may be susceptible to motor

Table 1 Characteristics of the study population according to outcomes at 3 months

	All patients ($n = 121$)	mRS = 0–1 ($n = 75$)	mRS = 2–6 ($n = 46$)	*P*-value
Age (mean ± SD)	63.4 ± 11.3	63.2 ± 10.5	63.8 ± 12.6	0.769
Sex, *n*(%)				0.490
Men	85(70.2)	51(68)	34(73.9)	
Female	36(29.8)	24(32)	12(26.1)	
Risk factor, n(%)				
Hypertension	61(50.8)	36(48.6)	25(54.3)	0.544
Diabetes	33(27.3)	14(18.7)	19(41.3)	0.007
Hyperlipidemia	17(14)	7(9.3)	10(21.7)	0.057
Atrial fibrillation	22(18.2)	16(21.3)	6(13)	0.251
Current smoking	31(25.6)	20(26.7)	11(23.9)	0.736
Previous coronary artery disease	14(11.6)	10(13.3)	4(8.7)	0.564
Previous stroke or TIA	11(9.1)	6(8.0)	5(10.9)	0.746
NIHSS on admission, (med, IQR)	4[3–5]	4[2–4]	4[3–5]	0.003
(mean ± SD)	3.6 ± 1.2	3.4 ± 1.2	4.0 ± 1.1	0.004
Onset to rt-PA time, (mean± SD)	143.1 ± 61.4	141.6 ± 57.9	145.6 ± 67.2	0.728
Blood glucose on admission, mg/dL	143.4 ± 52.6	134.7 ± 44.9	157.6 ± 61.0	0.019
Initial systolic blood pressure, mmHg	145.6 ± 26.3	145.4 ± 27.9	145.8 ± 23.5	0.924
Etiologic stroke subtypes, *n*(%)				0.302
Small vessel disease	25(20.7)	13(17.3)	12(26.1)	0.248
Large artery disease	36(29.8)	22(29.3)	14(30.4)	0.298
Cardiac embolism	34(28.1)	26(34.7)	8(17.4)	0.040
Undetermined etiology	26(21.5)	14(18.7)	12(26.1)	0.335
Lesions on pretreatment DWI, *n*(%)				0.317
Acute infarcts (+)	110(91.7)	67(89.3)	43(95.6)	
No lesions	10(8.3)	8(10.7)	2(4.4)	
Lesion patterns on DWI, *n*(%)				
Perforating artery infarcts	27(22.3)	12(16)	15(32.6)	0.033
Pial infarcts	51(42.1)	40(53.3)	11(23.9)	0.001
Borderzone infarcts	6(5)	5(6.7)	1(2.2)	0.406
Territorial infarcts	17(14)	10(13.3)	7(15.2)	0.772
Perforating artery infarcts plus	20(16.5)	8(10.7)	12(26.1)	0.027
Deep MCA infarcts (PAI + PAI plus)	47(38.8)	20(26.7)	27(58.7)	< 0.001
Angiographic findings of relevant artery, *n*(%)				0.383
No stenosis or occlusion	62(51.2)	42(56)	20(43.5)	
Stenosis (> 50%)	19(15.7)	10(13.3)	9(19.6)	
Occlusion	40(33.1)	23(30.7)	17(37)	
Steno-occlusive disease, *n*(%)	59(48.8)	33(44)	26(56.5)	0.181
END, *n*(%)	14(11.6)	3(4)	11(23.9)	0.002
Symptomatic ICH, *n*(%)	2(1.7)	1(1.3)	1(2.2)	1.000

TIA transient ischemic attack, *DWI* diffusion-weighted imaging, MCA middle cerebral artery, *PAI* perforating artery infarction, *END* early neurological deterioration, ICH intracranial hemorrhage

deficits, regardless of rt-PA thrombolysis. In some reports, patients with deep white matter or basal ganglia infarction have suffered from bad outcomes after thrombolysis or endovascular therapy [7, 22, 23]. Thus, even small lesions in this area could be critical to the outcome of mild ischemic stroke.

Second, END is an important factor associated with worse clinical outcome in minor strokes [9]. Several

Table 2 Multivariable analysis for unfavorable outcome at 90 days

	Unfavorable outcome (mRS score 2–6)		
	Adjusted OR	95% CI	*P*-value
Age - per 1 year	1.01	0.96–1.05	0.914
Men	1.95	0.69–5.48	0.205
Diabetes	3.41	1.06–10.9	0.039
Hyperlipidemia	2.92	0.81–10.5	0.102
Previous stroke or TIA	1.29	0.29–5.65	0.755
NIHSS on admission	2.11	1.35–3.30	0.001
Initial serum glucose	1.01	0.99–1.01	0.306
Cardiac embolism	0.48	0.16–1.46	0.195
Presence of deep MCA infarction	4.19	1.63–10.8	0.003
Steno-occlusive disease	1.6	0.63–3.72	0.351

Adjusted by age, sex and previous stroke

patients with infarcts in the perforator territory have END (29.1%) [13] and this rate was similar to that in patients with small vessel disease that received intravenous rt-PA therapy (33%) [24]. In our study, ENDs were more prevalent in Group A patients and were associated with unfavorable outcomes. These results may have important clinical implications. Previous study has shown that rt-PA use in acute lacunar stroke does not affect END [24]. Thus, special attention should be paid to patients with infarcts in the perforating territory, even when they show mild neurological deficits at the time of presentation and after rt-PA therapy.

Lastly, Group B was more likely to have cardiac embolism. This can be explained by a previous report that demonstrated a mild stroke caused by cardiac embolism could reveal small cortical lesions and lead to a high rate of neurological improvement [15]. However, Hao et al. [25] reported that in mild stroke, cardiac embolism was a predictor of death or disability at 3 months and that patients with small vessel occlusion had better outcomes. That study enrolled mild stroke patients within 30 days after stroke onset. There is a possibility that non-cardiac embolism patients with early worsening or early recurrence were excluded from that study, whereas we included patients treated with rt-PA therapy within 4.5 h. Further studies are needed to confirm whether cardiac embolism can be a protective factor in ischemic stroke with mild symptoms.

A significant strength of our study is that all patients underwent pretreatment MRI. DWI has the advantage of capturing small infarctions and detection of early ischemic changes in patients with acute mild ischemic stroke, unlike CT. Few studies on whether pretreatment DWI lesions pattern and arterial occlusion on MRA can predict outcome in mild stroke are available [21, 26]. To the best of our knowledge, this is the largest study to investigate the DWI findings in patients with mild stroke treated with rt-PA therapy.

The most notable limitation of our study is the uncontrolled, non-randomized design since this was a single hospital-based study. Limitations to using clinical

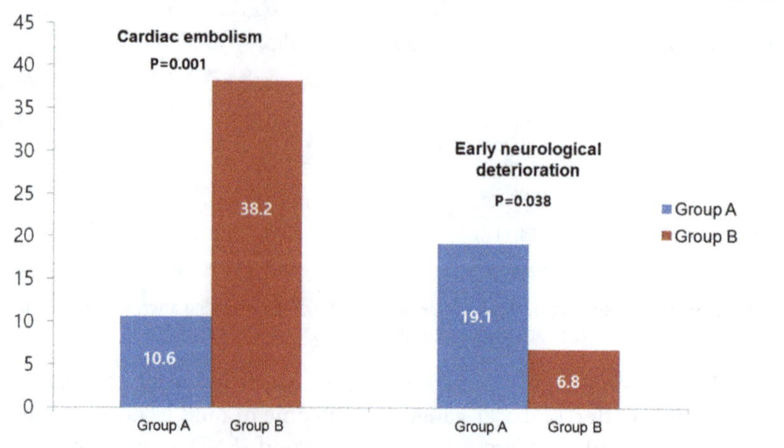

Fig. 3 Comparison of the general characteristics of group (**a**) and (**b**)

registry data may include the introduction of bias in patient selection including the imbalance of sex ratio in this study. Thus, generalizing the results of this study to other patient populations may be challenging.

Conclusions

We found that in spite of intravenous rt-PA treatment, approximately 40% of anterior circulation stroke patients with minor symptom had unfavorable outcomes at 3 months. Higher NIHSS scores, diabetes and deep MCA infarction with involvement of the perforating artery territory were associated with unfavorable outcomes after rt-PA therapy in patients with minor stroke. Brain MRI-DWI patterns assessed in the acute phase of mild stroke are useful to predict those patients at high risk of unfavorable outcome following rt-PA therapy.

Abbreviations

ACA: Anterior cerebral artery; CT: Computed tomography; DWI: Diffusion-weighted imaging; END: Early neurological deterioration; MCA: Middle cerebral artery; MRA: Magnetic resonance angiography; MRI: Magnetic resonance imaging; mRS: modified Rankin scale core; NIHSS: National Institutes of Health Stroke Scale; PAI: Perforating artery infarcts; rt-PA: recombinant tissue plasminogen activator; TOAST: Trial of Org 10,172 in Acute Stroke Treatment

Acknowledgements

Not applicable

Funding

This work was supported by the Dong-A University research fund.

Authors' contributions

DHK: conception and design, drafting the manuscript and revising it critically for important intellectual content. DSL: conception and design, acquisition of data and drafting the manuscript. HWN: acquisition of data, data analysis and drafting manuscript. JKC: conception and design, data collection and data interpretation. All authors have read and approved the final manuscript.

Competing interests

The authors declare that they have no competing interests.

References

1. Reeves M, Khoury J, Alwell K, Moomaw C, Flaherty M, Woo D, Khatri P, Adeoye O, Ferioli S, Kissela B, Kleindorfer D. Distribution of national institutes of health stroke scale in the Cincinnati/northern Kentucky stroke study. Stroke. 2013;44:3211–3.
2. Kim BJ, Park JM, Kang K, Lee SJ, Ko Y, Kim JG, Cha JK, Kim DH, Nah HW, Han MK, Park TH, Park SS, Lee KB, Lee J, Hong KS, Cho YJ, Lee BC, Yu KH, Oh MS, Kim DE, Ryu WS, Cho KH, Kim JT, Choi JC, Kim WJ, Shin DI, Yeo MJ, Sohn SI, Hong JH, Lee JS, Yoon BW, Bae HJ. Case characteristics, hyperacute treatment, and outcome information from the clinical research center for stroke-fifth division registry in South Korea. J Stroke. 2015;17:38–53.
3. Yu AY, Hill MD, Coutts SB. Should minor stroke patients be thrombolyzed? A focused review and future directions. Int J Stroke. 2015;10:292–7.
4. Emberson J, Lees KR, Lyden P, Blackwell L, Albers G, Bluhmki E, Brott T, Cohen G, Davis S, Donnan G, Grotta J, Howard G, Kaste M, Koga M, von Kummer R, Lansberg M, Lindley RI, Murray G, Olivot JM, Parsons M, Tilley B, Toni D, Toyoda K, Wahlgren N, Wardlaw J, Whiteley W, del Zoppo GJ, Baigent C, Sandercock P, Hacke W. Effect of treatment delay, age, and stroke severity on the effects of intravenous thrombolysis with alteplase for acute ischaemic stroke: a meta-analysis of individual patient data from randomised trials. Lancet. 2014;384:1929–35.
5. Romano JG, Smith EE, Liang L, Gardener H, Camp S, Shuey L, Cook A, Campo-Bustillo I, Khatri P, Bhatt DL, Fonarow GC, Sacco RL, Schwamm LH. Outcomes in mild acute ischemic stroke treated with intravenous thrombolysis: a retrospective analysis of the get with the guidelines-stroke registry. JAMA Neurol. 2015;72:423–31.
6. Bang OY, Lee PH, Heo KG, Joo US, Yoon SR, Kim SY. Specific DWI lesion patterns predict prognosis after acute ischaemic stroke within the MCA territory. J Neurol Neurosurg Psychiatry. 2005;76:1222–8.
7. Liu D, Scalzo F, Starkman S, Rao NM, Hinman JD, Kim D, Ali LK, Saver JL, Noorian AR, Ng K, Liang C, Sheth SA, Yoo B, Liu X, Liebeskind DS. DWI lesion patterns predict outcome in stroke patients with thrombolysis. Cerebrovasc Dis. 2015;40:279–85.
8. Sato S, Uehara T, Ohara T, Suzuki R, Toyoda K, Minematsu K, Factors associated with unfavorable outcome in minor ischemic stroke. Neurology. 2014;83:174–81.
9. Coutts SB, Modi J, Patel SK, Aram H, Demchuk AM, Goyal M, Hill MD. What causes disability after transient ischemic attack and minor stroke?: results from the CT and MRI in the triage of TIA and minor cerebrovascular events to identify high risk patients (CATCH) study. Stroke. 2012;43:3018–22.
10. Adams HP Jr, Bendixen BH, Kappelle LJ, Biller J, Love BB, Gordon DL, Marsh EE 3rd. Classification of subtype of acute ischemic stroke. Definitions for use in a multicenter clinical trial. TOAST trial of org 10172 in acute stroke treatment. Stroke. 1993;24:35–41.
11. Lee DK, Kim JS, Kwon SU, Yoo SH, Kang DW. Lesion patterns and stroke mechanism in atherosclerotic middle cerebral artery disease: early diffusion-weighted imaging study. Stroke. 2005;36:2583–8.
12. Hacke W, Kaste M, Fieschi C, von Kummer R, Davalos A, Meier D, Larrue V, Bluhmki E, Davis S, Donnan G, Schneider D, Diez-Tejedor E, Trouillas P. Randomised double-blind placebo-controlled trial of thrombolytic therapy with intravenous alteplase in acute ischaemic stroke (ECASS II). Second European-Australasian acute stroke study investigators. Lancet. 1998;352:1245–51.
13. Yamamoto N, Terasawa Y, Satomi J, Sakai W, Harada M, Izumi Y, Nagahiro S, Kaji R. Predictors of neurologic deterioration in patients with small-vessel occlusion and infarcts in the territory of perforating arteries. J Stroke Cerebrovasc Dis. 2014;23:2151–5.
14. Strbian D, Piironen K, Meretoja A, Sairanen T, Putaala J, Tiainen M, Artto V, Rantanen K, Happola O, Kaste M, Lindsberg PJ. Intravenous thrombolysis for acute ischemic stroke patients presenting with mild symptoms. Int J Stroke. 2013;8:293–9.
15. Strambo D, Zambon AA, Roveri L, Giacalone G, Di Maggio G, Peruzzotti-Jametti L, La Gioia S, Galantucci S, Comi G, Sessa M. Defining minor symptoms in acute ischemic stroke. Cerebrovasc Dis. 2015;39:209–15.
16. Zhu W, Churilov L, Campbell BC, Lin M, Liu X, Davis SM, Yan B. Does large vessel occlusion affect clinical outcome in stroke with mild neurologic deficits after intravenous thrombolysis? J Stroke Cerebrovasc Dis. 2014;23:2888–93.
17. Kohrmann M, Nowe T, Huttner HB, Engelhorn T, Struffert T, Kollmar R, Saake M, Doerfler A, Schwab S, Schellinger PD. Safety and outcome after thrombolysis in stroke patients with mild symptoms. Cerebrovasc Dis. 2009;27:160–6.
18. Legrand L, Naggara O, Turc G, Mellerio C, Roca P, Calvet D, Labeyrie MA, Baron JC, Mas JL, Meder JF, Touze E, Oppenheim C. Clot burden score on admission T2*-MRI predicts recanalization in acute stroke. Stroke. 2013;44:1878–84.
19. Saqqur M, Uchino K, Demchuk AM, Molina CA, Garami Z, Calleja S, Akhtar N, Orouk FO, Salam A, Shuaib A, Alexandrov AV. Site of arterial occlusion identified by transcranial doppler predicts the response to intravenous thrombolysis for stroke. Stroke. 2007;38:948–54.
20. Strbian D, Ringleb P, Michel P, Breuer L, Ollikainen J, Murao K, Seiffge DJ, Jung S, Obach V, Weder B, Eskandari A, Gensicke H, Chamorro A, Mattle HP, Engelter S, Leys D, Numminen H, Kohrmann M, Hacke W, Tatlisumak T. Ultra-early intravenous stroke thrombolysis: do all patients benefit similarly? Stroke. 2013;44:2913–6.
21. Roquer J, Rodriguez-Campello A, Cuadrado-Godia E, Vivanco-Hidalgo RM, Jimenez-Conde J, Perich X, Ois A. Acute brain MRI-DWI patterns and stroke recurrence after mild-moderate stroke. J Neurol. 2010;257:947–53.
22. Rosso C, Colliot O, Valabregue R, Crozier S, Dormont D, Lehericy S, Samson Y. Tissue at risk in the deep middle cerebral artery territory is critical to stroke outcome. Neuroradiology. 2011;53:763–71.
23. Kawano H, Hirano T, Inatomi Y, Terasaki T, Yonehara T, Uchino M. Presence of deep white matter lesions on diffusion-weighted imaging is a negative predictor of early dramatic improvement after intravenous tissue plasminogen activator thrombolysis. Cerebrovasc Dis. 2010;30:230–6.
24. Hwang YH, Seo JG, Lee HW, Park SP, Suh CK. Early neurological deterioration following intravenous recombinant tissue plasminogen activator therapy in patients with acute lacunar stroke. Cerebrovasc Dis. 2008;26:355–9.

10

Research on advanced intervention using novel bone marrOW stem cell (RAINBOW): a study protocol for a phase I, open-label, uncontrolled, dose-response trial of autologous bone marrow stromal cell transplantation in patients with acute ischemic stroke

Hideo Shichinohe[1,2*], Masahito Kawabori[1], Hiroaki Iijima[2], Tuyoshi Teramoto[2], Takeo Abumiya[1], Naoki Nakayama[1], Ken Kazumata[1], Shunsuke Terasaka[1], Teruyo Arato[2] and Kiyohiro Houkin[1]

Abstract

Background: Stroke is a leading cause of death and disability, and despite intensive research, few treatment options exist. However, a recent breakthrough in cell therapy is expected to reverse the neurological sequelae of stroke. Although some pioneer studies on the use of cell therapy for treating stroke have been reported, certain problems remain unsolved. Recent studies have demonstrated that bone marrow stromal cells (BMSCs) have therapeutic potential against stroke. We investigated the use of autologous BMSC transplantation as a next-generation cell therapy for treating stroke. In this article, we introduce the protocol of a new clinical trial, the Research on Advanced Intervention using Novel Bone marrOW stem cell (RAINBOW).

Methods/design: RAINBOW is a phase 1, open-label, uncontrolled, dose-response study, with the primary aim to determine the safety of the autologous BMSC product HUNS001–01 when administered to patients with acute ischemic stroke. Estimated enrollment is 6–10 patients suffering from moderate to severe neurological deficits. Approximately 50 mL of the bone marrow is extracted from the iliac bone of each patient 15 days or later from the onset. BMSCs are cultured with allogeneic human platelet lysate (PL) as a substitute for fetal calf serum and are labeled with superparamagnetic iron oxide for cell tracking using magnetic resonance imaging (MRI). HUNS001–01 is stereotactically administered around the area of infarction in the subacute phase. Each patient will be administered a dose of 20 or 50 million cells. Neurological scoring, MRI for cell tracking, ^{18}F–fuorodeoxyglucose positron emission tomography, and ^{123}I–Iomazenil singlephoton emission computed tomography will be performed for 1 year after the administration.

(Continued on next page)

* Correspondence: hshichi@med.hokudai.ac.jp
[1]Department of Neurosurgery, Hokkaido University Graduate School of Medicine, Sapporo, Japan
[2]Clinical Research and Medical Innovation Center, Hokkaido University Hospital, N14 W5, Kita-ku, Sapporo 060-8648, Japan

(Continued from previous page)

Discussion: This is a first-in-human trial for HUNS001–01 to the patients with acute ischemic stroke. We expect that intraparenchymal injection can be a more favorable method for cell delivery to the lesion and improvement of the motor function than intravenous infusion. Moreover, it is expected that the bio-imaging techniques can clarify the therapeutic mechanisms.

Keywords: Acute ischemic stroke, Bone marrow stromal cells, Cell therapy, Regenerative medicine, Intraparenchymal injection, Platelet lysate, Bio-imaging

Background

Since Azizi et al. published the first report on bone marrow stromal cell (BMSC) transplantation in 1998 [1], BMSCs have been considered as a promising cell source for central nervous system (CNS) regeneration. Some well-known advantages of BMSCs are the ease of their harvest, availability of autologous cells, absence of immunological rejection or tumorigenesis, and freedom from ethical problems [2]. Several articles have reported that BMSCs can survive in the host CNS, migrate to the lesion, and elicit neuroprotective effects when transplanted into animal models of CNS disease [3].

BMSCs originate from bone marrow mononuclear cells (BMMNCs). The floating cells are removed from BMMNCs, and only cells adhering to the floor of the flask are cultured for several weeks to obtain BMSCs [4]. A subpopulation of BMSCs, also termed mesenchymal stem cells, can differentiate into bone, cartilage, and fat. Moreover, there are many reports on their potential to differentiate into other lineages, including neural cells, via so-called transdifferentiation. Many researchers have reported how BMSCs could protect injured CNS. At first, their transdifferentiation to neuronal cells, endothelial cells, or pericyte was noticed. On the other hand, it has been known that they can promote neurogenesis, axonal elongation, vasculogenesis, and so on, due to their secretion of some growth factors or cytokines, so-called nursing effect [5, 6].

The first clinical trial using autologous BMSC therapy in patients with stroke was reported in 2005. Bang et al. showed the feasibility and safety of the therapy [7]. They adopted cell culture methods with fetal calf serum (FCS) and intravenous administration in the protocol. Regrettably, they reported no significant neurological recovery using the Barthel Index and modified Rankin Scale. We hypothesized that some unsolved problems regarding clinical application remained, including safety of the cell culture, suitable delivery routes, cell tracking after the transplantation, and monitoring the effects of intervention [8]. We aimed to solve these problems to develop the next generation of BMSC therapy for stroke. We hypothesize that xeno-free cell culture, direct cell administration near the lesion, and bioimaging for the therapeutic effects are indispensable for the next generation of BMSC therapy [8].

We have reported translational research on human BMSC transplantation in animal stroke models. Human BMSCs were cultured with human platelet lysate (hPL) instead of FCS [9, 10]. The cells were injected stereotactically into rat ischemic brains [9, 10]. In advance, the donor cells were labeled with superparamagnetic iron oxide (SPIO) for cell tracking using magnetic resonance imaging (MRI) [10]. After the transplantation, ^{18}F- fluorodeoxyglucose positron emission tomography (FDG-PET) and ^{123}I–Iomazenil singlephoton emission computed tomography (IMZSPECT) were performed to analyze cellular function and metabolism in the host brain [11, 12]. There were no differences in the surface markers and cell proliferation between cells culture in hPL and FCS [9]. Although a rotarod test showed that motor function deteriorated in rats suffering from permanent middle cerebral artery occlusion, a BMSC-hPL transplantation enhanced recovery of the motor function significantly [9]. MRI demonstrated that the SPIO-BMSCs aggressively migrated towards the lesion [10]. Moreover, FDG-PET and IMZ-SPECT showed that BMSC transplantation promoted recovery of the glucose utilization and the binding potential of iomazenil, respectively, in the peri-infarct area [11, 12]. Histological analysis supported the findings on MRI and showed an inclination for neural differentiation of donor cells [10, 13, 14].

We used these results to determine the optimal study design of our new clinical trial, Research on Advanced Intervention using Novel Bone marrOW stem cell (RAINBOW). The trial is a Phase I study to assess the potential benefits of autologous BMSC product (code name: HUNS001–01) administration to patients with acute ischemic stroke. We aim to evaluate its safety, feasibility, and efficacy. Autologous BMSC were cultured with allogeneic PL in the cell processing center (CPC) according to good manufacturing practice (GMP). The cells were labeled with SPIO. They were injected around the infarct stereotactically. After administration, we will perform MRI for cell tracking and FDG-PET and IMZ-SPECT for the analysis of the therapeutic effect. In addition, we hope that this study proves helpful in clarifying the therapeutic mechanisms. In the study, we expect that the findings of SPIO-labeling/MRI will help us to choose the suitable transplant location. About the therapeutic mechanisms, for instance, if MRI showed that the cluster of donor cells moved to SVZ, it might be an evidence for stimulation of endogenous neuronal regeneration. And FDG-PET and IMZ-SPECT may show the relation between the transplant location and the reaction of the host brain, for examples, brain metabolism may be increased in the contralateral hemisphere to the transplant location.

Methods/design

Study design

This study is an open-label, uncontrolled, dose-response, single-center, phase I clinical trial. The subjects will receive standard medication for 14 days after the onset of their stroke. The patients are then screened, and bone marrow harvest is performed as soon as possible. The BMSCs are cultured with allogeneic PL, and HUNS001–01 is manufactured from autologous BMSCs in the CPC. Once the preparation of HUNS001–01 is almost complete, the administration date is planned, and a second screening is performed 7 days before the administration. If the subject meets the requirements, HUNS001–01 (cell dose: 2×10^7 or 5×10^7 cells) is injected into the brain stereotactically. Follow-up is done for 1 year after the administration. The detailed trial flow is described in Fig. 1. This study is conducted in the Department of Neurosurgery, Hokkaido University Hospital, Sapporo, Japan. The trial was registered at The University Hospital Medical Information Network on February 22, 2017 (UMIN ID: UMIN000026130). The total study period is approximately 3 years, between March 2017 and August 2020.

Study population

Inclusion criteria (First screening; 14 days after the onset of stroke).

- Male or female subjects between 20 and 79 years old
- Informed consent within 14 days after the onset of stroke
- Clinical diagnosis of cerebral ischemic stroke in the internal carotid arterial region
- Subjects with a modified Rankin Scale (mRS) of 0 or 1 before the onset of stroke
- Subjects who can give informed consent; if insufficiently able, a legal representative is needed
- Subjects with moderate or severe neurological symptoms; National Institute of Health Stroke Scale (NIHSS) ≥ 6, (however, the partial score in both "Motor Arm" and "Motor Leg" must be ≥6)

(Second screening; 7 days before the administration of HUNS001–01).

- HUNS001–01 must be available within 74 days after the onset
- Subjects with moderate or severe neurological deficit; mRS ≥ 3

Exclusion criteria (First screening; 14 days after the onset of stroke)

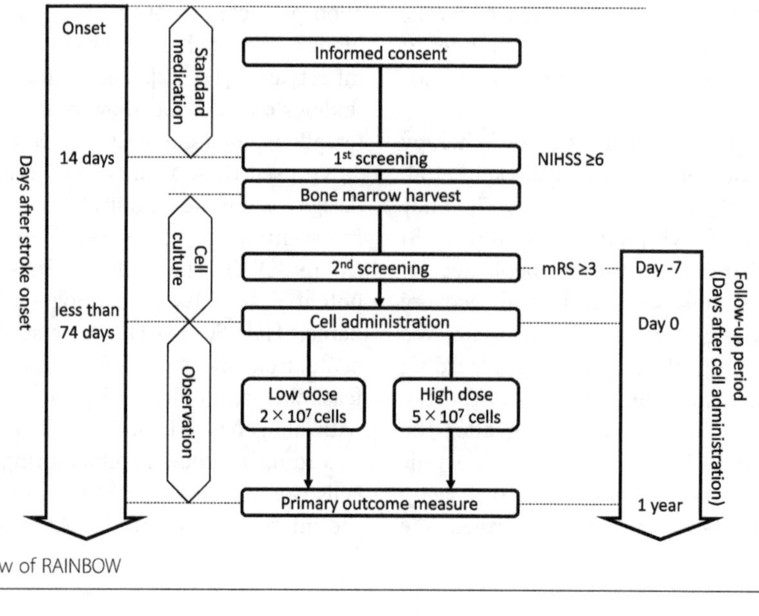

Fig. 1 The detailed trial flow of RAINBOW

- Occurrence of severe hemorrhagic transformation of ischemic stroke
- Subjects in a coma or a deep coma with a JCS-200 or JCS-300 score evaluated by the Japan Coma Scale
- Severe anemia (hemoglobin < 10.0 g/dL) or thrombocytopenia (platelet count < 100,000/mm^3)
- Severe heart disease (e.g., ischemic heart disease, heart failure)
- Significant abnormalities in laboratory tests:
  a. >3 × upper limit of normal (ULN) for alanine aminotransferase or aspartate aminotransferase.
  b. >1.5 × ULN for total bilirubin.
  c. >1.5 × ULN for serum creatinine
- Uncontrolled hypertension, despite antihypertensive therapy
- History of malignancy of any type
- Carriers of any of the following infectious diseases: Syphilis, hepatitis B virus (HBV), hepatitis C virus (HCV), human immunodeficiency virus (HIV)-1/2, human T cell leukemia virus (HTLV)-1, or parvovirus B19
- Subjects who are pregnant or want to have children
- History of seizure or administration of any antiepileptic drugs
- Contraindication for fosphenytoin sodium hydrate (Fostoin®, Eisai Co., Ltd., Tokyo, Japan)
- Serious allergy to any possible residues in the test product (e.g., any biomaterials used in manufacturing process, gentamicin sulfate, ferucarbotran) or any agents used for the administration of the test product or for inspections during the trial
- Contraindication for MRI (e.g., a pacemaker, metallic artificial heart valves, an implantable cardioverter defibrillator)
- Subjects who are inappropriate for this trial based on the judgment of the primary investigator or other investigators; for example, if other intracranial disorders were diagnosed due to history, symptoms, or neuroradiological findings during the trial, the primary investigator or other investigators will make a decision after reviewing the risks and benefits.

(Second screening; 7 days before the administration)

- Occurrence of severe hemorrhagic transformation of ischemic stroke
- Subjects in a coma or a deep coma with a JCS-200 or JCS-300 score evaluated by Japan Coma Scale
- Severe anemia (hemoglobin < 10.0 g/dL) or thrombocytopenia (platelet count < 100,000/mm^3)
- Severe heart disease (e.g., ischemic heart disease, heart failure)
- Significant abnormal laboratory tests:
  a. >3 × ULN for alanine aminotransferase or aspartate aminotransferase.
  b. >1.5 × ULN for total bilirubin.
  c. >1.5 × ULN for serum creatinine
- Uncontrolled hypertension, despite antihypertensive therapy
- Subjects who are inappropriate for this trial based on the judgment of the primary investigator or other investigators; for example, if other intracranial disorders were diagnosed due to history, symptoms, or neuroradiological findings during the trial, the primary investigator or other investigators will make a decision after reviewing the risks and benefits.

Sample size and statistical analysis

Since this trial is a phase I pilot study, each group is composed of three subjects to examine the safety of HUNS001–01 administration. The sample size of the trial was based on the traditional 3 + 3 dose escalation design. The first three subjects are included in the low-dose group (cell dose: 2 × 10^7 cells), and the following three patients are included in the high-dose group (cell dose: 5 × 10^7 cells). However, if the cultured BMSCs are inadequate for the high-dose group on 74 days after the onset of stroke, a subject could be moved to the low-dose group, if possible. In that case, the number of subjects will exceed six, and the last subject is the third subject in the high-dose group. The total number of subjects is limited to 10 if a third subject in the high-dose group is not accomplished.

Continuous data will be presented as means and standard deviations. Categorical data will be presented as absolute frequencies or relative percentages.

Characteristics of HUNS001–01

HUNS001–01 consists of plastic-adherent fibroblast-like cells. The phenotype of these cells is positivity for CD44, CD90, CD105, CD106, CD146, and CD 166, and negativity for CD19, CD34, and CD45. The expression of markers are consistent with the mesenchymal stromal cell phenotype according to the position statement of the International Society for Cellular Therapy (ISCT) [15].

Preparation of HUNS001–01

The cell source for HUNS001–01 is obtained by extracting approximately 50 mL of bone marrow from each subject. The bone marrow is brought to the CPC at Hokkaido University Hospital, and the following processes are performed in a closed operation system (CPWS System Cell Processing Work Station, Panasonic Healthcare Co., Tokyo, Japan). BMMNCs are isolated via density-gradient centrifugation with Ficoll-Hypaque® (Pharmacia, Uppsala, Sweden), and 1 × 10^7 cells are plated in a 175 cm^2 uncoated flask (Easy Flask 159,910;

Nunc) with 25 mL of αMEM with 10% hPL derived from healthy volunteers and 40 μg/mL of gentamicin sulfate. About the preparation of hPL, our previous report about safety and efficiency of hPL should be referred to [4]. After 24 h, nonadherent cells are removed by changing the medium. The culture medium is replaced 2 times a week. The BMSCs are passed two or three times for the subsequent procedure. In order to label the cells for MRI tracking, 1 μL/mL ferucarbotran (27.9 μg Fe/mL, Resovist®, Fuji lm RI Pharma Co., Ltd., Tokyo, Japan), a SPIO agent, is added into the culture medium and incubated with the BMSCs for 24 h before the cell injection procedure. The SPIO-labeled BMSCs in flasks are lifted using TrypLe Select® (a recombinant trypsin substitute, Gibco) and centrifuged. The supernatant is decanted and the cells are gently resuspended in Artcereb® (irrigation and perfusion solution used for cerebrospinal surgery; Otsuka Pharmaceutical Factory, Inc., Naruto, Japan) to a concentration of 5×10^7 cells/mL.

Intervention

On the day when HUNS001–01 is manufactured, the cell product will be administered to the subject. A dose of 2×10^7 cells (400 μL) will be administered in the low-dose group and a dose of 5×10^7 cells (1000 μL) will be administered in the high-dose group. HUNS001–01 is implanted using MRI stereotactic technique to define the target sites in the normal white matter around the lesion. The number of target sites is one or two in the low-dose group, and two or three in the high-dose group. The subject has a one or two burr-hole craniotomy under local anesthesia and sedation. Using 2.1-mm outer diameter stereotactic cannula, 200 to 500 μL of the product is injected over a period of 5 min at each site. The cannula is removed after 5 min after finishing the injection at each site. In the perioperative period, all subjects take fosphenytoin sodium hydrate to prevent epileptic seizure due to the procedure.

End point of the study

Primary end point

- Safety of HUNS001–01 administration for 1 year after the intervention: frequency of Adverse Event (AE)

Secondary end points

- Safety of HUNS001–01 administration for 30 days after the intervention: frequency of Adverse Event (AE)
- Safety of bone marrow aspiration: frequency of Adverse Event (AE)
- Frequency of the defects of HUNS001–01 at manufacturing
- Improvement of stroke symptoms for 1 year after the intervention using the following assessment scales:
  - ational Institute of Health Stroke Scale (NIHSS)
  - modified Rankin Scale (mRS)
  - Functional Independence Measure (FIM)
  - Barthel Index
  - Fugl-Meyer Assessment
- Improvement in lesion volume assessed by MRI analysis for 1 year after the intervention
- Assessment of cell distribution using MRI
- Assessment of possible functional shift for 1 year after the intervention using FDG-PET and IMZ-SPECT

Follow-up of study

The schedule of follow-up of study is as follows (Table 1):

- Vital signs, serological, and biochemical tests: Days 0, 1, 3, 7, 14, 30, 90, 180, 360
- Urinalysis: Days 30, 90, 180, 360
- Urine hCG-β (if needed): Days 90, 180, 360
- 12-lead electrocardiogram and chest X-ray examination: Days 1, 7, 30, 90, 360
- Neurological examination (NIHSS, mRS, FIM, Barthel Index, Fugl-Meyer Assessment): Days 1, 3, 7, 14, 30, 90, 180, 360
- MRI: Days 0, 3, 7, 14, 30, 90, 180, 360
- FDG-PET and IMZ-SPECT: Days 30, 90, 360

Data collection and monitoring

All data are collected by appointed staff members, who are approved by the Clinical Research and Medical Innovation Center, Hokkaido University Hospital. They are monitored by the Standard Operating Procedures (SOPs) of Good Clinical Practice (GCP) and the ICH guidelines.

Ethics and dissemination

This trial is conducted following the GCP guidelines and the principles of the Declaration of Helsinki. The data obtained in this study will be disseminated in peer-reviewed journals and presented at international scientific meetings.

Discussion

Subject screening

Current therapeutic strategies for ischemic stroke typically aim to improve blood flow in ischemic areas or to relieve neuronal damage through neuroprotective effects before the ischemic disorder is established. However, in

Table 1 The schedule of follow-up of study

	Screening			Follow up									
	1st screening	BM hervest	2nd screening	Pre-administration	Post-administration								
	Onset to14 days		Day −7 (±1)	Day 0		Day 1	Day 3	Day 7	Day 14	Day 30 (±3)	Day 90 (±30)	Day 180 (±30)	Day 360 (±30)
Informed consent	X												
Medical history	X												
Vital signs	X	X	X	X	X	X	X	X	X	X	X	X	X
Body weight and height	X												
Serological tests	X		X		X	X	X	X	X	X	X	X	X
Biochemical tests	X		X		X	X	X	X	X	X	X	X	X
Urinalysis	X		X							X	X	X	X
Urine hCG-β (If needed)	X									X	X	X	X
Infectious disease inspection	X												
12-lead electrocardiogram	X		X			X		X		X	X		X
Chest X-ray examination	X		X			X		X		X	X		X
Neurological examination	X		X			X		X		X	X	X	X
MRI	X		X	X	X		X	X	X	X	X	X	X
FDG-PET and IMZ-SPECT			X							X	X		X
Bone marrow harvest		X											
Cell product administration				X									
Concomitant medication	X	X	X	X	X	X	X	X	X	X	X	X	X
Adverse events	X	X	X	X	X	X	X	X	X	X	X	X	X

cell therapy, some strategies aim to resolve neurological disorders resulting from an established cerebral infarction. Autologous cell products, in particular, require time for tissue collection and manufacturing. If changes in a subject's condition are anticipated during the manufacturing period, appropriate screening at the start of the administration, as well as at the enrollment should be established.

In our trial, NIHSS score is assessed in the first screening on day 14 after the onset. The NIHSS is used for systematic assessment of potential symptoms and signs of stroke, and is designed primarily to assess symptoms and signs in the acute phase and to determine the severity of the disease. On the other hand, mRS, which is one of the disability measures, has been widely used as an efficacy endpoint in clinical trials all over the world. In our trial, mRS is examined in the second screening, 7 days before the administration. H, the NIHSS score on admission is inadequate for the first screening. Due to the weak correlation with the mRS score in chronic phase, possible dropouts are expected at the second screening. In fact, Kimura et al. reported that approximately half of the subjects with NIHSS scores of 7–10 at admission would have an mRS score of 0–2 at discharge [16]. We adopted the NIHSS on day 14 after the onset, but not on admission, as the first screening, because it has a stronger correlation with the mRS score and other outcome scales in the chronic phase [17].

In the trial, we enrolled patients who met the inclusion criteria of a total score of NIHSS ≥6, and a "Motor Arm" and "Motor Leg" score of NIHSS ≥6 at the first screening, since the improvement of injured motor function is an anticipated result of the administration of HUNS001–01.

Safety measures for intraparenchymal injection

Intraparenchymal injection is a technique to administer cells directly into the cerebral parenchyma. This technique can deliver numerous cells selectively to peri-infarct regions. Attention should be paid to possible complications of trepanation and cerebral puncture, such as epilepsy and hemorrhage due to cerebral injuries. In 2005, Kondziolka et al. reported a phase 2 trial with LBS-Neurons (human teratocarcinoma cell line origin, Layton BioScience, Inc.) [18]. They adopted the intraparenchymal cell transplantation technique for 14 patients with stroke. Serial evaluations demonstrated that one patient had a single seizure and one had an asymptomatic chronic subdural hematoma. In a recent report, Steinberg et al. described a phase 1/2A study, with SB623 cells (SanBio Inc., CA, USA) [19]. Eighteen patients with ischemic stroke underwent stereotactic transplantation in the chronic phase. In this trial, one patient had a single seizure and one had asymptomatic chronic subdural fluid collection.

In our protocol, all subjects will be taking fosphenytoin sodium hydrate to prevent epileptic seizures in the perioperative period. Moreover, we use a round head stereotactic cannula to prevent hemorrhagic events due to the procedure, while a thin and pointed cannula was used in the two previously mentioned trials.

The sample size of the trial was based on the traditional 3 + 3 dose escalation design. Indeed, it may be difficult to reach statistically significant differences with small number (6 to 10) of patients, but we think that such a small population can verify the safety. For examples, Savitz et al. reported the safety concerns of clinical trials about the stereotactic transplantation with LGE cells (Genvec Inc.) in only 5 stroke patients [20]. Because 2 patients had the adverse effects (the temporary worsening of motor deficits 3 weeks after transplantation and the seizures 1 week after transplantation), the trial was terminated by the FDA.

Administration dose

In our protocol, the administration dose was determined based on our own preclinical rodent study and prior clinical trials. In our preclinical safety study, immunodeficient rats received 1×10^6 BMSCs in the brain parenchyma. When the data was extrapolated, we determined that this is equivalent to an administration cell dose of 7×10^8 cells in humans. Because the highest dose used in the trial is 5×10^7 cells (high-dose group), which is one-fourteenth of the extrapolated dose, we concluded that this dose is adequate to investigate safety as the objects of the study.

Honmou et al. reported a phase 1/2 trial using autologous MSCs [21]. Twelve patients with acute cerebral infarction received an intravenous cell infusion (mean cell dose: 1×10^8 cells). They showed improvement in neurologic symptoms in 11 patients and concluded that intravenous administration of autologous MSCs may be effective for treatment of patients with acute cerebral infarction. In our previous study on cell delivery routes, however, we observed that intraparenchymal injection is a more favorable method for cell delivery to the lesion and improvement of the motor function than intravenous infusion [22]. When only one-third dose of BMSCs (1×10^6 cells) was delivered using intraparenchymal injection in a rat stroke model, the injured motor function was improved significantly compared with BMSC intravenous administration (3×10^6 cells). When we extrapolated data from the preclinical findings, we determined that one-third dose of BMSC (3.3×10^7 cells) would be more effective when administered via intraparenchymal injection than intravenous infusion. In our protocol, two doses of 2×10^7 and 5×10^7 cells were used. Thus, former is a lower dose of 3.3×10^7 cells, whereas the latter is an upper dose. The significance of dose-response relationships of cell products has not been established sufficiently. The low-dose group may be more effective because of a shorter cell culture period and earlier administration. Moreover, not only cell dose, but also administration site should be optimized. In our trial, these controversial variables may be solved using bioimaging methods, cell tracking using MRI, and assessment of functional shift using FDG-PET and IMZ-SPECT.

Time point of cell administration

In the protocol, we cannot provide the exact time point of cell administration. The autologous cells need a period for cell culture before the administration. We expect that the range of the period will be from 2 to 5 weeks, and then we will administer the cells as soon as possible. But the period may be prolonged due to some factors, for examples, aging of subjects. We set the dead line of the administration to 74 days after stroke onset, which means the culture period is set for maximum 60 days, because delayed cell administration may miss the therapeutic time window and the cells with too slow growth may be unhealthy or ineffective.

Abbreviations

AE: Adverse Event; BMMNC: Bone marrow mononuclear cell; BMSC: Bone marrow stromal cell; CNS: Central nervous system; CPC: Cell processing center; FCS: Fetal calf serum; FDG-PET: ^{18}F- fluorodeoxyglucose positron emission tomography; FIM: Functional Independence Measure; GCP: Good clinical practice; GMP: Good manufacturing practice; HBV: Hepatitis B virus; HCV: Hepatitis C virus; HIV: Human immunodeficiency virus; hPL: Human platelet lysate; HTLV: Human T cell leukemia virus; IMZSPECT: ^{123}I–Iomazenil singlephoton emission computed tomography; ISCT: International society for cellular therapy; JCS: Japan coma scale; MRI: Magnetic resonance imaging; mRS: Modified rankin scale; NIHSS: National institute of health stroke scale; RAINBOW: Research on advanced intervention using novel bone marrow stem cell; SOP: Standard Operating Procedure; SPIO: Superparamagnetic iron oxide; ULN: Upper limit of normal; UMIN: The university hospital medical information network

Acknowledgements

The authors thank Dr. Shigeru Takamoto and his staffs in Japanese Red Cross, Hokkaido Block Blood Center as suppliers of human platelet concentrate, and the staffs at CPC in Hokkaido University Hospital.

Funding

The study was supported by Initiative for Accelerating Regulatory Science in Innovative Drug, Medical Device, and Regenerative Medicine (Funds from Ministry of Health, Labour and Welfare in Japan) and Research Project for Practical Applications of Regenerative Medicine (Funds from Japan Agency for Medical Research and Development).

Authors' contributions

MK is the principal investigator, responsible for conception, design, and processing of the trial. KH had the original concept of the trial. HS designed the trial and wrote/reviewed all protocol versions. TA1, NN, KK and ST reviewed all protocol versions and contributed by start-up of the trial. TT and TA2 participated in the protocol validity and conducting of this trial. HI devised the statistical plan. All authors read and approved the final manuscript.

Competing interests

All authors declare that they have no competing interests.

References

1. Azizi SA, Stokes D, Augelli BJ, DiGirolamo C, Prockop DJ. Engraftment and migration of human bone marrow stromal cells implanted in the brains of albino rats–similarities to astrocyte grafts. Proc Natl Acad Sci U S A. 1998; 95(7):3908–13.
2. Abe K, Yamashita T, Takizawa S, Kuroda S, Kinouchi H, Kawahara N. Stem cell therapy for cerebral ischemia: from basic science to clinical applications. J Cereb Blood Flow Metab. 2012;32(7):1317–31.
3. Bliss T, Guzman R, Daadi M, Steinberg GK. Cell transplantation therapy for stroke. Stroke. 2007;38(2 Suppl):817–26.
4. Tan C, Shichinohe H, Wang Z, Hamauchi S, Abumiya T, Nakayama N, Kazumata K, Ito T, Kudo K, Takamoto S, et al. Feasibility and efficiency of human bone marrow Stromal cell culture with Allogeneic platelet Lysate-supplementation for cell therapy against stroke. Stem Cells Int. 2016;2016:6104780.
5. Shichinohe H, Kuroda S, Sugiyama T, Ito M, Kawabori M, Nishio M, Takeda Y, Koike T, Houkin K. Biological features of human bone marrow Stromal cells (hBMSC) cultured with animal protein-free medium-safety and efficacy of clinical use for Neurotransplantation. Transl Stroke Res. 2011;2(3):307–15.
6. Shichinohe H, Ishihara T, Takahashi K, Tanaka Y, Miyamoto M, Yamauchi T, Saito H, Takemoto H, Houkin K, Kuroda S. Bone marrow stromal cells rescue ischemic brain by trophic effects and phenotypic change toward neural cells. Neurorehabil Neural Repair. 2015;29(1):80–9.
7. Bang OY, Lee JS, Lee PH, Lee G. Autologous mesenchymal stem cell transplantation in stroke patients. Ann Neurol. 2005;57(6):874–82.
8. Shichinohe H, Houkin K. Cell therapy for stroke: review of previous clinical trials and introduction of our new trials. Neurol Med Chir (Tokyo). 2016; 56(10):592–6.
9. Sugiyama T, Kuroda S, Takeda Y, Nishio M, Ito M, Shichinohe H, Koike T. Therapeutic impact of human bone marrow stromal cells (hbmsc) expanded by animal serum-free medium for cerebral infarct in rats. Neurosurgery. 2011;68(6):1733–42.
10. Ito M, Kuroda S, Sugiyama T, Shichinohe H, Takeda Y, Nishio M, Koike T, Houkin K. Validity of bone marrow stromal cell expansion by animal serum-free medium for cell transplantation therapy of cerebral infarct in rats-a serial MRI study. Trans Stroke Res. 2011;2(3):294–306.
11. Miyamoto M, Kuroda S, Zhao S, Magota K, Shichinohe H, Houkin K, Kuge Y, Tamaki N. Bone marrow stromal cell transplantation enhances recovery of local glucose metabolism after cerebral infarction in rats: a serial 18F-FDG PET study. J Nucl Med : official Publi, Soc Nucl Med. 2013;54(1):145–50.
12. Saito H, Magota K, Zhao S, Kubo N, Kuge Y, Shichinohe H, Houkin K, Tamaki N, Kuroda S. 123I-iomazenil single photon emission computed tomography visualizes recovery of neuronal integrity by bone marrow stromal cell therapy in rat infarct brain. Stroke. 2013;44(10):2869–74.
13. Shichinohe H, Yamauchi T, Saito H, Houkin K, Kuroda S. Bone marrow stromal cell transplantation enhances recovery of motor function after lacunar stroke in rats. Acta Neurobiol Exp (Wars). 2013;73(3):354–63.
14. Tan C, Shichinohe H, Abumiya T, Nakayama N, Kazumata K, Hokari M, Hamauchi S, Houkin K. Short-, middle- and long-term safety of superparamagnetic iron oxide-labeled allogeneic bone marrow stromal cell transplantation in rat model of lacunar infarction. Neuropathology. 2015; 35(3):197–208.
15. Dominici M, Le Blanc K, Mueller I, Slaper-Cortenbach I, Marini F, Krause D, Deans R, Keating A, Prockop D, Horwitz E. Minimal criteria for defining multipotent mesenchymal stromal cells. The International Society for Cellular Therapy position statement. Cytotherapy. 2006;8(4):315–7.
16. Kimura K, Kazui S, Minematsu K, Yamaguchi T. Japan multicenter stroke Investigator's C: analysis of 16,922 patients with acute ischemic stroke and transient ischemic attack in Japan. A hospital-based prospective registration study. Cerebrovasc Dis. 2004;18(1):47–56.
17. Lyden P, Lu M, Jackson C, Marler J, Kothari R, Brott T, Zivin J. Underlying structure of the National Institutes of Health stroke scale: results of a factor analysis. NINDS tPA stroke trial investigators. Stroke. 1999;30(11):2347–54.
18. Kondziolka D, Steinberg GK, Wechsler L, Meltzer CC, Elder E, Gebel J, Decesare S, Jovin T, Zafonte R, Lebowitz J, et al. Neurotransplantation for patients with subcortical motor stroke: a phase 2 randomized trial. J Neurosurg. 2005;103(1):38–45.
19. Steinberg GK, Kondziolka D, Wechsler LR, Lunsford LD, Coburn ML, Billigen JB, Kim AS, Johnson JN, Bates D, King B, et al. Clinical outcomes of transplanted modified bone marrow-derived Mesenchymal stem cells in stroke: a phase 1/2a study. Stroke. 2016;47(7):1817–24.
20. Savitz SI, Dinsmore J, Wu J, Henderson GV, Stieg P, Caplan LR. Neurotransplantation of fetal porcine cells in patients with basal ganglia infarcts: a preliminary safety and feasibility study. Cerebrovasc Dis. 2005; 20(2):101–7.
21. Honmou O, Houkin K, Matsunaga T, Niitsu Y, Ishiai S, Onodera R, Waxman SG, Kocsis JD. Intravenous administration of auto serum-expanded autologous mesenchymal stem cells in stroke. Brain. 2011;134(Pt 6):1790–807.
22. Kawabori M, Kuroda S, Sugiyama T, Ito M, Shichinohe H, Houkin K, Kuge Y, Tamaki N. Intracerebral, but not intravenous, transplantation of bone marrow stromal cells enhances functional recovery in rat cerebral infarct: an optical imaging study. Neuropathology. 2012;32(3):217–26.

Elevated blood viscosity is associated with cerebral small vessel disease in patients with acute ischemic stroke

Seung Hoon Song[1], Jeong Hee Kim[1], Joon Hwa Lee[1], Yeo-Min Yun[2], Dong-Hee Choi[3] and Hahn Young Kim[1*]

Abstract

Background: Increased level of blood viscosity, which is one of the major factors that determine blood rheology, has been reported as a risk factor or predictor for cerebrovascular events. We investigated how blood viscosity is associated with acute stroke and chronic radiological manifestations of cerebral small vessel disease, and how blood viscosity changes after stroke.

Methods: We prospectively enrolled consecutive patients with acute ischemic stroke. Whole blood viscosities at a low or high shear rate were measured using a scanning capillary tube viscometer, and were referred to as diastolic blood viscosity (DBV) and systolic blood viscosity (SBV), respectively. Correlations between blood viscosity and acute stroke etiology or chronic radiological manifestations of cerebral small vessel disease were investigated. The temporal profiles of blood viscosity at the onset of stroke and follow-up at 1 and 5 weeks were investigated.

Results: Of the 127 patients admitted with acute ischemic stroke, 63 patients were included in the final analyses. DBV at the onset of stroke was significantly higher in small artery occlusion (SAO) stroke than in other stroke subtypes ($p = 0.037$). DBV showed a significant positive correlation with the number of chronic lacunes ($r = 0.274$, $p = 0.030$). The temporal profiles of DBV in SAO stroke showed a transient decrease due to the hydration therapy after 1 week and recurrent elevation at 5 week follow-up ($p = 0.009$).

Conclusions: Our study suggests that elevated DBV may play a role in the development of acute and chronic manifestations of cerebral small vessel disease. The recurring elevation of DBV in SAO stroke indicates that sufficient hydration and additional therapeutic interventions targeting blood viscosity may be needed in patients with SAO stroke.

Keywords: Blood viscosity, Small vessel disease, Small artery occlusion, Lacunes, Ischemic stroke

Background

Increased fibrinogen level, whole blood viscosity, and plasma viscosity, which are major factors that determine blood rheology, have been reported as risk factors or predictors for various cardio- or cerebrovascular events [1–11]. Whole blood viscosity can be determined through the complex interactions of blood constituents, including red blood cells, white blood cells, platelets, fibrinogen, and other plasma proteins [12, 13]. Whole blood viscosity measured at a high shear rate of 300 s^{-1} or more is referred to as systolic blood viscosity (SBV) [14, 15]. Blood viscosity at a high shear rate represents the frictional characteristics of fast blood flow, defined as having a velocity of over 30 cm/s in a vessel with a large diameter [13]. In the high blood flow state, the inertia force representing the kinetic energy is much larger than the viscous force that arises from the blood viscosity [15]. Therefore, blood flow is predominantly determined by the inertia force rather than the viscous force [15]. Meanwhile, the whole blood viscosity measured at a low shear rate of 5 s^{-1} or less is referred to as diastolic blood viscosity (DBV) [14, 15]. In the low blood flow

* Correspondence: hykimmd@gmail.com
[1]Department of Neurology, Research Institute of Medical Science, Konkuk University School of Medicine, Konkuk University Medical Center, Seoul, Republic of Korea
Full list of author information is available at the end of the article

state, in which the blood flows through a vessel with a smaller diameter or through the distal part of an occluded vascular segment, blood viscosity becomes a critical factor for determining the tissue perfusion status [13]. Therefore, DBV may be attributed more to the pathophysiology of small vessel disease than SBV. In the case of coronary microvascular dysfunction without definite occlusion of the main coronary artery, i.e. microvascular angina, increased blood viscosity may play a key role in the deterioration of tissue perfusion at a microvascular level [16]. A comparable microvascular dysfunction in the brain may be chronic cerebral ischemia due to cerebral small vessel disease [17, 18]. Radiological manifestations, such as white matter hyperintensities, lacunes, and microbleeds, are known consequences of impaired microvascular perfusion in the brain and chronic radiological markers for cerebral small vessel disease [19, 20].

The role of blood viscosity has been reported in the stroke population [1–7]. Previous studies, which included stroke subtype in the scope of their studies, have suggested that the blood viscosity measured in small artery occlusion (SAO) stroke was higher than in other stroke subtypes, such as large artery atherosclerosis (LAA) and/or cardioembolism (CE) [2–4]. Based on these previous studies, we hypothesized that blood viscosity may be closely associated with acute or chronic manifestations of cerebral small vessel disease. We first questioned how blood viscosity is related to different etiologies leading to acute stroke. Second, we asked how blood viscosity is associated with the chronic radiological manifestations of cerebral small vessel disease. Third, we asked if there is an abnormality in blood viscosity in relation to acute stroke, how it changes after acute stroke. For the first two questions, we investigated which stroke subtype at the onset of index stroke and which chronic radiological manifestations, including white matter hyperintensities, lacunes, and microbleeds, are correlated with blood viscosity in patients with acute ischemic stroke. For the last question, the temporal profiles of blood viscosity at both stroke onset and follow-up were investigated.

Methods

Patients and blood sampling

We prospectively enrolled consecutive acute ischemic stroke patients who had been admitted within 3 days of the onset of stroke, from July 2013 to February 2014. Acute ischemic stroke was confirmed by diffusion-weighted magnetic resonance imaging (MRI) in all patients. To minimize the diluting effect on blood viscosity by hydration therapy, the blood samples used to measure the baseline blood viscosity levels were obtained during the initial blood sampling procedure in the emergency room prior to any medical intervention including hydration therapy. Follow-up measurements of blood viscosity were performed twice, at 1 week and 5 weeks after the baseline measurement. To minimize the transient diluting effect by oral hydration, the samples for the follow-up measurement were obtained under fasting state. Patients were instructed not to eat or drink anything, including water, after taking their evening pills until blood sampling was performed early the next morning. Blood samples from patients diagnosed with stroke mimic during the same study period were used with permission, for comparison with those from patients with acute ischemic stroke. This study was approved by the institutional review board of the Konkuk University Hospital. Written informed consent was obtained from each patient.

Clinical evaluation

The vascular risk factors and laboratory findings affecting blood viscosity including hemoglobin, hematocrit, white blood cells, platelets, blood protein, fibrinogen, D-dimer, BUN/Cr (blood urea nitrogen-to-creatinine) ratio, and lipid profiles were investigated. The patients were considered to have hypertension if they were on medication for hypertension or had a blood pressure of ≥140/90 mmHg on repeated measurement. Similarly, the patients were considered to have diabetes mellitus if they were on medication for diabetes or had a fasting blood sugar ≥126 mg/dl; and to have hyperlipidemia if they were on lipid-lowering medications or had an overnight fasting cholesterol level ≥220 mg/dl or low-density lipoprotein cholesterol level ≥140 mg/dl. Smoking was defined by the current smoking status. The stroke subtype was classified according to the modified Trial of Org 10172 in Acute Stroke Treatment classification [21].

Blood viscosity measurement

A scanning capillary tube viscometer (BVD-PR01, BioVisco Inc., Korea) was used to measure whole blood viscosity [15]. The scanning capillary tube viscometer simultaneously measures the SBV and DBV, which correspond to the whole blood viscosities at high and low shear rates, respectively [15]. Samples containing 3 mL whole blood were collected in a vacutainer containing ethylenediaminetetraacetic acid (EDTA) anticoagulant and stored in a refrigerator at 4 °C until measurement. All the measurements were performed within 24 h of the collection. The whole blood viscosity was measured over a wide range of shear rates, ranging from 1 to 1000 s^{-1}. In the low shear rate range of 5 s^{-1} or less, a whole blood viscosity level of 1 s^{-1} was selected as the DBV for our study. In the high shear rate range of 300 s^{-1} or more, a whole blood viscosity level of 300 s^{-1} was selected as the SBV for our study.

Radiological evaluation

T1-weighted, T2-weighted, fluid attenuation inversion recovery (FLAIR), and T2* gradient-echo images were obtained using a 3 T MR system (Signa HDx; GE Medical Systems, Milwaukee, WI, USA). The T1- and T2-weighted images were obtained during the same imaging session at the same orientation and slice position: matrix, 128; field of view, 280 × 280 mm; section thickness, 5 mm; intersection space, 2 mm. The radiological manifestations associated with small vessel disease in the brain, such as white matter hyperintensities, lacunes, and microbleeds were subsequently defined. The severity of white matter hyperintensities on FLAIR images were assessed by a scale of periventricular hyperintensity (PVH) and deep white matter hyperintensity (DWMH) according to the Fazekas scale [22]. Lacunes were distinguished from white matter ischemic changes as small distinct lesions (<15 mm in diameter) with a low signal on T1-weighted images, a high signal on T2-weighted images, and perilesional gliotic changes on FLAIR images [23]. Lacunes usually had a hyperintense rim around the cavity on FLAIR images, unlike Virchow Robin spaces or white matter ischemic changes. Acute lacunar infarctions that presented as an index stroke when enrolling patients, were not included in the analysis. Only previous chronic lacunes were included, regardless of whether they were symptomatic or asymptomatic. A microbleed was defined as a small, homogenous, round signal loss lesion (<10 mm in diameter) on T2* gradient-echo images [23].

Statistical analysis

The differences in vascular risk factors or laboratory findings were assessed using a chi square test for dichotomized variables, and either an independent *t* test, Mann-Whitney *U* test, or analysis of variance (ANOVA) with a Tukey's post-hoc test for continuous variables, where appropriate. The association between SAO stroke and the laboratory variables was assessed using a calculation of crude or adjusted odds ratios with 95% confidence intervals through uni- or multivariate logistic models. The associations among the laboratory findings, including DBV, SBV, hematocrit, and fibrinogen levels were analyzed using a Pearson correlation. The associations between laboratory and radiological findings were also analyzed using a Pearson correlation. Differences were considered statistically significant at p values of < 0.05. All statistical analyses were performed using SPSS version 17.0.

Results

Patient enrollment

Of the 127 consecutive patients with acute ischemic stroke admitted during the study period from July 2013 to February 2014, samples for blood viscosity measurement were obtained from 70 patients (Fig. 1). In order to homogenize the study population, 16 patients with a stroke onset of more than 3 days, 4 patients whose stroke was not confirmed by diffusion-weighted MRI, 6 patients with stroke of other determined etiology, and 7 patients with severe medical or neurological status were excluded. Of the 94 patients eligible for the study, 24 patients refused to provide written informed consent. Seven samples were discarded due to either technical errors or poor quality. Thus, data from 63 patients were analyzed in our study. Sixteen patients were included in the stroke mimic group, which was comprised of 7 patients with non-specific dizziness, 5 patients with transient weakness without a vascular cause, 3 patients with vestibular neuronitis, and 1 patient with hypochondriasis. Patients with

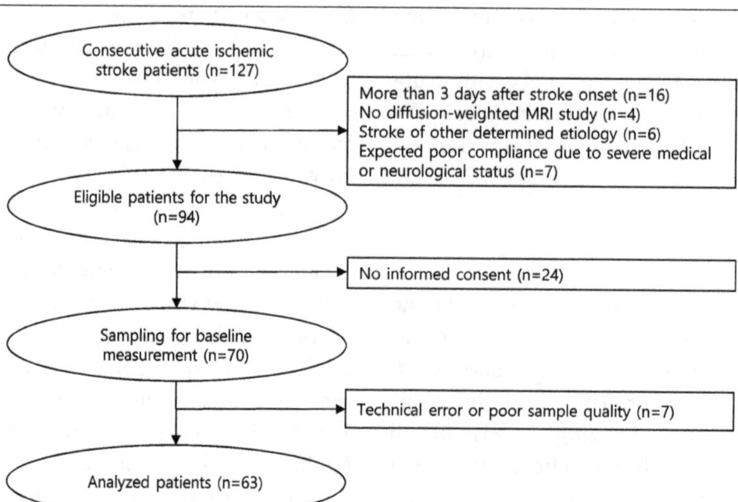

Fig. 1 Patient enrollment flow chart

suspected transient ischemic attack (TIA) were not included in the stroke mimic group because TIA can be also influenced by blood viscosity.

Demographic and clinical characteristics of patients

The clinical demographics, radiological findings, and laboratory findings of patients are presented in Table 1. The most frequent stroke subtype was SAO ($n = 25$, 39.7%) followed by LAA ($n = 23$, 36.5%), CE ($n = 12$, 19.0%), and cryptogenic stroke (Cryp; $n = 3$, 4.8%). The prevalence of vascular risk factors, except for atrial fibrillation, were not different among the stroke subtypes (Table 1).

Blood viscosity, hematocrit, and blood fibrinogen level

The DBV and SBV were significantly correlated with each other ($r = 0.456$, $p < 0.001$). The DBV was significantly correlated with hematocrit ($r = 0.421$, $p = 0.001$; Fig. 2a) and the SBV with blood fibrinogen level ($r = 0.340$, $p = 0.01$; Fig. 2d).

Blood viscosity and stroke subtypes

The baseline DBV was 274.7 ± 70.9 mP in SAO, followed by 258.9 ± 46.5 mP in Cryp, 252.0 ± 57.5 mP in CE, and 214.5 ± 75.9 mP in LAA stroke subtypes. The baseline DBV in SAO was significantly higher than that in other stroke subtypes ($p = 0.037$). In addition, the post-hoc test revealed that the baseline DBV in SAO was significantly

Table 1 Clinical demographics, radiological findings, and laboratory findings for the 63 patients included in the study

	Total (*n* = 63)				
	SAO (*n* = 25, 39.7%)	LAA (*n* = 23, 36.5%)	CE (*n* = 12, 19.0%)	Cryp (*n* = 3, 4.8%)	*P* value
Blood viscosity (mean ± sd)					
Diastolic blood viscosity, mP	274.7 ± 70.9	214.5 ± 75.9	252.0 ± 57.5	258.9 ± 46.5	0.037*
Systolic blood viscosity, mP	45.2 ± 16.0	38.1 ± 12.4	40.0 ± 4.9	39.0 ± 4.7	0.273
Clinical findings					
Age, years (mean ± sd)	62.7 ± 12.9	67.0 ± 15.5	71.2 ± 11.6	63.3 ± 7.5	0.335
Male, *n* (%)	19 (76)	13 (57)	7 (58)	2 (67)	0.513
Hypertension, *n* (%)	16 (64)	16 (70)	5 (42)	3 (100)	0.207
Diabetes, *n* (%)	6 (24)	7 (30)	3 (25)	0 (0)	0.716
Hyperlipidemia, *n* (%)	6 (24)	3 (13)	1 (8)	0 (0)	0.484
Atrial fibrillation, *n* (%)	0 (0)	0 (0)	9 (75)	0 (0)	<0.001
Smoking, *n* (%)	14 (56)	8 (35)	2 (17)	0 (0)	0.053
Radiological findings, median (IQR)					
PVH, Fazekas scale	1 (1–2)	1 (1–2)	1 (1–3)	2 (0–2)	0.872
DWMH, Fazekas scale	1 (0–1.5)	1 (0–2)	1 (0–2.75)	1 (0–1)	0.834
Number of chronic lacunes	1 (0–3)	0 (0–2)	1 (0–2.75)	1 (0–2)	0.255
Number of microbleeds	0 (0–2.5)	0 (0–1)	1 (0–2)	0 (0–2)	0.869
Laboratory findings (mean ± sd)					
Hemoglobin, g/dL	14.9 ± 1.8	13.9 ± 1.9	13.6 ± 1.7	13.7 ± 1.9	0.129
Hematocrit, %	43.4 ± 5.2	40.9 ± 5.0	39.8 ± 4.4	40.0 ± 5.0	0.135
White blood cells, 10^3/μL	7.2 ± 2.0	7.6 ± 2.9	9.5 ± 3.6	6.8 ± 2.6	0.110
Platelets, 10^3/μL	238 ± 56	227 ± 48	233 ± 80	199 ± 40	0.700
Total protein, gm/dL	7.1 ± 0.5	7.0 ± 0.4	7.2 ± 0.5	7.2 ± 0.1	0.429
Fibrinogen, mg/dL	323 ± 78	335 ± 71	357 ± 70	215 ± 44	0.099
D-dimer, μg/dL	0.44 ± 0.32	0.75 ± 0.92	1.51 ± 1.93	0.28 ± 0.10	0.038**
BUN/Cr ratio	19.0 ± 4.6	23.1 ± 8.2	21.1 ± 5.3	17.3 ± 5.1	0.115
Total cholesterol, mg/dL	176 ± 36	177 ± 28	155 ± 56	140 ± 32	0.192
Low-density lipoprotein, mg/dL	109 ± 32	108 ± 22	94 ± 50	80 ± 30	0.319
Triglycerides, mg/dL	127 ± 61	116 ± 80	70 ± 60	60 ± 35	0.078

Abbreviations: *SAO* small artery occlusion, *LAA* large artery atherosclerosis, *CE* cardioembolism, *Cryp* cryptogenic stroke, *sd* standard deviation, *IQR* interquartile range, *PVH* periventricular hyperintensity, *DWMH* deep white matter hyperintensity, *BUN/Cr* blood urea nitrogen-to-creatinine

*, $p = 0.021$, SAO vs. LAA in the post-hoc test; **, $p = 0.027$, SAO vs. CE in the post-hoc test

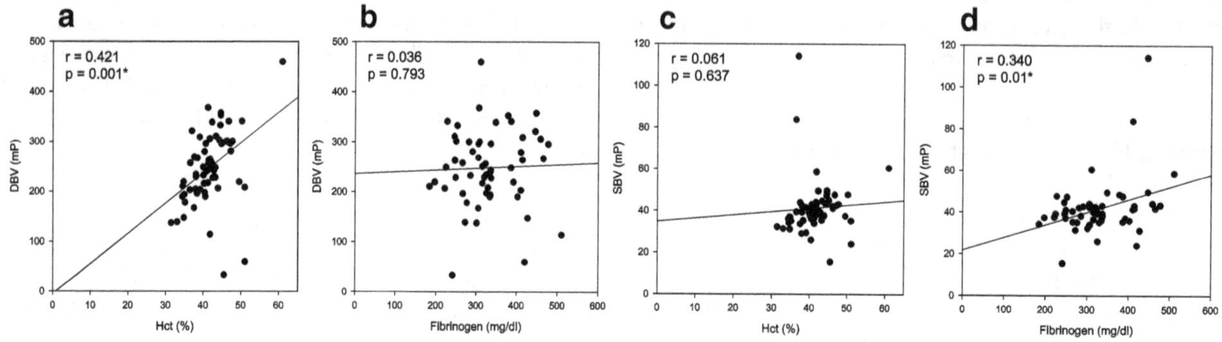

Fig. 2 The correlation of diastolic blood viscosity with hematocrit **a** and blood fibrinogen level **b**. The correlation of systolic blood viscosity with hematocrit **c** and blood fibrinogen level **d**. *, $p < 0.05$; *DBV*, diastolic blood viscosity; *SBV*, systolic blood viscosity; *Hct*, hematocrit

higher compared to that of LAA ($p = 0.021$; Table 1 and Fig. 3a). Among laboratory variables which were significantly associated with SAO stroke in the univariate analysis, such as DBV, hemoglobin, and hematocrit, only DBV was still significant in the multivariate analysis adjusted for multiple vascular risk factors, including age, sex, hypertension, diabetes, hyperlipidemia, atrial fibrillation, and smoking (p = 0.033; Table 2). The DBV in the stroke mimic group was 240.8 ± 38.1 mP. Laboratory findings affecting blood viscosity were not different among the stroke subtypes, except for elevated D-dimer level in CE (Table 1). The baseline SBV, hematocrit, blood fibrinogen level, and BUN/Cr ratio were not different among the stroke subtypes (Fig. 3b, c, d and e).

Blood viscosity and chronic radiological manifestations of cerebral small vessel disease

The correlations between the major determinants of blood viscosity such as the DBV, SBV, hematocrit, and blood fibrinogen level and the chronic radiological manifestations of cerebral small vessel disease such as white matter hyperintensities, lacunes, and microbleeds, were investigated in all the patients regardless of the stroke subtype. A statistically significant correlation was observed between the DBV and the number of chronic lacunes ($r = 0.274$, $p = 0.030$; Fig. 4a). The DBV showed trends for positive correlation with the severity of PVH ($r = 0.135$, $p = 0.291$; Fig. 4a) or the number of microbleeds ($r = 0.145$, $p = 0.256$; Fig. 4a), although neither reached statistical significance. The SBV, hematocrit, and blood fibrinogen level were not significantly correlated with any of the radiological manifestations (Fig. 4b, c, and d).

Temporal blood viscosity profiles

The follow-up blood viscosity was measured in 41 out of the 63 patients (65.1%). The patients who were followed up and those who were not followed up were not

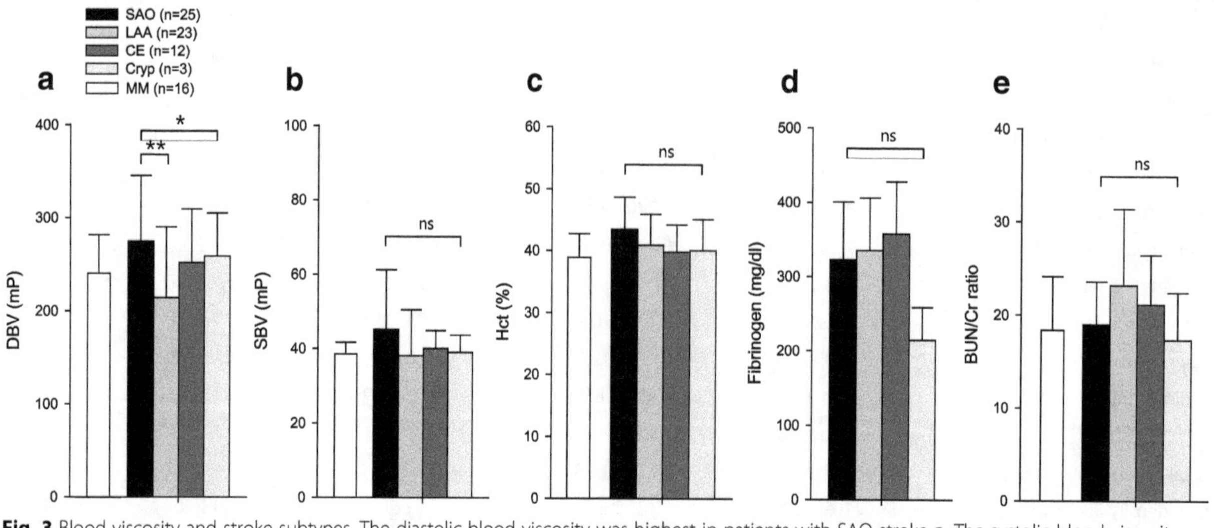

Fig. 3 Blood viscosity and stroke subtypes. The diastolic blood viscosity was highest in patients with SAO stroke **a**. The systolic blood viscosity, hematocrit, blood fibrinogen level, and BUN/Cr ratio were not different among the stroke subtypes **b**, **c**, **d**, and **e**. *$p < 0.05$ on ANOVA; **$p < 0.05$ on the post-hoc test; ns, not significant; *SAO*, small artery occlusion; *LAA*, large artery atherosclerosis; *CE*, cardioembolism; *Cryp*, cryptogenic stroke; *MM*, stroke mimic; *DBV*, diastolic blood viscosity; *SBV*, systolic blood viscosity; *Hct*, hematocrit; *BUN*, blood urea nitrogen

Table 2 Crude and adjusted odds ratios for the association with small artery occlusion stroke

	Univariate analysis		Multivariate analysis	
	Crude OR (95% CI)	*P* value	Adjusted OR (95% CI)**	*P* value
Diastolic blood viscosity (per 1mP)	1.01 (1.00–1.02)	0.023*	1.01 (1.00–1.02)	0.033*
Systolic blood viscosity (per 1mP)	1.05 (0.99–1.12)	0.099	1.05 (0.99–1.10)	0.111
Hemoglobin (per 1 g/dL)	1.42 (1.04–1.94)	0.026*	1.27 (0.87–1.85)	0.223
Hematocrit (per 1%)	1.14 (1.01–1.28)	0.032*	1.09 (0.94–1.25)	0.252
Fibrinogen (per 1 mg/dL)	1.00 (0.99–1.01)	0.560	1.00 (0.99–1.01)	0.604
BUN/Cr ratio (per 1)	0.90 (0.80–1.01)	0.069	0.90 (0.79–1.02)	0.104

Abbreviations: *OR* odds ratio, *CI* confidence interval, *BUN/Cr* blood urea nitrogen-to-creatinine
*, $p < 0.05$; **, adjusted for multiple vascular risk factors including age, sex, hypertension, diabetes, hyperlipidemia, atrial fibrillation, and smoking

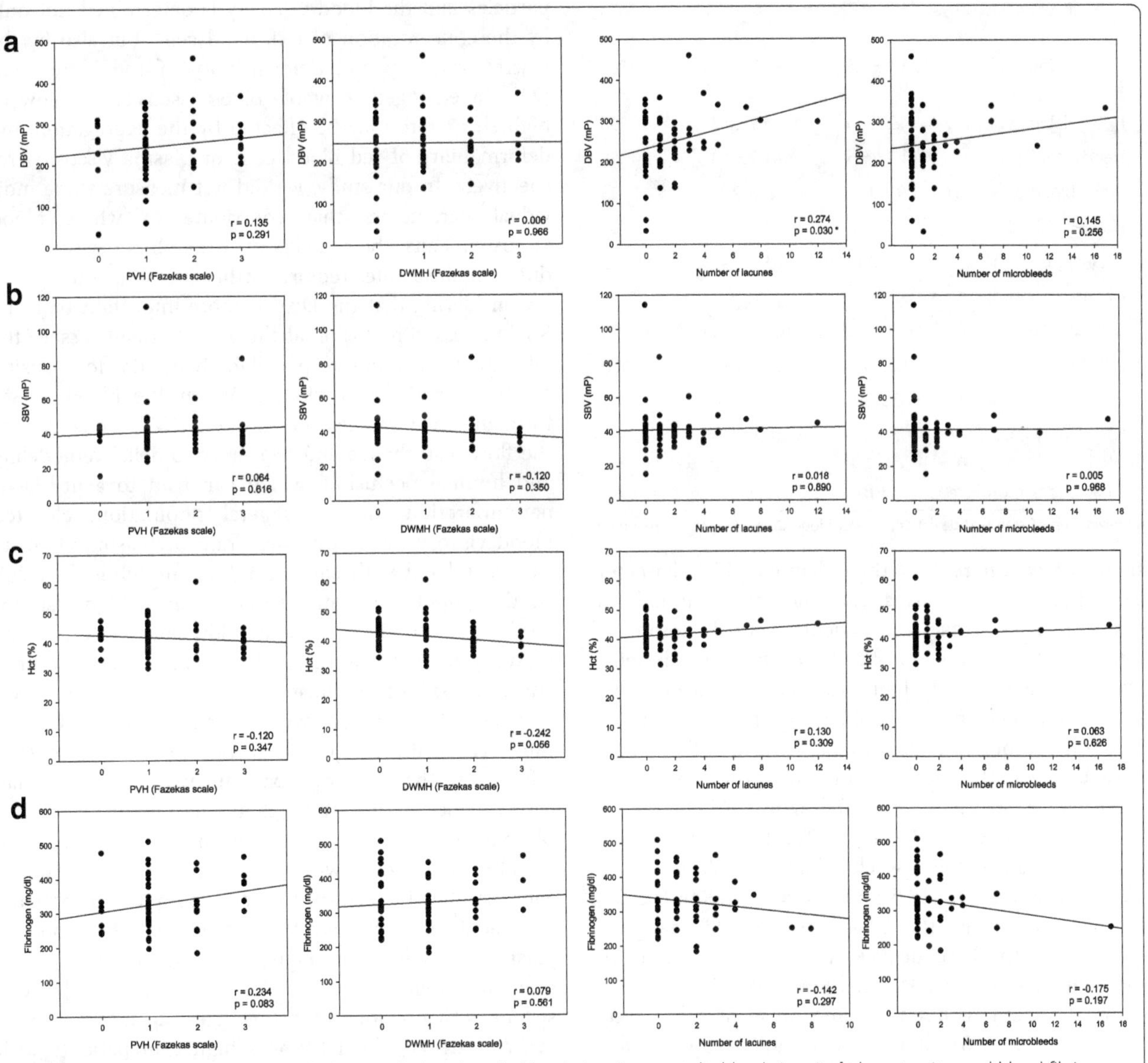

Fig. 4 Correlation between laboratory findings, including diastolic blood viscosity **a**, systolic blood viscosity **b**, hematocrit **c**, and blood fibrinogen level **d**, and chronic radiological manifestations of cerebral small vessel disease. *, $p < 0.05$; *DBV*, diastolic blood viscosity; *SBV*, systolic blood viscosity; *Hct*, hematocrit; *PVH*, periventricular hyperintensity; *DWMH*, deep white matter hyperintensity

Table 3 Comparison of demographics for patients followed-up and not-followed-up

	Followed-up patients ($n = 41$)	Not-followed-up patients ($n = 22$)	P value
Clinical findings			
Age, years (mean ± sd)	65.1 ± 13.6	67.5 ± 13.7	0.496
Male, n (%)	25 (61.0)	16 (72.7)	0.415
Hypertension, n (%)	29 (70.7)	11 (50.0)	0.169
Diabetes, n (%)	12 (29.3)	4 (18.2)	0.382
Hyperlipidemia, n (%)	6 (14.6)	4 (18.2)	0.729
Atrial fibrillation, n (%)	6 (14.6)	3 (13.6)	1.000
Smoking, n (%)	15 (36.6)	9 (40.9)	0.790
Laboratory findings (mean ± sd)			
Diastolic blood viscosity, mP	258.9 ± 72.5	226.6 ± 71.3	0.623
Systolic blood viscosity, mP	41.4 ± 9.5	41.3 ± 18.1	0.284
Hemoglobin, g/dL	14.2 ± 2.0	14.4 ± 1.7	0.598
Hematocrit, %	41.5 ± 5.5	41.9 ± 4.3	0.333
White blood cells, 10^3/μL	7.9 ± 3.1	7.5 ± 2.2	0.133
Platelets, 10^3/μL	228 ± 48	237 ± 73	0.104
Total protein, gm/dL	7.1 ± 0.4	6.9 ± 0.4	0.943
Fibrinogen, mg/dL	332 ± 71	325 ± 87	0.591
D-dimer, μg/dL	0.78 ± 1.25	0.63 ± 0.38	0.105
BUN/Cr ratio	21.0 ± 7.2	20.4 ± 5.0	0.500
Total cholesterol, mg/dL	167 ± 39	178 ± 36	0.943
Low-density lipoprotein, mg/dL	102 ± 34	109 ± 30	0.760
Triglycerides, mg/dL	117 ± 81	92 ± 40	0.091

Abbreviations: sd standard deviation, *BUN/Cr* blood urea nitrogen-to-creatinine

significantly different in their demographic characteristics (Table 3). To investigate the role of blood viscosity in SAO stroke, the patients were dichotomized into the SAO and non-SAO groups. The baseline DBV was significantly higher in the SAO group than in the non-SAO group (274.7 ± 70.9 mP and 229.8 ± 70.0 mP, respectively; $p = 0.016$; Fig. 5a). The difference between the DBVs of the two groups was seen to decrease at the 1-week follow-up (SAO, 232.7 ± 54.9 mP; non-SAO, 216.2 ± 48.0 mP; $p = 0.394$) and increase again at the 5-week follow-up (SAO, 273.2 ± 48.9 mP; non-SAO, 218.6 ± 65.4 mP; $p = 0.009$; Fig. 5a). In the SAO group, the DBV was elevated again and returned to the baseline level at the stroke onset. On the other hand, the DBV in the non-SAO group was seen to remain within the same range at the 1-week follow-up. The SBV at the 5-week follow-up was also significantly higher in the SAO group than in the non-SAO group (42.0 ± 4.3 mP and 36.1 ± 6.9 mP, respectively; $p = 0.005$; Fig. 5b).

Discussion

Role of blood viscosity in SAO stroke

The whole blood viscosity at a low shear rate, equivalent to the DBV in our study, is dependent on the aggregation of red blood cells in the lumen of small vessels [12, 13]. Both hematocrit and fibrinogen play key roles in the aggregation of red blood cells [12, 13]. In our study, the DBV was correlated with hematocrit, while the SBV was correlated with the blood fibrinogen level. These findings appear consistent with the hypothesis that at a low shear rate, the red blood cells form a rouleaux and the blood viscosity is predominantly determined by a function of the concentration and aggregation properties of the red blood cells [24]. At a high shear rate, equivalent to the SBV in our study, the red blood cells move as free particles and the blood viscosity is determined not only by the concentration of red blood cells, but also by the plasma viscosity and deformability of red blood cells [24]. Taken together, whole blood viscosity at a low or high shear rate may be affected by the aggregation and deformability of red blood cells or plasma viscosity, respectively. In our study, we did not measure these individual parameters that contribute to whole blood viscosity. Thus, their effects on whole blood viscosity at different shear rates require further investigation.

Considering that the DBV is more important than the SBV for tissue perfusion at the level of small vessels, the DBV may be more responsible than SBV for causing cerebral small vessel disease. When the blood passes through small vessels, an elevated DBV can aggravate the flow disturbance and trigger endothelial remodeling and luminal occlusion, which can lead to acute lacunar infarction. In the general population, elevated blood viscosity at a low shear rate or plasma viscosity was correlated with silent cerebral infarction [11, 25]. In the population with stroke or at a high risk for stroke, the blood viscosity at a low shear rate and the plasma viscosity were both elevated [1]. Another study of patients with stroke showed that the blood viscosity was elevated over the entire range of shear rates, especially at low shear rates [6]. A more specific study that included patients with cerebral small vessel disease reported that the blood viscosity, plasma viscosity, and blood fibrinogen level were all elevated in patients with acute lacunar infarction [7]. More studies in relation to stroke subtypes in patients with acute ischemic stroke showed that the blood or plasma viscosity was higher in patients with SAO than in patients with LAA or CE stroke [2–4]. Consistent with previous reports suggesting hyperviscosity in SAO stroke, the DBV was higher in patients with SAO than in those with other stroke subtypes in our study. Taken together, elevated DBV at the onset of stroke can impair microvascular tissue perfusion and

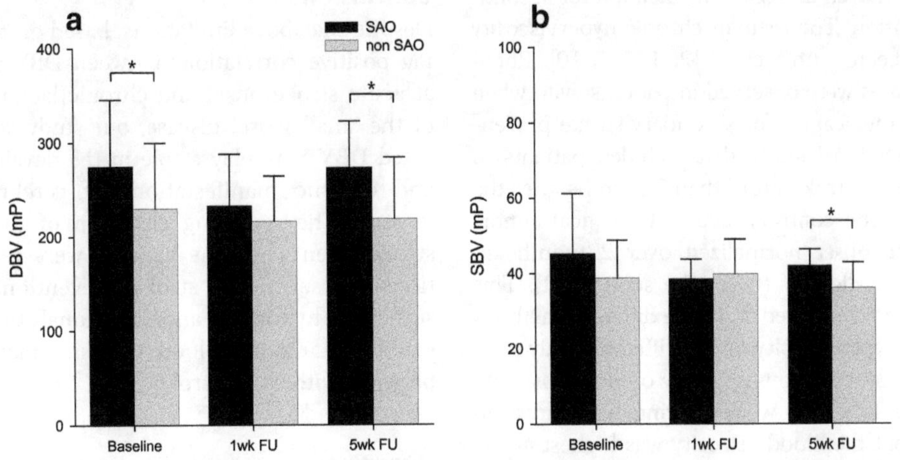

Fig. 5 Temporal profiles of blood viscosity in SAO and non-SAO stroke. The baseline diastolic blood viscosity was higher in the SAO group than that in the non-SAO group **a**. The difference between the two groups was seen to decrease at the 1-week follow-up, and increase at the 5-week follow-up **a**. The systolic blood viscosity in the SAO group was higher than that in the non-SAO group at the 5-weeks follow-up **b**. *$p < 0.05$; *DBV*, diastolic blood viscosity; *SBV*, systolic blood viscosity; *SAO*, small artery occlusion

may be associated with the pathomechanisms involved in SAO stroke.

Association between blood viscosity and chronic radiological manifestations of cerebral small vessel disease

The elevated blood viscosity at stroke onset may indicate not only that acute hyperviscosity triggers stroke, but also that underlying chronic hyperviscosity is present prior to stroke. White matter hyperintensities, lacunes, and microbleeds are various chronic radiological manifestations of cerebral small vessel disease [17–20]. Therefore, we hypothesized that if the blood viscosity at stroke onset is also associated with white matter hyperintensities, lacunes, or microbleeds in patients with acute ischemic stroke, the elevated blood viscosity at stroke onset might have been present prior to stroke onset.

The pathomechanisms of lacunes and white matter hyperintensities are intimately related, and acute small subcortical infarctions can progress to chronic lacunes or white matter hyperintensities [19]. Ischemia and chronic leakage of fluid and macromolecules are known to be the main pathophysiologies attributed to the development of white matter lesions [26]. More complicated pathologies of white matter lesions, including cerebral ischemia, ependymal loss, demyelination, and microcytic infarction have also been reported [17, 26, 27]. The pathophysiology of microbleeds is a leakage of red blood cells through the loosened blood-brain barrier caused by bleeding-prone small vessel disease related to hypertension or cerebral amyloid angiopathy [19]. Consistent with previous studies suggesting that blood or plasma viscosity is associated with white matter hyperintensities [11, 14, 25, 28, 29], the severity of PVH in our study showed trends for positive correlation with the DBV or blood fibrinogen level, although neither reached statistical significance. Similar to previous studies that have indicated an association between the elevated plasma viscosity and lacunar infarction [3, 11], we observed a significant positive correlation between the DBV and the number of chronic lacunes. Based on this result, the elevated blood viscosity at stroke onset may indicate hyperviscosity not only in the acute period but also in the period prior to stroke onset. A prospective observational study is needed to confirm this hypothesis.

Recurrent blood hyperviscosity in SAO stroke

To investigate the hyperviscosity in SAO stroke, stroke subtypes were dichotomized into SAO and non-SAO groups. The DBV at stroke onset was significantly higher in the SAO group than in the non-SAO group. However, this discrepancy decreased after 1 week, as the DBV decreased more dramatically in the SAO group than in the non-SAO group. Dehydration leading to the elevation of blood viscosity is considered to be one of the major factors responsible for triggering acute ischemic stroke [3, 4, 30]. Although the DBV was higher in SAO stroke than in other stroke subtypes in our study, the BUN/Cr ratio, which generally reflects the hydration status [31], was not elevated in SAO stroke compared to that in other stroke subtypes. The elevation of DBV in SAO stroke may be caused not only by dehydration, but also by other factors determining blood viscosity. The decrease in the DBV at the 1-week follow-up may be mainly due to the hydration therapy given after admission. In the SAO group, the DBV measured at the 5-week follow-up, when the hydration therapy was terminated, showed a recurrent elevation even under the medication for secondary stroke prevention. The issue of chronic hyperviscosity after stroke has been controversial [2, 4, 5, 7, 10]. Rheological abnormalities were observed in patients even when they were under medication for secondary stroke prevention in a cross-sectional study that included patients in the chronic phase of stroke more than 3 months after the onset [5, 10]. On the contrary, acute rheological abnormalities at stroke onset normalized over 2 months in another study, regardless of the stroke subtype [2]. This discrepancy may have resulted from the different methods used to measure hyperviscosity or the different study populations. A recent serial follow-up study of blood viscosity measured at 100 s^{-1} for 2 weeks during the admission period showed that the blood viscosity was highest at the date of admission and decreased over the following 2 weeks [4]. While a serial follow-up for 2 weeks was performed during the admission period [4], the follow-up at 5 weeks in our study was performed at the outpatient clinic when the hydration therapy had already been terminated. Therefore, the results of our study may reflect the chronic status of blood viscosity after stroke, and are likely unrelated to the hydration therapy administered during admission. The recurrent elevation of the DBV in SAO stroke suggests that chronic hyperviscosity may be a persistent underlying pathomechanim of SAO stroke.

Limitations of our study

Our study has several limitations. First, the number of patients included in our study is too small and the statistical power to support our conclusion is relatively weak. Second, a cross-sectional study design was used to investigate the role of blood viscosity in acute stroke onset or chronic radiological manifestations of cerebral small vessel disease. However, our results provide the rationale for future prospective observational studies that might confirm the cause-effect relationship. Third, follow-up of the blood viscosity was not performed in all the patients for various reasons. The number of patients lost to follow-up was relatively high ($n = 22$, 34.9%). Although there were no statistically significant differences in the baseline clinical and laboratory profiles of the patients who were followed-up and those who were not, baseline DBV showed some non-significant differences (followed-up, 258.9 ± 72.5 mP; not-followed-up, 226.6 ± 71.3 mP; $p = 0.623$). This might have led to some selection bias. Fourth, the blood viscosity can be easily influenced by hydration therapy using fluids or drinking water. In order to minimize the transient diluting effect by hydration, samples for the baseline and follow-up measurements were obtained before the hydration therapy and in a fasting state, respectively.

Conclusions

Despite the above limitations, based on the results showing positive correlations between DBV and SAO stroke at acute stroke onset and chronic lacunar manifestation of the small vessel disease, our study suggests that elevated DBV may play a role in the development of acute and chronic manifestations of cerebral small vessel disease. The recurring elevation of the DBV in SAO stroke, even when the patients were receiving medications for secondary stroke prevention, indicates that sufficient hydration and additional therapeutic interventions targeting blood viscosity may be needed in patients with SAO stroke.

Abbreviations

ANOVA: Analysis of variance; BUN/Cr: Blood urea nitrogen-to-creatinine; CE: Cardioembolism; Crypt: Cryptogenic stroke; DBV: Diastolic blood viscosity; DWMH: Deep white matter hyperintensity; EDTA: Ethylenediaminetetraacetic acid; FLAIR: Fluid attenuation inversion recovery; LAA: Large artery atherosclerosis; MRI: Magnetic resonance imaging; PVH: Periventricular hyperintensity; SAO: Small artery occlusion; SBV: Systolic blood viscosity; TIA: Transient ischemic attack

Acknowledgements

Not applicable.

Funding

This work was supported by a Konkuk University Medical Center Research Grant 2014.

Authors' contributions

SHS and HYK drafted the manuscript and participated in the general management of the study. SHS, JHK, and JHL interpreted the imaging studies. YM and DHC helped to draft the manuscript. All authors reviewed and approved the final manuscript.

Competing interests

All authors declare that they have no competing interests.

Author details

[1]Department of Neurology, Research Institute of Medical Science, Konkuk University School of Medicine, Konkuk University Medical Center, Seoul, Republic of Korea. [2]Department of Laboratory Medicine, Konkuk University School of Medicine, Konkuk University Medical Center, Seoul, Republic of Korea. [3]Department of Medical Science, Konkuk University School of Medicine, Seoul, Republic of Korea.

References

1. Coull BM, Beamer N, de Garmo P, Sexton G, Nordt F, Knox R, Seaman GV. Chronic blood hyperviscosity in subjects with acute stroke, transient ischemic attack, and risk factors for stroke. Stroke. 1991;22:162–8.
2. Fisher M, Meiselman HJ. Hemorheological factors in cerebral ischemia. Stroke. 1991;22:1164–9.
3. Grotemeyer KC, Kaiser R, Grotemeyer KH, Husstedt IW. Association of elevated plasma viscosity with small vessel occlusion in ischemic cerebral disease. Thromb Res. 2014;133:96–100.
4. Furukawa K, Abumiya T, Sakai K, Hirano M, Osanai T, Shichinohe H, Nakayama

N, Kazumata K, Hida K, Houkin K. Increased blood viscosity in ischemic stroke patients with small artery occlusion measured by an electromagnetic spinning sphere viscometer. J Stroke Cerebrovasc Dis. 2016;25:2762–9.
5. Szapary L, Horvath B, Marton Z, Alexy T, Demeter N, Szots M, Klabuzai A, Kesmarky G, Juricskay I, Gaal V, et al. Hemorheological disturbances in patients with chronic cerebrovascular diseases. Clin Hemorheol Microcirc. 2004;31:1–9.
6. Ott EO, Lechner H, Aranibar A. High blood viscosity syndrome in cerebral infarction. Stroke. 1974;5:330–3.
7. Tsuda Y, Satoh K, Kitadai M, Takahashi T. Hemorheologic profiles of plasma fibrinogen and blood viscosity from silent to acute and chronic cerebral infarctions. J Neurol Sci. 1997;147:49–54.
8. Folsom AR, Peacock JM, Nieto FJ, Rosamond WD, Eigenbrodt ML, Davis CE, Wu KK. Plasma fibrinogen and incident hypertension in the Atherosclerosis Risk in Communities (ARIC) Study. J Hypertens. 1998;16:1579–83.
9. Briley DP, Giraud GD, Beamer NB, Spear EM, Grauer SE, Edwards JM, Clark WM, Sexton GJ, Coull BM. Spontaneous echo contrast and hemorheologic abnormalities in cerebrovascular disease. Stroke. 1994;25:1564–9.
10. Kowal P, Marcinkowska-Gapinska A. Hemorheological changes dependent on the time from the onset of ischemic stroke. J Neurol Sci. 2007;258:132–6.
11. Aono Y, Ohkubo T, Kikuya M, Hara A, Kondo T, Obara T, Metoki H, Inoue R, Asayama K, Shintani Y, et al. Plasma fibrinogen, ambulatory blood pressure, and silent cerebrovascular lesions: the Ohasama study. Arterioscler Thromb Vasc Biol. 2007;27:963–8.
12. Grotta J, Ostrow P, Fraifeld E, Hartman D, Gary H. Fibrinogen, blood viscosity, and cerebral ischemia. Stroke. 1985;16:192–8.
13. Cho YI, Cho DJ, Rosenson RS. Endothelial shear stress and blood viscosity in peripheral arterial disease. Curr Atheroscler Rep. 2014;16:404.
14. Noh HJ, Seo SW, Jeong Y, Park JE, Kim GH, Noh Y, Cho H, Kim HJ, Yoon CW, Ye BS, et al. Blood viscosity in subcortical vascular mild cognitive impairment with versus without cerebral amyloid burden. J Stroke Cerebrovasc Dis. 2014;23:958–66.
15. Kim H, Cho YI, Lee DH, Park CM, Moon HW, Hur M, Kim JQ, Yun YM. Analytical performance evaluation of the scanning capillary tube viscometer for measurement of whole blood viscosity. Clin Biochem. 2013;46:139–42.
16. Crea F, Camici PG, Bairey Merz CN. Coronary microvascular dysfunction: an update. Eur Heart J. 2014;35:1101–11.
17. Pantoni L. Cerebral small vessel disease: from pathogenesis and clinical characteristics to therapeutic challenges. Lancet Neurol. 2010;9:689–701.
18. Mok V, Kim JS. Prevention and management of cerebral small vessel disease. J Stroke. 2015;17:111–22.
19. Norrving B. Evolving concept of small vessel disease through advanced brain imaging. J Stroke. 2015;17:94–100.
20. Kim BJ, Lee SH. Prognostic impact of cerebral small vessel disease on stroke outcome. J Stroke. 2015;17:101–10.
21. Adams Jr HP, Bendixen BH, Kappelle LJ, Biller J, Love BB, Gordon DL, Marsh 3rd EE. Classification of subtype of acute ischemic stroke. Definitions for use in a multicenter clinical trial. TOAST. Trial of Org 10172 in acute stroke treatment. Stroke. 1993;24:35–41.
22. Fazekas F, Chawluk JB, Alavi A, Hurtig HI, Zimmerman RA. MR signal abnormalities at 1.5 T in Alzheimer's dementia and normal aging. AJR Am J Roentgenol. 1987;149:351–6.
23. Lee JH, Kim YJ, Moon Y, Cho HJ, Kim HY. Acute simultaneous multiple lacunar infarcts: a severe disease entity in small artery disease. Eur Neurol. 2012;67:303–11.
24. Cecchi E, Marcucci R, Poli D, Antonucci E, Abbate R, Gensini GF, Prisco D, Mannini L. Hyperviscosity as a possible risk factor for cerebral ischemic complications in atrial fibrillation patients. Am J Cardiol. 2006;97:1745–8.
25. Li RY, Cao ZG, Li Y, Wang RT. Increased whole blood viscosity is associated with silent cerebral infarction. Clin Hemorheol Microcirc. 2015;59:301–7.
26. Kim KW, Macfall JR, Payne ME. Classification of white matter lesions on magnetic resonance imaging in elderly persons. Biol Psychiatry. 2008;64:273–80.
27. Chen YF, Wang H, Chu Y, Huang YC, Su MY. Regional quantification of white matter hyperintensity in normal aging, mild cognitive impairment, and Alzheimer's disease. Dement Geriatr Cogn Disord. 2006;22:177–84.
28. Wada M, Takahashi Y, Iseki C, Kawanami T, Daimon M, Kato T. Plasma fibrinogen, global cognitive function, and cerebral small vessel disease: results of a cross-sectional study in community-dwelling Japanese elderly. Intern Med. 2011;50:999–1007.
29. Schneider R, Ringelstein EB, Zeumer H, Kiesewetter H, Jung F. The role of plasma hyperviscosity in subcortical arteriosclerotic encephalopathy (Binswanger's disease). J Neurol. 1987;234:67–73.
30. Mucke S, Grotemeyer KH, Stahlhut L, Husstedt IW, Evers S. The influence of fluid intake on stroke recurrence—a prospective study. J Neurol Sci. 2012;315:82–5.
31. Schrock JW, Glasenapp M, Drogell K. Elevated blood urea nitrogen/creatinine ratio is associated with poor outcome in patients with ischemic stroke. Clin Neurol Neurosurg. 2012;114:881–4.

Hemoglobin concentration does not impact 3-month outcome following acute ischemic stroke

Kartavya Sharma[1,2,3*], Daniel J. Johnson[1], Brenda Johnson[2], Steven M. Frank[1] and Robert D. Stevens[1,2,4]

Abstract

Background: There is uncertainty regarding the effect of anemia and red blood cell transfusion on functional outcome following acute ischemic stroke. We studied the relationship of hemoglobin parameters and red cell transfusion with post stroke functional outcome after adjustment for neurological severity and medical comorbidities.

Methods: Retrospective cohort study of 536 patients discharged with a diagnosis of ischemic stroke from a tertiary care hospital between January 2012 and April 2015. Hemoglobin level at hospital admission, lowest recorded value during hospitalization (nadir), delta hemoglobin (admission minus nadir), red cell transfusion during hospitalization were noted. Charlson Comorbidity Index (CCI) was computed as a summary measure of medical comorbidities. A multivariable logistic regression model was used to determine risk-adjusted odds of unfavorable outcome, defined as a modified Rankin Score of > 2.

Results: Anemia was present on hospital admission in 31% of patients. Forty five percent of patients had unfavorable outcome. In the univariable analysis increasing age, admission National Institutes of Health Stroke Scale (NIHSS), CCI, nadir hemoglobin, delta hemoglobin and blood transfusion were associated with unfavorable outcome. In the multivariable model, only increasing age, CCI and NIHSS remained associated with unfavorable outcome. No quadratic association was found on repeating the model to identify a possible U-shaped relationship of hemoglobin with outcome.

Conclusions: Our findings contradict prior observational studies and highlight an area of clinical equipoise regarding the optimal management of anemia in patients hospitalized for ischemic stroke. This uncertainty could be addressed with appropriately designed clinical trials.

Keywords: Ischemic stroke, Anemia, Hemoglobin, Transfusion, Disability, Mortality, Charlson comorbidity index

Background

Anemia is a frequent comorbid or complicating factor in patients with ischemic stroke, yet the influence of hemoglobin (Hb) concentration on stroke outcome is a matter of considerable uncertainty. Increases in mortality following ischemic stroke have been associated with abnormally low Hb level [1–5] as well as abnormally high Hb level [6], or both high and low levels in the same cohort [7]. Observational studies have suggested an unfavorable impact of admission anemia on long term post-stroke functional outcome [3, 7]. However, one study found this association only in a subgroup of patients with less severe strokes [8] and another large cohort study with meta-analysis did not find any association with functional outcome [2].

Several factors may contribute to these differences in findings. First, Hb-related exposure/predictor variables are not consistently reported across studies. For example, dynamic assessments of anemia after ischemic stroke, such as the decrease in Hb or the nadir Hb, were shown to be independently predictive of worse outcome in one report [9], however most studies have not evaluated anemia in this way. Second, statistical models vary widely across studies particularly regarding the use of multivariable approaches, and in the selection of covariates used in the

* Correspondence: ksharma@kumc.edu
[1]Department of Anesthesiology and Critical Care Medicine, Johns Hopkins University School of Medicine, Baltimore, USA
[2]Department of Neurology, Johns Hopkins University School of Medicine, Baltimore, USA
Full list of author information is available at the end of the article

multivariable models. For example, it is plausible that red blood cell (RBC) transfusion will modify any presumed impact of anemia on stroke pathophysiology, yet RBC transfusion is not consistently adjusted for across studies. Lastly, anemia can be regarded as a marker of underlying medical illnesses which can influence outcome independently of any direct mechanistic effect on the ischemic brain. Variability in study results may therefore reflect unmeasured or unreported confounders (e.g. acquired immune deficiency syndrome, malignancy, malnutrition and liver failure) which can influence Hb level, functional outcome or both.

To clarify these effects, we examined the relationship of Hb indices including admission, nadir, discharge and change in Hb level with 3-month functional outcome in a large hospital-based stroke registry, adjusting for RBC transfusion and for medical comorbidities using the comprehensive Charlson Comorbidity Index (CCI).

Methods

We queried the Johns Hopkins Hospital stroke registry, a prospective database, for patients aged 18 and above who were discharged with a diagnosis of ischemic stroke between Jan 1st 2012 and Apr 30th 2015. For patients admitted more than once with acute ischemic stroke, we considered only the earliest hospitalization. Out of a total of 802 patients, modified Rankin Scale (mRS) at 3 months was available for 536 patients. These patients were cross-referenced against a separate Blood Product Utilization Database established by one of the co-investigators (SMF). Predictor variables were clinical characteristics including pre-admission CCI, laboratory values and record of blood product transfusions during the hospitalization. Anemia was defined as per the World Health Organization as a serum Hb of < 13 g/dL in men and < 12 g/dL in women [10]. The principal outcome variable was unfavorable functional status defined as mRS > 2 at 3 months follow up.

Statistical analyses: Exploratory univariable analysis was performed to determine strength of the association between potential predictors and the principal outcome variable. Nominal logistic regression was used for continuous variables and Pearson's chi-squared test for categorical variables. Covariates having a P value < 0.1 on univariable analysis were used in a multiple logistic regression model with unfavorable outcome as the dependent variable. Of note, despite having no association on univariable testing ($P = 0.59$), intravenous tissue plasminogen activator (tPA) administration was included in the multivariable models because of its well-established efficacy in improving stroke outcomes. We tested using separate models, the following Hb indices as continuous variables for strength of association with outcome: admission, nadir, last recorded serum Hb concentration, as well as delta (difference between admission and nadir) Hb. In secondary analyses, we repeated our model to address two issues. First, to investigate a possible quadratic relationship of Hb with outcome, we included Hb squared as a continuous variable. Second, instead of linear or quadratic Hb values, we used anemia as a categorical predictor (Hb < 12 g/dl for women and < 13 g/dl for men) [10]. P value threshold was set at ≤0.05 for statistical significance. Analyses were performed using JMP®, Version 12.1 (SAS Institute Inc., Cary, NC).

Results

A total of 536 patients were included in the study. Patient characteristics and hemoglobin parameters are provided in Table 1. The prevalence of anemia on admission was 31% in the study sample. The proportion of anemic women (38%) was significantly higher than men (26%), $P = 0.002$. During the hospitalization, the prevalence of anemia increased to 59% based on nadir Hb values.

Three-month unfavorable outcome, defined as a mRS > 2, was noted in 243 (45%) patients, of whom 34 (6%) died within the 3-month follow up period. In the univariable analysis, greater age, higher NIHSS score, CCI, lower nadir Hb, larger delta Hb, and RBC transfusion were associated with unfavorable outcome (Table 2). In the multivariable model, age, CCI and NIHSS remained associated with worse outcome (Table 2). However, the associations of nadir or delta Hb and RBC transfusion with unfavorable outcome were not significant in the risk-adjusted analysis (Table 3). Modeling performed with admission Hb as a dichotomized value (anemia vs no anemia) did not reveal significant association on multivariable analysis (Table 3). In post hoc analyses using only death as the outcome of interest, Hb indices were again not associated with mortality. There was no quadratic relationship of Hb with mortality or functional outcome (models not shown).

Discussion

In this large cohort of patients admitted to a tertiary care center with ischemic stroke, anemia was present on admission in nearly one third of cases. Moreover, anemia developed after admission in 28% of patients who were initially hospitalized without anemia. Nevertheless, in carefully risk adjusted models, neither anemia on admission nor anemia during hospitalization, nor any Hb-associated variable, nor RBC transfusion was significantly associated with functional status at 3 months. Taken in the context of other published studies, the results illustrate an area of significant uncertainty in the evaluation and management of patients with ischemic stroke.

Putative mechanisms for how anemia may influence the pathophysiology and outcome of ischemic stroke

Table 1 Patient characteristics ($N = 536$)

Characteristic	No. (%) of Patients
Female	244 (45.5)
Age, mean (SD), y	62 (15)
Admission NIHSS score	
Median (IQR)	3 (5)
Mean (SD)	5.2 (5.5)
NIHSS < 10	450 (84)
Hemoglobin parameters	
Admission Hb, mean (SD), g/dl	13.2 (1.9)
Nadir Hb, mean (SD), g/dl	11.7 (2.3)
Delta Hb, median (IQR), g/dl	1.1 (1.9)
Charlson Comorbidity Index, median (IQR)	3 (3)
Body mass index ≥30	58 (11)
Congestive heart failure	66 (12)
Hypertension	90 (17)
Diabetes mellitus	157 (29)
Renal disease	63 (12)
Liver disease	14 (3)
HIV positive	6 (1)
Intravenous alteplase administered	39 (7)
Length of stay, median (IQR)	3 (5)
Red blood cell transfusion	28 (5)
3-month modified Rankin scale score	
0	98 (18)
1	90 (17)
2	105 (20)
3	121 (23)
4	68 (13)
5	20 (4)
6	34 (6)

Abbreviations: *HIV* human immunodeficiency virus, *IQR* interquartile range, *NIHSS* National Institutes of Health stroke scale, *SD* standard deviation

include reduction of oxygen carrying capacity to the penumbral regions [11], the generation of a hyperkinetic thrombogenic state especially in acute blood loss [12] and the association with a proinflammatory state [13]. However, findings from studies looking at the association of Hb with functional outcome after stroke have been inconsistent. Tanne et al. reported significantly increased odds of combined death and disability (Barthel Index < 75) at 1 year in patients with anemia [7]. Similarly, Milionis et al. reported significantly increased odds of poor functional status measured with mRS at 3 months and 1 year in anemic vs non-anemic patients [3]. In contrast, Hao et al. found no association between anemia and measures of disability in their cohort and meta-analysis of similar studies published in the period 2007–2013 [2].

Increased mortality in anemic patients has been demonstrated in studies with follow up periods ranging from 1 month to 3 years [1–5]. This seemingly intuitive relationship has not borne out uniformly. Furlan et al. noted no association of low Hb with 7-day and 30-day mortality but slight increase in 90-day mortality [6]. Some caveats bear mentioning when interpreting these data. Two of these large cohort studies did not incorporate stroke severity as a covariate influencing mortality [4, 5]. There also seems to be publication bias favoring reports with increased odds of mortality in anemic patients with stroke [5, 14].

Some data suggest that both low and high Hb may be linked with increased mortality. In the study by Furlan et al., abnormally high Hb was robustly associated with increased mortality at all follow up intervals [6]. Tanne et al. found increased mortality rates at both low and high Hb concentrations [7]. Thrombogenic effects and compromised collateral flow have been postulated as mechanisms worsening outcomes in patients with supranormal serum Hb values. An alternative explanation would be that both extremes of Hb concentration are biomarkers of systemic medical comorbidities which are the true drivers of

Table 2 Univariable and multivariable predictors of unfavorable outcome (mRS > 2)

	Univariable Analysis[a]		Multivariable analysis[b]	
	OR (95% CI)	P Value	Adjusted OR (95% CI)	P value
Age	1.02 (1.01–1.04)	< 0.001	1.02 (1.01–1.04)	0.001
NIHSS score	1.26 (1.19–1.33)	< 0.001	1.30 (1.23–1.39)	< 0.001
IV alteplase use	0.84 (0.42–1.61)	0.59	0.19 (0.07–0.46)	< 0.001
Charlson Comorbidity Index	1.30 (1.17–1.44)	< 0.001	1.25 (1.11–1.41)	< 0.001
Nadir Hb	0.82 (0.76–0.89)	< 0.001	0.99 (0.89–1.10)	0.84
Delta Hb	1.40 (1.20–1.60)	< 0.001		
Anemia during hospitalization	1.60 (1.15–2.33)	0.006		
Red blood cell transfusion	2.67 (1.21–6.31)	0.013	1.45 (0.49–4.40)	0.50

Abbreviations: *CI* Confidence interval, *OR* Odds ratio, *Hb* Hemoglobin
[a]Odds ratios are per unit change for continuous variables (Age,y; NIHSS score; Charlson Comorbidity Index; Nadir Hb, g/dl; Delta Hb, g/dl; Body Mass Index)
[b]Only one multivariable model shown here. Results for models with other Hb indices shown in Table 3.

Table 3 Unadjusted and adjusted odds ratios for unfavorable outcome with different hemoglobin variables

	OR (95% CI)	P value	Adjusted OR[a] (95% CI)	P value
Admission Hb	0.96 (0.88–1.05)	0.47	1.05 (0.94–1.17)	0.34
Nadir Hb	0.82 (0.76–0.89)	< 0.001	0.99 (0.89–1.1)	0.84
Last Hb	0.82 (0.76–0.89)	< 0.001	0.98 (0.88–1.09)	0.75
Delta Hb	1.40 (1.20–1.60)	< 0.001	1.14 (0.97–1.34)	0.09
Nadir Hb in patients with NIHSS < 10	0.86 (0.79–0.94)	0.002	0.99 (0.88–1.1)	0.93
Anemia during hospitalization	1.60 (1.15–2.33)	0.006	0.83 (0.5–1.3)	0.41

Abbreviations: *Hb* hemoglobin
[a]Models were adjusted for age, NIHSS, Charlson Comorbidity Index, delta Hb and red blood cell transfusion

mortality. Indeed, we did not find any such quadratic association of mortality with Hb parameters.

It has been also been postulated that with increasing severity of stroke, the relative impact of anemia on outcome may become insignificant due to the extent of neurological injury [8, 9, 15]. Sico et al. reported an association of low hematocrit (< 30%) with combined outcome of death and discharge to hospice in patients with mild to moderate stroke (NIHSS < 10) but not in those with more severe strokes [8]. In another set of studies, Kellert et al. implicated post-admission drop in Hb levels in worsening functional outcome in thrombolysed patients admitted to the stroke unit, but found no such association in their neurological intensive care unit patients with more severe illness [9, 15]. In our cohort, however, there was no association of Hb parameters with mortality or functional outcome in the subgroup of patients with NIHSS < 10 ($n = 450$, Table 3).

Strengths of this study include the relatively large sample size, adjustment for stroke severity and the use of the CCI as a summary measure for comorbidity information. Due to the large number of conditions that may be covariant with anemia and mortality, a summary measure provides the convenience of a single number that adequately captures information from individual comorbidities [16]. The CCI has been in extensive use in administrative databases and has been validated as a prognostic indicator in ischemic stroke as well [17, 18]. Consistent use of such a measure will be useful in comparing and pooling data across studies in future. Limitations of the study include the retrospective design and potential selection bias due to exclusion of patients with missing mRS data. We did not have documented pre-stroke mRS for the study patients. Change in mRS would certainly be a more accurate outcome measure than post-stroke value alone. Lastly, we could not extract information about mechanism of stroke in our patients. It is entirely plausible that different stroke subtypes may be differentially affected by abnormal hemoglobin levels.

In summary, in our cohort of patients with ischemic stroke, admission, nadir or change in Hb were not predictive of 3-month functional outcome. It is possible that mild to moderate anemia, other than being a marker of illness, does not materially affect prognosis from ischemic stroke. Perhaps the central nervous system adaptation to chronic anemia may be protective in the setting of acute ischemia, similar to the neuroprotective effect of hypoxic preconditioning in a rodent model of ischemic stroke [19]. Another potentially important factor is the intrinsic biological heterogeneity in populations of patients with ischemic stroke [20]. An emerging body of research is demonstrating that variance in the risk, presentation and outcomes of ischemic stroke is determined to a significant degree by underlying genetic factors [21], suggesting that anemia and RBC transfusion could have differential effects depending on underlying (and yet insufficiently characterized) patient-specific characteristics.

Inconsistent results from available studies suggest a state of clinical equipoise regarding the optimal management of anemia in patients with acute ischemic stroke. Resolving this uncertainty could involve 3 linked strategies. First, prospective studies are needed with sample sizes adequately powered to answer primary hypotheses. Such studies must use carefully designed modeling approaches that control for a range of potential confounders and focus on functional outcomes in addition to mortality. Consistency in the use of comorbidity summary measures and outcome measures may enable pooling of data across studies to overcome the limitations of sample size. Second, research is needed to discover and validate sensitive and specific biomarkers to guide management of anemia (e.g. timing of transfusion, optimal Hb cutoffs) in stratified subsets or individuals with ischemic stroke. Third, carefully designed and adequately powered randomized controlled trials (preferably biomarker-guided) are warranted to address primary questions on the role of higher versus lower Hb management thresholds in ischemic stroke populations.

Conclusion

Our study demonstrated no association of hemoglobin parameters with mortality and 3-month functional outcome, which contradicts prior observational evidence. This uncertainty could be addressed with appropriately designed clinical trials.

Abbreviations

CCI: Charlson Comorbidity Index; CI: Confidence interval; Hb: Hemoglobin; HIV: Human immunodeficiency virus; IQR: Interquartile range; mRS: Modified rankin scale; NIHSS: National Institutes of Health Stroke Scale; OR: Odds ratio; RBC: Red blood cell; SD: Standard deviation; tPA: Tissue plasminogen activator

Authors' contributions

Conception: KS, RDS, SMF; Data acquisition: KS, BJ, RDS, SMF, DJJ; Analysis and interpretation of data: KS, RDS, SMF, DJJ; Manuscript drafting: KS, RDS, SMF; All authors were involved in critical revision of the manuscript and approved the final manuscript.

Competing interests

Steven M. Frank has received compensation from Haemonetics and Medtronic for serving on their advisory boards. The rest of the authors (KS, DJ, BJ, RS) declare that they have no conflict of interest.

Author details

[1]Department of Anesthesiology and Critical Care Medicine, Johns Hopkins University School of Medicine, Baltimore, USA. [2]Department of Neurology, Johns Hopkins University School of Medicine, Baltimore, USA. [3]Department of Neurology, University of Kansas Medical Center, Mailstop 2012, 3901 Rainbow Blvd, Kansas City, KS 66160, USA. [4]Department of Neurosurgery, Johns Hopkins University School of Medicine, Baltimore, USA.

References

1. Nybo M, Kristensen SR, Mickley H, Jensen JK. The influence of anaemia on stroke prognosis and its relation to N-terminal pro-brain natriuretic peptide. Eur J Neurol. 2007;14:477–82. https://doi.org/10.1111/j.1468-1331.2006.01591.x.
2. Hao Z, Wu B, Wang D, Lin S, Tao W, Liu M. A cohort study of patients with anemia on admission and fatality after acute ischemic stroke. J Clin Neurosci. 2013;20:37–42. https://doi.org/10.1016/j.jocn.2012.05.020.
3. Milionis H, Papavasileiou V, Eskandari A, D'Ambrogio-Remillard S, Ntaios G, Michel P. Anemia on admission predicts short- and long-term outcomes in patients with acute ischemic stroke. Int J Stroke. 2015;10:224–30. https://doi.org/10.1111/ijs.12397.
4. Huang WY, Chen IC, Meng L, Weng WC, Peng TI. The influence of anemia on clinical presentation and outcome of patients with first-ever atherosclerosis-related ischemic stroke. J Clin Neurosci. 2009;16:645–9. https://doi.org/10.1016/j.jocn.2008.08.014.
5. Barlas RS, Honney K, Loke YK, McCall SJ, Bettencourt-Silva JH, Clark AB, et al. Impact of hemoglobin levels and Anemia on mortality in acute stroke: analysis of UK regional registry data, systematic review, and meta-analysis. J Am Heart Assoc. 2016;5 https://doi.org/10.1161/jaha.115.003019.
6. Furlan JC, Fang J, Silver FL. Acute ischemic stroke and abnormal blood hemoglobin concentration. Acta Neurol Scand. 2016;134:123–30. https://doi.org/10.1111/ane.12521.
7. Tanne D, Molshatzki N, Merzeliak O, Tsabari R, Toashi M, Schwammenthal Y. Anemia status, hemoglobin concentration and outcome after acute stroke: a cohort study. BMC Neurol. 2010;10:22. https://doi.org/10.1186/1471-2377-10-22.
8. Sico JJ, Concato J, Wells CK, Lo AC, Nadeau SE, Williams LS, et al. Anemia is associated with poor outcomes in patients with less severe ischemic stroke. J Stroke Cerebrovasc Dis. 2013;22:271–8. https://doi.org/10.1016/j.jstrokecerebrovasdis.2011.09.003.
9. Kellert L, Martin E, Sykora M, Bauer H, Gussmann P, Diedler J, et al. Cerebral oxygen transport failure?: decreasing hemoglobin and hematocrit levels after ischemic stroke predict poor outcome and mortality: STroke: RelevAnt impact of hemoGlobin, hematocrit and transfusion (STRAIGHT)–an observational study. Stroke. 2011;42:2832–7. https://doi.org/10.1161/strokeaha.110.606665.
10. Fagnoul D, Combes A, De Backer D. Extracorporeal cardiopulmonary resuscitation. Curr Opin Crit Care. 2014;20:259–65. https://doi.org/10.1097/mcc.0000000000000098.
11. Dexter F, Hindman BJ. Effect of haemoglobin concentration on brain oxygenation in focal stroke: a mathematical modelling study. Br J Anaesth. 1997;79:346–51.
12. Kim JS, Kang SY. Bleeding and subsequent anemia: a precipitant for cerebral infarction. Eur Neurol. 2000;43:201–8. doi: 8176
13. Ferrucci L, Guralnik JM, Woodman RC, Bandinelli S, Lauretani F, Corsi AM, et al. Proinflammatory state and circulating erythropoietin in persons with and without anemia. Am J Med. 2005;118:1288. https://doi.org/10.1016/j.amjmed.2005.06.039.
14. Li Z, Zhou T, Li Y, Chen P, Chen L. Anemia increases the mortality risk in patients with stroke: a meta-analysis of cohort studies. Sci Rep. 2016;6:26636. https://doi.org/10.1038/srep26636.
15. Kellert L, Herweh C, Sykora M, Gussmann P, Martin E, Ringleb PA, et al. Loss of penumbra by impaired oxygen supply? Decreasing hemoglobin levels predict infarct growth after acute ischemic stroke: stroke: Relevant impact of hemoglobin, hematocrit and transfusion (STRAIGHT) - an observational study. Cerebrovasc Dis Extra. 2012;2:99–107. https://doi.org/10.1159/000343731.
16. Austin SR, Wong Y-N, Uzzo RG, Beck JR, Egleston BL. Why summary comorbidity measures such as the Charlson comorbidity index and Elixhauser score work. Med Care. 2015;53:e65–72. https://doi.org/10.1097/MLR.0b013e318297429c.
17. Goldstein LB, Samsa GP, Matchar DB, Horner RD. Charlson index comorbidity adjustment for ischemic stroke outcome studies. Stroke. 2004;35:1941–5. https://doi.org/10.1161/01.STR.0000135225.80898.1c.
18. Tessier A, Finch L, Daskalopoulou SS, Mayo NE. Validation of the Charlson comorbidity index for predicting functional outcome of stroke. Arch Phys Med Rehabil. 2008;89:1276–83. https://doi.org/10.1016/j.apmr.2007.11.049.
19. Wacker BK, Perfater JL, Gidday JM. Hypoxic preconditioning induces stroke tolerance in mice via a cascading HIF, sphingosine kinase, and CCL2 signaling pathway. J Neurochem. 2012;123:954–62. https://doi.org/10.1111/jnc.12047.
20. Rostanski SK, Marshall RS. Precision medicine for ischemic stroke. JAMA Neurol. 2016;73:773–4. https://doi.org/10.1001/jamaneurol.2016.0087.
21. Falcone GJ, Malik R, Dichgans M, Rosand J. Current concepts and clinical applications of stroke genetics. Lancet Neurol. 2014;13:405–18. https://doi.org/10.1016/s1474-4422(14)70029-8.

13

The hemorrhagic transformation index score: a prediction tool in middle cerebral artery ischemic stroke

Mikhail N. Kalinin[1,2*], Dina R. Khasanova[1,2] and Murat M. Ibatullin[1,3]

Abstract

Background: We aimed to develop a tool, the hemorrhagic transformation (HT) index (HTI), to predict any HT within 14 days after middle cerebral artery (MCA) stroke onset regardless of the intravenous recombinant tissue plasminogen activator (IV rtPA) use. That is especially important in the light of missing evidence-based data concerning the timing of anticoagulant resumption after stroke in patients with atrial fibrillation (AF).

Methods: We retrospectively analyzed 783 consecutive MCA stroke patients. Clinical and brain imaging data at admission were recorded. A follow-up period was 2 weeks after admission. The patients were divided into derivation (DC) and validation (VC) cohorts by generating Bernoulli variates with probability parameter 0.7. Univariate/multivariate logistic regression, and factor analysis were used to extract independent predictors. Validation was performed with internal consistency reliability and receiver operating characteristic (ROC) analysis. Bootstrapping was used to reduce bias.

Results: The HTI was composed of 4 items: Alberta Stroke Program Early CT score (ASPECTS), National Institutes of Health Stroke Scale (NIHSS), hyperdense MCA (HMCA) sign, and AF on electrocardiogram (ECG) at admission. According to the predicted probability (PP) range, scores were allocated to ASPECTS as follows: 10–7 = 0; 6–5 = 1; 4–3 = 2; 2–0 = 3; to NIHSS: 0–11 = 0; 12–17 = 1; 18–23 = 2; >23 = 3; to HMCA sign: yes = 1; to AF on ECG: yes = 1. The HTI score varied from 0 to 8. For each score, adjusted PP of any HT with 95% confidence intervals (CI) was as follows: 0 = 0.027 (0.011–0.042); 1 = 0.07 (0.043–0.098); 2 = 0.169 (0.125–0.213); 3 = 0.346 (0.275–0.417); 4 = 0.571 (0.474–0.668); 5 = 0.768 (0.676–0.861); 6 = 0.893 (0.829–0.957); 7 = 0.956 (0.92–0.992); 8 = 0.983 (0.965–1.0). The optimal cutpoint score to differentiate between HT-positive and negative groups was 2 (95% normal-based CI, 1–3) for the DC and VC alike. ROC area/sensitivity/specificity with 95% normal-based CI for the DC and VC were 0.85 (0.82–0.89)/0.82 (0.73–0.9)/0.89 (0.8–0.97) and 0.83 (0.78–0.88)/0.8 (0.66–0.94)/0.87 (0.73–1.0) respectively. McDonald's categorical omega with 95% bias-corrected and accelerated CI for the DC and VC was 0.81 (0.77–0.84) and 0.82 (0.76–0.86) respectively.

Conclusions: The HTI is a simple yet reliable tool to predict any HT within 2 weeks after MCA stroke onset regardless of the IV rtPA use.

Keywords: Stroke, Middle cerebral artery, Complication, Hemorrhage, Prognosis, Hemorrhagic transformation

* Correspondence: ninilak@gmail.com
[1]Department of Neurology and Neurosurgery for Postgraduate Training, Kazan State Medical University, Kazan, Russia
[2]Department of Neurology, Interregional Clinical Diagnostic Center, 12A Karbyshev St, Kazan 420101, Russia
Full list of author information is available at the end of the article

Table 1 Variables with Missing Values

	Missing, *n* (%)	Valid, *n*
Cholesterol, total	107 (13.7)	676
LVEF	80 (10.2)	703
AST	61 (7.8)	722
Bilirubin, total	55 (7)	728
Fibrinogen	41 (5.2)	742
Albumin	37 (4.7)	746
Protein, total	18 (2.3)	765
Sodium	11 (1.4)	772
Potassium	10 (1.3)	773
Prothrombin time	5 (0.6)	778
ALT	4 (0.5)	779
Urea	2 (0.3)	781
Hematocrit	2 (0.3)	781
Hemoglobin	1 (0.1)	782

Note: *ALT* stands for Alanine transaminase, *AST* Aspartate transaminase, and *LVEF* Left ventricular ejection fraction (echocardiography, Simpson method)

Background

Hemorrhagic transformation (HT), either asymptomatic (AHT) or symptomatic (SHT), is considered to be a notorious complication of acute ischemic stroke (AIS), associated with limited treatment options and long-term adverse outcomes [1]. It seems reasonable that efforts should be directed towards preventing HT before it occurs. Fortunately, it is more predictable than other types of intracranial hemorrhage.

In AIS patients, the incidence of HT induced by intravenous recombinant tissue plasminogen activator (IV rtPA) is reported to be 4.5–39.6% for AHT and 5.2–7.3% for SHT. In contrast, the rate of spontaneous AHT and SHT ranges from 13% to 43% and from 0.6% to 20% respectively [2, 3]. Although the proportion of AIS patients treated with IV rtPA is relatively small (4.7–21.4%) [4], the majority of authors have focused on searching HT

Table 2 MI Specification

Software package	IBM SPSS Statistics, v.24; Armonk, NY
Random number generator	Mersenne twister
Imputation method	Fully conditional specification (MCMC)
Model type	Linear regression, no interaction terms
Number of iterations	100
Predictors	All collected data, including missing variables
Restrictions	Extrema of source data
Number of imputations	15
Quality of MI	No pattern on MCMC convergence charts FMI, RIV, RE (Table 4)

Note: *FMI* stands for Fraction of missing information, *MCMC* Markov chain Monte Carlo, *RE* Relative efficiency, and *RIV* Relative increase in variance

Table 3 Baseline Characteristics in the DC and VC

	DC (n = 535)	VC (n = 248)	*p*-Value
Clinical data, median (IQR)			
Age (y)	71 (60–78)	69 (61–77)	0.924
DBP (mm Hg)	90 (80–100)	100 (80–100)	0.025
Height (m)	1.65 (1.6–1.72)	1.65 (1.58–1.71)	0.063
Male sex, *n* (%)	289 (54)	125 (50.4)	0.346
NIHSS	8 (4–16)	8 (4–16)	0.574
Pulse rate (bpm)	78 (74–83)	78 (74–85)	0.155
SBP (mm Hg)	160 (140–180)	160 (140–180)	0.19
Time from onset (h)	5.5 (2–11)	6 (2.5–11)	0.265
Temperature (°C)	36.6 (36.4–36.6)	36.6 (36.5–36.6)	0.194
Weight (kg)	78 (68–88)	76.7 (68–85)	0.476
Stroke cause, *n* (%)			
Large-artery atherosclerosis	212 (39.6)	109 (44)	0.252
Cardioembolism	225 (42.1)	101 (40.7)	0.725
Small-vessel occlusion	79 (14.8)	33 (13.3)	0.587
Other determined etiology	7 (1.3)	1 (0.4)	0.241
Undetermined etiology	12 (2.2)	4 (1.6)	0.562
Risk factors, *n* (%)			
Acute myocardial infarction	25 (4.7)	8 (3.2)	0.348
AF history	210 (39.3)	94 (37.9)	0.719
Alcohol abuse	62 (11.6)	29 (11.7)	0.966
Atherosclerosis	528 (98.7)	248 (100)	0.07
Bleeding history	41 (7.7)	27 (10.9)	0.136
Chronic heart failure	62 (11.6)	28 (11.3)	0.903
Chronic liver failure	5 (0.9)	7 (2.8)	0.045
Chronic renal failure	20 (3.7)	11 (4.4)	0.642
Coronary artery disease	191 (35.7)	89 (35.9)	0.96
Diabetes mellitus	142 (26.5)	69 (27.8)	0.707
Dyslipidemia	216 (40.4)	103 (41.5)	0.759
Hypertension	497 (92.9)	230 (92.7)	0.937
Malignancy	10 (1.9)	4 (1.6)	0.801
Seizures at onset	10 (1.9)	3 (1.2)	0.502
Previous TIA/stroke	221 (41.3)	116 (46.8)	0.151
Brain CT, *n* (%)			
ASPECTS, median (IQR)	8 (6–9)	8 (6–9)	0.708
HMCA sign	141 (26.4)	66 (26.6)	0.939
Leukoaraiosis	347 (64.9)	168 (67.7)	0.429
Left hemispheric stroke	286 (53.5)	122 (49.2)	0.266
Right hemispheric stroke	234 (43.7)	122 (49.2)	0.154
Bihemispheric stroke	15 (2.8)	4 (1.6)	0.314
Blood tests, median (IQR)			
Albumin (g/L), n = 513/233	41.1 (38.6–43.1)	40.7 (38.8–42.9)	0.612
ALT (IU/L), n = 531/248	20 (14–28)	19 (13.2–29.8)	0.48

Table 3 Baseline Characteristics in the DC and VC *(Continued)*

AST (IU/L), *n* = 495/227	24 (19–31)	23 (19–32)	0.939
APTT (s)	32 (28.8–35.3)	31.9 (28.7–34.5)	0.299
Bilirubin, total (μmol/L), *n* = 497/231	11.5 (8.3–17)	11.5 (8–16.1)	0.699
Cholesterol, total (mmol/L), *n* = 467/209	5.1 (4.3–5.9)	5.2 (4.3–6.1)	0.286
Creatinine (μmol/L)	90.6 (79.3–106)	90 (77.4–108)	0.851
Fibrinogen (g/L), *n* = 502/240	3.2 (2.6–4)	3.2 (2.6–4.2)	0.985
Glucose (mmol/L)	6.8 (5.9–8.3)	6.8 (5.9–8.1)	0.998
Hematocrit, *n* = 534/247	0.43 (0.38–0.46)	0.42 (0.37–0.45)	0.08
Hemoglobin (g/L), *n* = 535/247	141 (128–153)	139 (124–150)	0.12
INR	1.04 (0.96–1.15)	1.05 (0.98–1.15)	0.361
Platelet count (×10^9 cells/L)	245 (199–306)	249.5 (201–301)	0.865
Protein, total (g/L), *n* = 523/242	67.9 (64.4–71.7)	68.4 (64.7–72.7)	0.159
Potassium (mmol/L), *n* = 530/243	4 (3.7–4.3)	4 (3.7–4.3)	0.223
PT (s), *n* = 531/247	12 (10.9–14.8)	12 (11.2–15.3)	0.408
RBC (×10^{12} cells/L)	4.63 (4.28–4.97)	4.55 (4.14–4.93)	0.032
Sodium (mmol/L), *n* = 530/242	139.5 (138–141.3)	139.1 (137–141)	0.164
Urea (mmol/L), *n* = 533/248	6 (4.7–7.7)	5.7 (4.6–7.6)	0.403
WBC (×10^9 cells/L)	7.9 (6.5–9.7)	7.6 (6.3–9.5)	0.285
ECG, *n* (%)			
AF rhythm	164 (30.7)	77 (31)	0.911
HR (bpm), median (IQR)	79 (67–91)	80 (68–96)	0.157
Normal ECG	26 (4.9)	10 (4)	0.607
Other ECG changes	259 (48.4)	121 (48.8)	0.921
LVEF (%), *n* = 486/217, median (IQR)	57 (50–60)	57 (50–61)	0.993
Chest X-ray, *n* (%)			
Aortic atherosclerosis	462 (86.4)	217 (87.5)	0.661
Cardiomegaly	401 (75)	207 (83.5)	0.008
Normal chest X-ray	28 (5.2)	13 (5.2)	0.996
Pleural effusion	62 (11.6)	20 (8.1)	0.134
Pneumonia	48 (9)	23 (9.3)	0.891
Pulmonary congestion	215 (40.2)	109 (44)	0.32
Antithrombotic medication, *n* (%)			
Anticoagulant	28 (5.2)	14 (5.6)	0.812
Antiplatelet	390 (73)	201 (81)	0.014
Anticoagulant + antiplatelet	66 (12.3)	17 (6.9)	0.02
IV rtPA	51 (9.5)	16 (6.5)	0.152
Outcome, *n* (%)			
Any HT	126 (23.6)	60 (24.2)	0.844
SHT	69 (12.9)	29 (11.7)	0.636
HI-1	22 (4.1)	4 (1.6)	0.069
HI-2	82 (15.3)	38 (15.3)	0.999
PH-1	9 (1.7)	4 (1.6)	0.944
PH-2	13 (2.4)	14 (5.6)	0.022
Death	34 (6.4)	19 (7.7)	0.499
Malignant cerebral edema	32 (6)	14 (5.6)	0.852
Dependency	325 (60.7)	147 (59.3)	0.695

Note: *APTT* stands for Activated partial thromboplastin time, *DBP* Diastolic blood pressure, *INR* International normalized ratio, *PT* Prothrombin time, *RBC* Red blood cells, *SBP* Systolic blood pressure, and *WBC* White blood cells

predictors coupled with IV rtPA over the past decade. As a result, a variety of predictive clinical scores have emerged [5–9].

On the other hand, there is a lack of tools for making an accurate HT prediction in AIS patients who are not eligible for IV rtPA. That is especially important in the light of missing evidence-based data concerning the timing of anticoagulant resumption after AIS in patients with atrial fibrillation (AF). Recommendations on the initiation of anticoagulation are currently based on consensus opinion, in what is known as the "1–3–6–12 day rule" [10]. Therefore, the two-week timeframe following the AIS onset is the most critical for developing HT. In this instance, an accurate prediction of HT could make a difference in decision making to reinstitute anticoagulation. The middle cerebral artery (MCA) is by far the largest cerebral artery and is the vessel most commonly affected by cerebrovascular accident.

Given the background, we aimed to develop a simple and yet reliable instrument called the hemorrhagic transformation index (HTI) to predict any HT within 14 days after AIS onset in the MCA territory regardless of the use of IV rtPA.

Methods

Patients

Using prospectively collected clinical and radiological databases, we retrospectively identified 783 consecutive patients with AIS in the MCA territory who were admitted to the stroke unit of the Interregional Clinical Diagnostic Center, Kazan, Russia, within 12 h after onset between January 2013 and May 2016. The exclusion criteria were: involvement of other vascular territories; AIS following any surgery or endovascular procedure within 1 month; brain ischemic lesions due to an intracranial tumor, infection, cerebral venous thrombosis, subarachnoid hemorrhage, and arteriovenous malformation/fistula. In total, 1361 AIS patients were admitted over the specified period. The sample was drawn from the local Caucasian population.

Table 4 Univariate Analysis in the DC Using the MI Dataset

	Any HT (n = 126)	No HT (n = 409)	OR (95% CI)	p-Value	FMI	RIV	RE
Clinical data, median (IQR)							
Age (y)	74 (62–79)	70 (60–77)	1.016 (0.998–1.034)	0.077	0	0	1
DBP (mm Hg)	90 (80–100)	90 (80–100)	0.992 (0.979–1.005)	0.217	0	0	1
Height (m)	1.65 (1.6–1.7)	1.66 (1.6–1.73)	0.983 (0.961–1.006)	0.138	0	0	1
Male sex, n (%)	60 (47.6)	229 (56)	0.715 (0.479–1.066)	0.1	0	0	1
NIHSS	20 (14–23)	6 (3–10)	1.253 (1.206–1.302)	<0.001	0	0	1
Pulse rate (bpm)	80 (74–88)	78 (72–80)	1.037 (1.021–1.053)	<0.001	0	0	1
SBP (mm Hg)	155 (140–180)	160 (140–179)	0.999 (0.992–1.006)	0.683	0	0	1
Temperature (°C)	36.6 (36.4–36.7)	36.6 (36.4–36.6)	1.658 (0.904–3.041)	0.102	0	0	1
Weight (kg)	76 (65–90)	79.5 (70–87)	0.998 (0.986–1.01)	0.759	0	0	1
Risk factors, n (%)							
Acute myocardial infarction	16 (12.6)	9 (2.2)	6.39 (2.75–14.851)	<0.001	0	0	1
AF history	81 (63.8)	129 (31.6)	3.808 (2.508–5.783)	<0.001	0	0	1
Alcohol abuse	11 (8.7)	51 (12.5)	0.664 (0.335–1.316)	0.241	0	0	1
Atherosclerosis	124 (97.6)	404 (99)	0.409 (0.09–1.853)	0.246	0	0	1
Bleeding history	9 (7.1)	32 (7.8)	1.116 (0.518–2.405)	0.78	0	0	1
Chronic heart failure	24 (18.4)	38 (9.3)	0.441 (0.253–0.768)	0.004	0	0	1
Chronic liver failure	1 (0.8)	4 (1)	0.802 (0.89–7.237)	0.844	0	0	1
Chronic renal failure	7 (5.5)	13 (3.2)	1.772 (0.691–4.543)	0.233	0	0	1
Coronary artery disease	56 (44.1)	135 (33.1)	1.595 (1.062–2.395)	0.024	0	0	1
Diabetes mellitus	39 (30.7)	103 (25.2)	1.312 (0.847–2.034)	0.224	0	0	1
Dyslipidemia	41 (32.3)	175 (42.9)	0.635 (0.417–0.967)	0.034	0	0	1
Hypertension	118 (92.9)	379 (92.9)	0.997 (0.459–2.166)	0.994	0	0	1
Malignancy	4 (3.1)	6 (1.5)	2.179 (0.605–7.846)	0.233	0	0	1
Previous TIA/stroke	51 (40.2)	170 (41.7)	0.939 (0.626–1.41)	0.763	0	0	1
Seizures at onset	0 (0)	10 (2.5)	–	0.075[a]	0	0	1
Brain CT, n (%)							
ASPECTS, median (IQR)	4 (1–6)	8 (7–9)	0.499 (0.44–0.567)	<0.001	0	0	1
HMCA sign	88 (69.3)	54 (13.2)	14.792 (9.213–23.749)	<0.001	0	0	1
Leukoaraiosis	87 (68.5)	260 (63.7)	1.238 (0.809–1.894)	0.325	0	0	1
Left hemispheric stroke	73 (58)	213 (52)	1.291 (0.863–1.931)	0.214	0	0	1
Right hemispheric stroke	53 (42)	181 (44.3)	0.898 (0.6–1.344)	0.602	0	0	1
Bihemispheric stroke	0 (0)	15 (3.7)	–	0.028[a]	0	0	1
Stroke cause, n (%)							
Large-artery atherosclerosis	41 (32.5)	171 (41.8)	0.671 (0.441–1.023)	0.064	0	0	1
Cardioembolism	79 (62.7)	146 (35.7)	3.028 (2.002–4.58)	<0.001	0	0	1
Small-vessel occlusion	0 (0)	79 (19.3)	–	<0.001[a]	0	0	1
Other determined etiology	1 (0.8)	6 (1.5)	0.537 (0.064–4.506)	0.567	0	0	1
Undetermined etiology	5 (4)	7 (1.7)	2.373 (0.74–7.612)	0.146	0	0	1
LVEF (%), n = 120/366, median (IQR)	55 (46.25–59)	58 (53–61.25)	0.957 (0.938–0.975)	<0.001	0.026	0.027	0.998
Chest X-ray, n (%)							
Aortic atherosclerosis	114 (89.8)	348 (85.3)	1.512 (0.801–2.85)	0.203	0	0	1
Cardiomegaly	109 (85.8)	292 (71.6)	2.406 (1.398–4.141)	0.002	0	0	1
Normal chest X-ray	3 (2.4)	25 (6.1)	0.371 (0.11–1.249)	0.109	0	0	1

Table 4 Univariate Analysis in the DC Using the MI Dataset *(Continued)*

Pleural effusion	25 (19.7)	37 (9.1)	2.458 (1.414–4.271)	0.001	0	0	1
Pneumonia	21 (16.5)	27 (6.6)	2.796 (1.52–5.143)	0.001	0	0	1
Pulmonary congestion	78 (61.4)	137 (33.6)	3.149 (2.085–4.755)	<0.001	0	0	1
ECG, *n* (%)							
AF rhythm	70 (55.1)	94 (23)	4.102 (2.699–6.236)	<0.001	0	0	1
HR (bpm), median (IQR)	90 (73–107)	75 (65.25–88)	1.034 (1.023–1.045)	<0.001	0	0	1
Normal ECG	3 (2.4)	23 (5.6)	0.405 (0.12–1.372)	0.146	0	0	1
Other changes	68 (53.5)	191 (46.8)	1.309 (0.878–1.952)	0.186	0	0	1
Blood tests, median (IQR)							
Albumin (g/L), *n* = 122/391	40.4 (38.4–42.8)	41.2 (38.7–43.2)	0.957 (0.905–1.012)	0.124	0.026	0.026	0.998
ALT (IU/L), *n* = 126/404	19 (15–29)	20 (14–27.5)	1.001 (0.992–1.01)	0.849	0.001	0.001	1
APPT (s)	31.7 (28.1–35.1)	32.2 (29–35.4)	0.993 (0.97–1.015)	0.52	0	0	1
AST (IU/L), *n* = 120/375	27 (20.4–32)	23 (18–30.3)	1.001 (0.995–1.008)	0.697	0.031	0.032	0.998
Bilirubin, total (μmol/L), *n* = 117/380	14.04 (9.3–19.6)	10.9 (8.1–15.4)	1.043 (1.018–1.068)	0.001	0.067	0.071	0.996
Creatinine (μmol/L)	89 (77.7–104.9)	91 (79.9–106.7)	0.998 (0.991–1.006)	0.638	0	0	1
Cholesterol, total (mmol/L), *n* = 113/354	4.8 (4–5.8)	5.2 (4.4–5.9)	0.805 (0.676–0.96)	0.016	0.038	0.039	0.998
Fibrinogen (g/L), *n* = 121/381	3.5 (2.7–4.4)	3.11 (2.6–3.9)	1.266 (1.087–1.475)	0.002	0.04	0.041	0.997
Glucose (mmol/L)	7.5 (6.4–9.7)	6.6 (5.8–7.9)	1.061 (1.009–1.117)	0.021	0	0	1
Hematocrit, *n* = 126/407	0.43 (0.38–0.46)	0.42 (0.38–0.46)	0.993 (0.958–1.029)	0.679	0	0	1
Hemoglobin (g/L)	141 (127–152)	141 (128.625–153)	0.997 (0.987–1.006)	0.515	0	0	1
INR	1.06 (0.98–1.15)	1.04 (0.95–1.12)	0.919 (0.467–1.808)	0.808	0	0	1
Platelet count ($\times 10^9$ cells/L)	236 (186–286)	248 (206–309)	0.998 (0.995–1)	0.048	0	0	1
Potassium (mmol/L), *n* = 126/404	4 (3.7–4.3)	4 (3.6–4.2)	1.247 (0.862–1.802)	0.241	0.009	0.009	0.999
Protein, total (g/L), *n* = 126/397	67.6 (64–71.2)	68 (64.8–71.7)	0.987 (0.953–1.021)	0.444	0.006	0.006	1
PT (s), *n* = 126/405	12.2 (11.3–13.8)	11.8 (10.8–16.1)	0.976 (0.932–1.022)	0.305	0.002	0.002	1
RBC ($\times 10^{12}$ cells/L)	4.64 (4.23–5.01)	4.63 (4.3–4.97)	0.941 (0.664–1.332)	0.73	0	0	1
Sodium (mmol/L), *n* = 126/404	139.3 (138–141.9)	139.5 (138–141.3)	1.015 (0.957–1.077)	0.624	0.011	0.011	0.999
Urea (mmol/L), *n* = 126/406	6.36 (5.2–8.5)	5.81 (4.5–7.3)	1.089 (1.02–1.161)	0.01	0	0	1
WBC ($\times 10^9$ cells/L)	8.8 (6.6–11.4)	7.8 (6.5–9.3)	1.145 (1.071–1.225)	<0.001	0	0	1
Antithrombotic medication, *n* (%)							
Anticoagulant	5 (4)	23 (5.6)	0.693 (0.258–1.863)	0.468	0	0	1
Antiplatelet	68 (54)	322 (78.7)	0.317 (0.208–0.483)	<0.001	0	0	1
Anticoagulant + antiplatelet	29 (23)	37 (9.1)	3.006 (1.76–5.132)	<0.001	0	0	1
IV rtPA	24 (19)	27 (6.6)	3.329 (1.842–6.015)	<0.001	0	0	1

Note: [a]Perfect predictor. Instead of BLR, Pearson χ^2 test was used

Table 5 Multivariate Analysis (DC, *n* = 535)

	Coefficient	Bias	Bootstrap SE	OR (95% BCa CI)	*p*-Value
ASPECTS	−0.472	−0.026	0.092	0.62 (0.52–0.75)	<0.001
AF on ECG	1.157	0.029	0.405	3.18 (1.47–6.66)	0.002
Male sex	0.88	0.055	0.381	2.41 (1.12–5.15)	0.027
NIHSS	0.135	0.004	0.029	1.15 (1.08–1.21)	<0.001
HR on ECG (bpm)	0.027	0.001	0.008	1.03 (1.01–1.04)	0.001
HMCA sign	1.041	0.001	0.346	2.83 (1.44–5.45)	0.002
INR	−3.304	−0.179	0.92	0.04 (0.01–0.22)	<0.001

Note: *SE* stands for Standard error

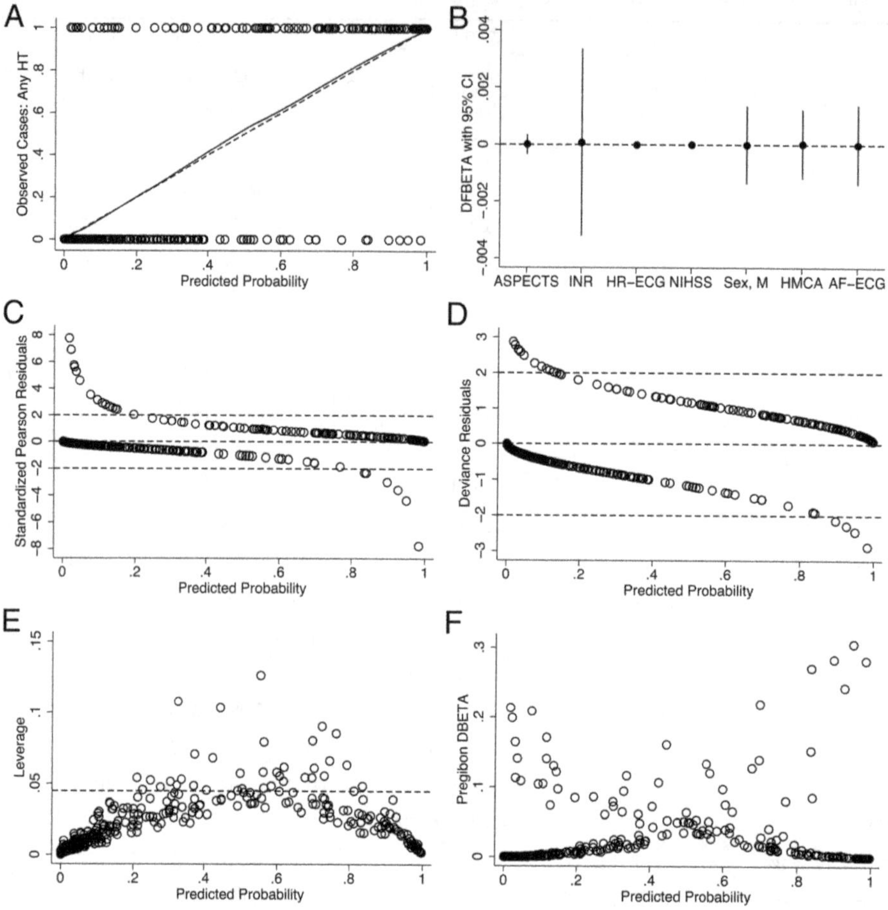

Fig. 1 Multivariate BLR Model Diagnostics. **a** LOWESS graph, bandwidth = 0.8. Each hollow circle is an individual observation. **b** Influence of each individual observation on the coefficient estimate (dfbeta). **c** Standardized Pearson residuals. **d** Deviance residuals. **e** Leverage. The dashed line corresponds to the 3-fold leverage mean. **f** Pregibon's influential statistics (dbeta)

The eligible patients received diagnostic tests and treatment in accordance with current national stroke guidelines. The permissible hospital length of stay was at least 14 days, which was determined by the state mandatory medical insurance standard for AIS patients.

Clinical baseline variables, including age, sex, risk factors, pre-admission medication, stroke subtype according to the Trial of ORG 10172 in Acute Stroke Treatment classification, NIHSS score, vital signs, blood tests, electrocardiogram (ECG), echocardiogram, and chest X-ray findings at admission were extracted from the medical charts. The NIHSS score was routinely and systematically assessed by neurologists. The time of AIS onset was documented as described by the patient or witness; if unknown, it was considered to be the last time the patient was seen well. In-hospital antithrombotic medication was logged for 14 consecutive days; the log was withdrawn earlier if HT occurred.

Imaging protocol

Brain non-contrast computed tomography (CT) was performed using a multidetector CT scanner (Aquilion 64; Toshiba Medical Systems, Otawara, Japan). All CT scans were obtained with 0.5 mm slice thickness; the technical parameters were as follows: 120 kVp, 300 mA, rotation time 0.75 s, matrix size 512 × 512, helical scan mode, total scan time 9.7 s, reconstruction interval 5 mm. Window levels and widths were optimized for gray/white matter distinction. The Alberta Stroke Program Early CT score (ASPECTS), hyperdense MCA (HMCA) sign, and leukoaraiosis were routinely and systematically recorded at admission by radiologists. The HMCA sign was assessed by measurements of absolute attenuation of the affected and normal vessels. Absolute density of the affected MCA of >43 Hounsfield units and the MCA ratio of >1.2 on a non-contrast CT scan were regarded as the positive HMCA sign [11]. Diffuse hypodense areas involving the periventricular and/or centrum semiovale white matter were considered as leukoaraiosis. A follow-up CT scan was routinely done on hospitalization day 7 and 14 or at any time if required by a treating neurologist. All patients had at least one follow-up CT scan.

Table 6 Derivation of the HTI Score

	PP Range[a]	Allocated Points
ASPECTS		
10–7	0.1–0.2	0
6–5	0.2–0.3	1
4–3	0.3–0.4	2
2–0	>0.4	3
NIHSS		
0–11	0.1–0.2	0
12–17	0.2–0.3	1
18–23	0.3–0.4	2
>23	>0.4	3
INR		
>1.82	<0.1	0
1.26–1.82	0.1–0.2	1
≤1.25	>0.2	2
HR on ECG (bpm)		
40–68	0.1–0.2	0
69–112	0.2–0.3	1
113–147	0.3–0.4	2
>147	>0.4	3
AF on ECG	0.2–0.3	1
HMCA sign	0.2–0.3	1
Male sex	0.2–0.3	1

Note: [a]Holding all other variables constant at their observed values

Outcome measures

The outcome was retrospectively revised based on prospectively collected data. Any HT on a follow-up CT scan within 14 days after AIS onset was taken into account. A hemorrhage was considered symptomatic if it was not seen on a previous CT scan and there had subsequently been either a suspicion of hemorrhage or any decline in neurologic status [12]. According to the ECASS I trial [13], HT was further classified into hemorrhagic infarction type 1 (HI-1), or type 2 (HI-2), or parenchymal hematoma type 1 (PH-1), or type 2 (PH-2).

Statistical analysis

Multinomial logistic regression with relative risk ratio (RRR) estimation was used to highlight the AHT and SHT association with poor outcomes (death, malignant edema, and dependency defined as the modified Rankin scale of >2 at discharge); the baseline category was the HT-negative group.

The intraclass correlation coefficient (ICC) was computed to assess inter-rater agreement for the ASPECTS and NIHSS. In order to calculate the ICC for the NIHSS, the same set of video files with NIHSS examination from six patients with different stroke severity was demonstrated to seven neurologists who regularly admitted patients to our stroke unit. The ICC for the ASPECTS was obtained in the similar manner: the identical pool of brain non-contrast CT scans from 33 patients with different ischemic burden was presented to four radiologists, who regularly evaluated brain CT scans at admission. Each doctor was evaluated separately and independently; the NIHSS and ASPECTS reference manuals were available on request. He or she had a chance to make any corrections during the evaluation process, but was not allowed to do so after his or her assessment had been completed.

A preliminary data analysis showed that 14 variables in 39.21% of observations were missing (Table 1).

The data were not missing completely at random (Little's test: $\chi^2(1706)$, 2336.69; $p < 0.001$). However, the omissions did occur accidentally because some tests were not available at the time of patient's admission or the results were lost. Moreover, the missing variables correlated with other collected data. Therefore, it was reasonable to assume that the data were missing at random and multiple imputation (MI) was an appropriate technique to manage the absent values (Table 2).

After obtaining the imputed data, the observations were divided into derivation (DC) and validation (VC) cohorts by generating Bernoulli variates with probability parameter 0.7.

Descriptive statistics included median with interquartile range (IQR) and percentage for continuous (the distribution was not normal) and categorical data respectively. The NIHSS and ASPECTS were treated as continuous variables because of multiple categories. Lists of univariate and multivariate HT predictors were obtained by fitting a binary logistic regression (BLR) model. Variables with univariate p-value ≤0.25 were further included in multivariate analysis, whereas only items with p-value <0.05 were kept in the multivariate BLR equation. Once the list of HT predictors was obtained by fitting a multivariate BLR model, we dropped the MI dataset because the included variables had no missing values in the source data.

In order to proceed with exploratory (EFA) and confirmatory (CFA) factor analysis, the Bartlett's test of sphericity, Kaiser-Meyer-Olkin measure, and Doornik-Hansen test were carried out to check for patterned relationships between the HTI items, data sufficiency, and multivariate normality respectively. EFA by means of principal factor (PF) and principal component factor (PCF) techniques was performed with varimax and promax rotations to assess dimensionality of the HTI items and to extract variables with shared variance; an eigenvalue cut-off was 1.0. CFA with maximum likelihood estimation was applied to select the final model; goodness of fit was assessed with the Satorra-Bentler scaled χ^2 test to adjust for data non-normality.

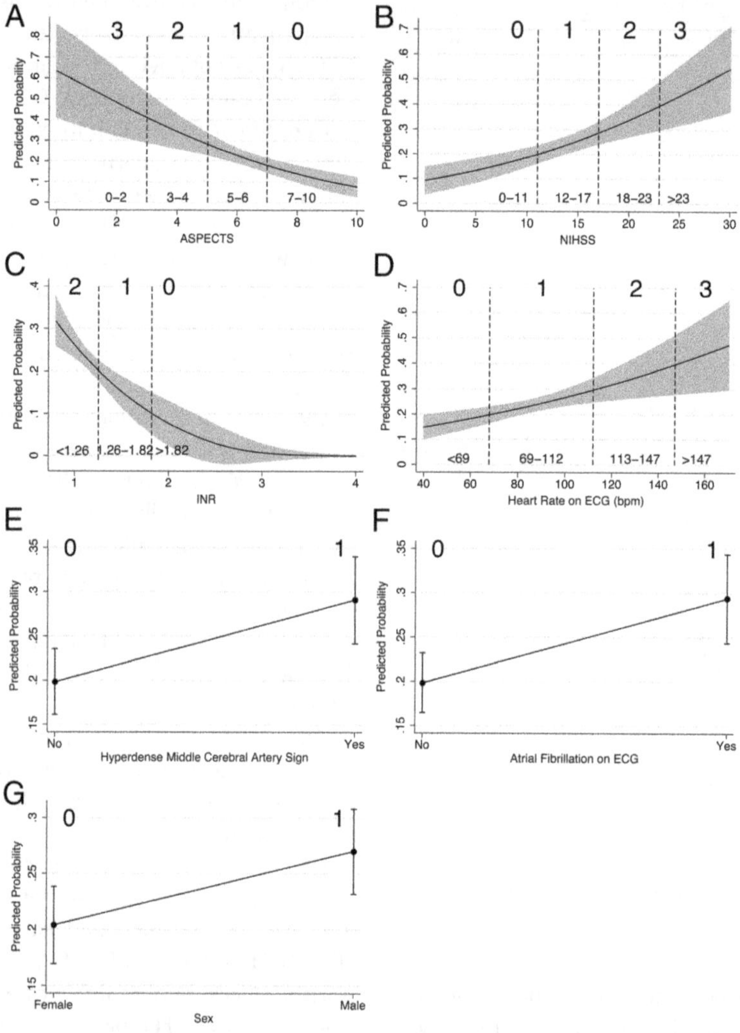

Fig. 2 Derivation of HTI Score. **a** ASPECTS. **b** NIHSS. **c** INR. **d** HR on ECG. **e** HMCA sign. **f** AF on ECG. **g** Sex. Grey areas and capped lines represent 95% CI. Numbers at the top indicate HTI scores; at the bottom, units of variables. The confounders are held constant at their observed values

HTI internal consistency reliability (ICR) was evaluated with the ordinal α, Guttman λ_2 and λ_4 bounds, Raykov's ρ, McDonald's ω, and greatest lower bound [14, 15]. The values ≥0.7 were considered to be reliable. As the model included ordinal and dichotomous variables, a polychoric correlation matrix was used for EFA and ICR analysis except for McDonald's categorical ω. The latter was computed by using the Green and Yang method [16].

The DC and VC were compared by using the Mann-Whitney U and Pearson χ^2 tests for continuous and categorical variables respectively. The equality of kernel density estimate (KDE) for predicted probability (PP) of any HT between the multivariate BLR model and HTI score as well as for HTI scores between the DC and VC was evaluated with the two-sample Kolmogorov-Smirnov test.

Receiver operating characteristic (ROC) analysis was conducted to assess prognostic performance. The optimal cutpoint score to distinguish between HT-positive and negative groups was defined with the Youden index. Based on the VC appraisal, the predictive ability of the HTI was compared with several alternative tools by testing the area under the ROC curve (AUC) of each score against the HTI one. For each comparison, the Šidák-adjusted *p*-value was reported. The AUC equality was evaluated by using the DeLong algorithm [17].

Whenever possible, bootstrapping was performed with 1000 samples and computing either adjusted for ties bias-corrected and accelerated (BCa) or normal-based (NB) confidence intervals (CI) to reduce sampling bias, overfitting, and prediction errors.

Results

Overall, HT occurred in 186 (23.8%) out of 783 cases, whereas SHT was determined in 98 (12.5%). HI-1 was established in 26 (3.3%); HI-2, 120 (15.3%); PH-1, 13 (1.7%); and PH-2, 27 (3.4%) observations. Patients with

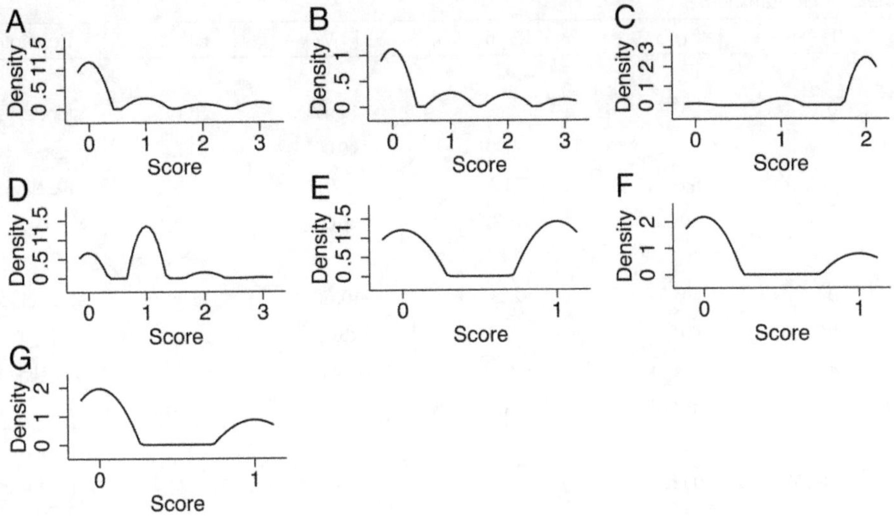

Fig. 3 KDE for HTI Items. Kernel = Epanechnikov for all items. **a** ASPECTS; bandwidth = 0.1899. **b** NIHSS; bandwidth = 0.1899. **c** INR; bandwidth = 0.116. **d** HR on ECG; bandwidth = 0.1528. **e** Sex; bandwidth = 0.1278. **f** HMCA sign; bandwidth = 0.113. **g** AF on ECG; bandwidth = 0.1182

any HT were more likely to have a poor outcome: death (AHT: RRR, 4.8; 95% CI, 2.2–10.6; $p < 0.001$; SHT: RRR, 11.7; 95% CI, 6–22.6; $p < 0.001$), malignant edema (AHT: RRR, 16.7; 95% CI, 5.6–49.2; $p < 0.001$; SHT: RRR, 52.1; 95% CI, 19.6–138.9; $p < 0.001$), and dependency (AHT: RRR, 4.4; 95% CI, 2.5–7.7; $p < 0.001$; SHT: RRR, 30.4; 95% CI, 9.5–97.1; $p < 0.001$).

There was no difference between AHT and SHT groups with regard to timing ($p = 0.08$): the former, median day 2 (IQR, 1–4); the latter, median day 2 (IQR, 1–3). The median AIS onset time was 6 h (IQR, 2–11). Just under half of all cases (346; 44.2%) were admitted within the 4.5-h therapeutic window; in total, 67 (8.6%) patients were treated with IV rtPA.

The ICC was 0.95 (95% CI, 0.85–0.99; $p < 0.001$) and 0.78 (95% CI, 0.59–0.88; $p < 0.001$) for the NIHSS and ASPECTS respectively, which indicated excellent inter-rater agreement. There was no difference between the DC and VC (Table 3).

Univariate analysis was summarized in Table 4.

Multivariate analysis

Although univariate p-values for leukoaraiosis and international normalized ratio (INR) were above our acceptable threshold, we included them in the multivariate analysis because some authors had proposed them as risk factors [18, 19]. As a result of fitting a multivariate BLR model, seven variables were kept in the final equation (Table 5).

Swapping AF on ECG for the AF history variable increased the Bayesian and Akaike information criteria by 1.18, which slightly favored the initial model. Overall, the multivariate BLR model was statistically significant (Wald test: $\chi^2(7)$, 87.76; $p < 0.001$; −2log-likelihood,

Table 7 Factor/Component Loadings and Uniqueness in EFA of the HTI Items

	No Rotation			Varimax Rotation		Promax Rotation		Uniqueness	
	F1	C1	C2	C1	C2	C1	C2	PF	PCF
ASPECTS	0.84	0.86		0.9		0.9		0.29	0.17
HR on ECG	0.34	0.43	−0.6		0.73		0.75	0.89	0.45
INR			0.56		−0.54		−0.58	0.99	0.68
NIHSS	0.83	0.86		0.89		0.89		0.32	0.18
Male sex	−0.33	−0.43			−0.4		−0.39	0.89	0.76
HMCA sign	0.81	0.84	0.36	0.91		0.91		0.35	0.18
AF on ECG	0.56	0.65	−0.59		0.83		0.82	0.69	0.23
Eigenvalue	2.58	2.98	1.38	NA	NA	NA	NA	NA	NA
Variance, %	82.8	42.5	19.76	37.56	24.7	39.33	28.1	NA	NA

Note: Empty cells indicate that absolute factor or component loading value is <0.3. *C1* stands for Component 1, *C2* Component 2, *F1* Factor 1, and *NA* Not applicable

Table 8 CFA. Goodness of Fit Statistics

	F1-V4	F1-V5	F1-V6	F1-V7	F2	Description
Likelihood ratio						
χ^2(2/5/9/14/13)	0.5	56.17	87.26	103.66	18.19	Model vs. saturated
p-value	0.78	<0.001	<0.001	<0.001	0.15	
χ^2(6/10/15/21/21)	594.14	664.18	711.01	727.4	727.4	Baseline vs. saturated
p-value	<0.001	<0.001	<0.001	<0.001	<0.001	
Satorra-Bentler test						
χ^2(2/5/9/14/13)	0.4	50.96	82.63	100.31	18.08	Model vs. saturated
p-value	0.82	<0.001	<0.001	<0.001	0.16	
χ^2(6/10/15/21/21)	475.75	574.14	649.06	684.79	684.79	Baseline vs. saturated
p-value	<0.001	<0.001	<0.001	<0.001	<0.001	
Population error						
RMSEA	<0.001	0.138	0.127	0.109	0.027	Root mean squared error of approximation
90% CI	0–0.056	0.107–0.172	0.104–0.153	0.09–0.13	0–0.054	
p-close	0.932	<0.001	<0.001	<0.001	0.909	Probability RMSEA ≤0.05
RMSEA-SB	<0.001	0.131	0.124	0.107	0.027	Satorra-Bentler RMSEA
Information criteria						
AIC	3726.82	4682.79	5446.18	6121.68	6038.21	Akaike information criterion
BIC	3778.21	4747.02	5523.26	6211.6	6132.42	Bayesian information criterion
Baseline comparison						
CFI	1	0.92	0.89	0.87	0.99	Comparative fit index
TLI	1	0.84	0.81	0.81	0.99	Tucker-Lewis index
CFI-SB	1	0.92	0.88	0.87	0.99	Satorra-Bentler CFI
TLI-SB	1	0.84	0.81	0.81	0.99	Satorra-Bentler TLI
Size of residuals						
SRMR	0.01	0.08	0.08	0.08	0.03	Standardized root mean squared residual
CD	0.83	0.83	0.83	0.83	0.96	Coefficient of determination

Note: *F1-V4* indicates one-factor model with 4 variables (ASPECTS, NIHSS, HMCA sign, and AF on ECG), *F1-V5* one-factor model with 5 variables (4 previous variables + HR on ECG), *F1-V6* one-factor model with 6 variables (5 previous variables + sex), *F1-V7* one-factor model with 7 variables (6 previous variables + INR), and *F2* two-factor model with factor 1 (ASPECTS, NIHSS, and HMCA sign) and factor 2 (AF on ECG, INR, sex, and HR on ECG)

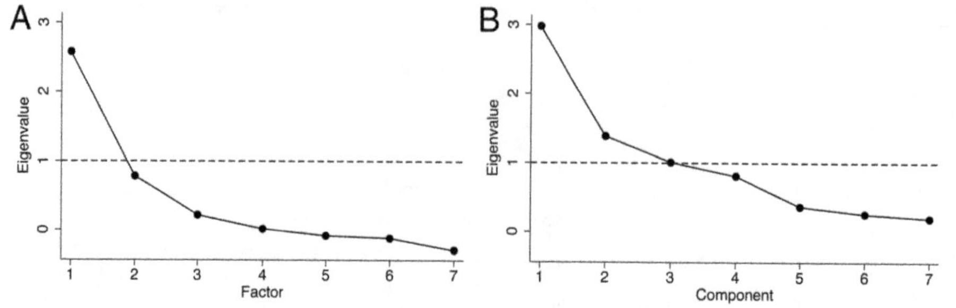

Fig. 4 Scree Plot. EFA by using (**a**) PF and (**b**) PCF methods

Table 9 BLR Coefficients, Bias, and Bootstrap SE for the HTI (DC, n = 535)

	Crude			Adjusted[a]		
	Coefficient	Bias	Bootstrap SE	Coefficient	Bias	Bootstrap SE
HTI, overall	0.941	0.012	0.085	1.03	0.027	0.109
HTI items						
ASPECTS	0.815	0.031	0.165	0.914	0.047	0.188
NIHSS	0.958	0.02	0.175	1.053	0.038	0.201
HMCA sign	1.157	−0.005	0.336	1.214	0.008	0.347
AF on ECG	1.115	0.002	0.317	1.214	0.031	0.403

Note: [a]Confounders (sex, INR, and HR on ECG) were measured in allocated points (Table 6)

271.93; Cox-Snell pseudo-R^2, 0.44; Nagelkerke pseudo-R^2, 0.67). It explained variance of 78.4% (variance of latent variable, y^* = 11.13; error, ε = 3.29) and fitted the data well (Hosmer-Lemeshow goodness of fit test for 10 groups: $\chi^2(8)$, 6.87; p = 0.551). Neither significant interactions nor polynomial terms were found.

There was no specification error (Pregibon's link test: linear predicted value, $p < 0.001$; linear predicted value squared, p = 0.54). Assumption of linearity between independent variables and log odds was confirmed by the LOWESS graph. Multicollinearity was not an issue: the extrema of the variance inflation factor were 1.01 and 2.29.

Although standardized Pearson and deviance residuals exceeded 2 in a few observations, their leverage and Pregibon's influential statistics (dbeta) turned out to be very small. Moreover, removing those observations did not significantly change the equation coefficients. Influence of each individual observation on the coefficient estimate (not adjusted for the covariate pattern), dfbeta, was not strong. However, the most sensitive was the INR variable (Fig. 1).

Model sensitivity, specificity, positive and negative predictive values were 76.2%, 95.6%, 84.2%, and 92.9% respectively. The model accurately classified 91% of the observations, whereas the equation without any independent variables classified correctly only 76.5% of the cases.

Based on PP tables and plots, we divided each predictor into categories and allocated them points according to the PP range in order to draw the HTI score. Given the Doornik-Hansen test ($\chi^2(14)$, 3665.64; $p < 0.001$), the distribution of the newly derived HTI items was not multivariate normal (Table 6; Figs. 2 and 3).

Factor analysis

The Bartlett's test of sphericity ($\chi^2(21)$, 721.74; $p < 0.001$) and the Kaiser-Meyer-Olkin measure of 0.71 demonstrated that the HTI items did have patterned relationships and were sufficient for EFA. PF EFA established a unidimensional scale, i.e. there was only one factor that explained a cumulative variance of 82.8%. By means of PCF EFA, the factor was discovered to consist of cerebral (ASPECTS, NIHSS, and HMCA sign) and extracerebral (resting heart rate (HR) on ECG, AF on ECG, sex, and INR) components as we called them. However, the resting HR on ECG, INR, and sex variables showed high uniqueness values and low factor loadings; therefore, we had to drop them. The final 4-item HTI was strongly supported by subsequent CFA (Tables 7 and 8; Fig. 4).

Once the HTI was definitively established, crude PP of any HT was computed for each score by using BLR. Although the dropped items were no longer a part of the HTI, we put them into the BLR equation for confounding adjustment. Unsurprisingly, the confounders exerted only a minor influence on the overall HTI OR by increasing it up to 12% and had no significant effect on the OR of the separate HTI items (Tables 9, 10 and 11; Fig. 5).

KDE for PP of any HT was equal between the multivariate BLR model and HTI score (D = 0.184; p = 0.371). Thus, the HTI score was considered as a surrogate for the multivariate BLR model (Fig. 6).

Table 10 OR for the HTI (DC, n = 535)

	Crude		Adjusted[a]		Crude vs. Adjusted[b]	
	OR (95% BCa CI)	p-Value	OR (95% BCa CI)	p-Value	$\chi^2(1)$	p-Value
HTI, overall	2.56 (2.19–3.02)	<0.001	2.80 (2.32–3.39)	<0.001	4.03	0.045
HTI items						
ASPECTS	2.26 (1.64–3.07)	<0.001	2.49 (1.75–3.54)	<0.001	2.4	0.121
NIHSS	2.61 (1.88–3.7)	<0.001	2.87 (1.91–4.15)	<0.001	1.91	0.167
HMCA sign	3.18 (1.71–6.24)	0.001	3.37 (1.73–6.89)	<0.001	0.33	0.565
AF on ECG	3.05 (1.71–5.88)	<0.001	3.37 (1.55–7.4)	0.003	0.27	0.605

Note: [a]Confounders (sex, INR, and HR on ECG) were measured in allocated points (Table 6). [b]Wald test was performed

Table 11 PP of Any HT for Each HTI Score

HTI Score	Crude		Adjusted[a]	
	PP (95% CI)	*p*-Value	PP (95% CI)	*p*-Value
0	0.03 (0.015–0.044)	<0.001	0.027 (0.011–0.042)	0.001
1	0.073 (0.047–0.099)	<0.001	0.07 (0.043–0.098)	<0.001
2	0.168 (0.126–0.21)	<0.001	0.169 (0.125–0.213)	<0.001
3	0.34 (0.274–0.407)	<0.001	0.346 (0.275–0.417)	<0.001
4	0.569 (0.479–0.66)	<0.001	0.571 (0.474–0.668)	<0.001
5	0.772 (0.686–0.858)	<0.001	0.768 (0.676–0.861)	<0.001
6	0.897 (0.838–0.955)	<0.001	0.893 (0.829–0.957)	<0.001
7	0.957 (0.925–0.989)	<0.001	0.956 (0.92–0.992)	<0.001
8	0.983 (0.967–0.998)	<0.001	0.983 (0.965–1.0)	<0.001

Note: [a]Confounders (sex, INR, and HR on ECG) were held constant at their observed values

ICR and ROC analysis

Given multiple reliability tests, HTI ICR was considered to be fair enough for the DC and VC alike. There was also no difference in the AUC ($\chi^2(1)$, 0.01; p = 0.93) and KDE for the HTI scores (D = 0.02; p = 1.0) between both cohorts (Table 12; Fig. 7).

Taking into account that alternative scores had been developed in AIS patients with slightly different clinical settings, the HTI prognostic performance was considered to be at least non-inferior to the competitors (Tables 13 and 14).

Discussion

The incidence of HT showed in our study echoes the rate reported in literature. We have also reaffirmed the concept that AHT is not clinically innocuous. The study unequivocally reiterates infarct size, stroke severity, large-artery occlusion, and cardioembolism defined by ASPECTS, NIHSS, HMCA sign, and AF respectively are well-established independent HT predictors [20, 21]. In our HTI score, we use the presence of AF on ECG at admission rather than AF history for the reason discussed in the Results. However, other known predictors – platelet count, cholesterol level, age, hypertension, renal failure, hyperglycemia, and leukoaraiosis – have shown no independent association with any HT in our cohort; similar results were obtained by other authors [22–26]. The mechanism of this association needs to be explored.

Although women tend to be more likely HT-positive in our univariate BLR model, multivariate analysis reveals the opposite. It seems there is still controversy about the sex propensity for developing HT [27].

Accelerated HR at rest is known to be associated with an increased risk of stroke especially recurrent [28]. Since AIS commonly induces change in cardiovascular responses, post-stroke HR at admission could be a potential marker to identify patients at risk for short-term deterioration and long-term poor outcomes [29]. To the best of our knowledge, we have not found any literature, concerning HR correlations with HT. Here, we report that the more the HR is accelerated on ECG (but not the pulse rate), the more likely HT can occur.

Hypercoagulability at AIS onset measured by INR and other tests is known to be associated with an increased thrombotic tendency. As long as the hypercoagulable state persists, both arterial and venous thromboembolic recurrences can be expected. The association of these coagulation abnormalities with HT is not always clear [30]. As we have shown here, the less the INR, the higher the risk of HT.

Having identified seven independent variables in our multivariate analysis, we applied the PP range followed by factor analysis to assigned HTI scores and to regroup HTI variables into a limited set of clusters based on shared variance. We assume probability is more intuitive for interpreting than OR. In contrast, authors of other predictive tools allocated scores based on OR changes only [5–9, 31–33]. While BLR analyzes effects of each individual predictor on the dependent variable, factor analysis isolating constructs and concepts treats the model as a whole [34]. Thus, it helped us to avoid overfitting.

Among the compared predictive tools, the SPAN-100 and HeRS were derived from the cohorts, which were

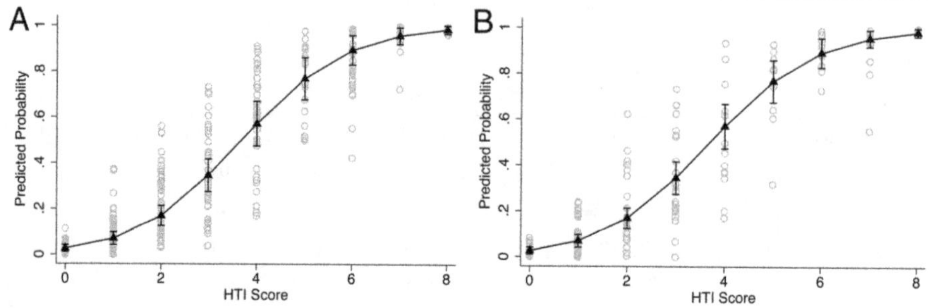

Fig. 5 Calibration Plot. The scatterplots display PP of any HT for individual observations obtained from multivariate analysis (Table 5) and arranged by the HTI score: (**a**) The DC, (**b**) The VC. The superimposed connected line graph drawn from the DC demonstrates PP of any HT for each HTI score with 95% CI adjusted for sex, INR, and HR on ECG (Table 11). The confounders are held constant at their observed values

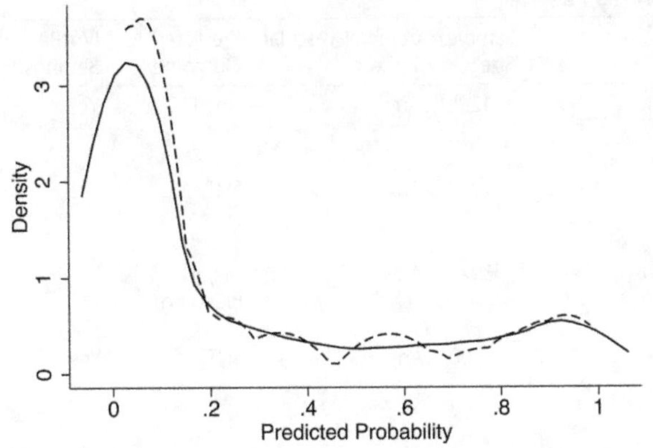

Fig. 6 KDE for PP of Any HT. Kernel = Epanechnikov, bandwidth = 0.0623. The solid line represents the multivariate BLR model (Table 5); the dashed line, the HTI score (Table 11)

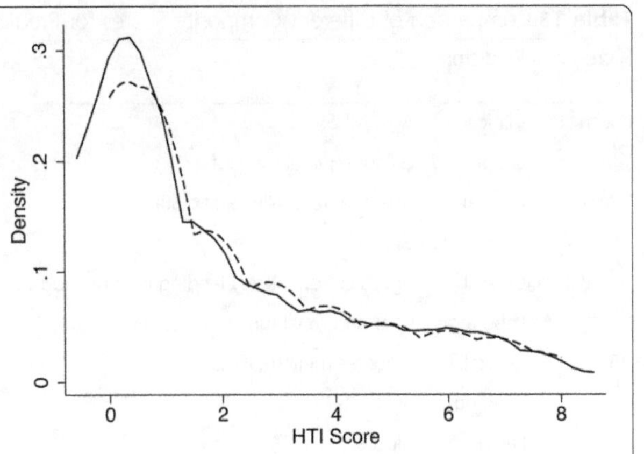

Fig. 7 KDE for HTI Scores. Kernel = Epanechnikov, bandwidth = 0.5697. The solid line represents the DC; the dashed line, the VC

very similar in clinical settings to ours (Table 13). As to the former, we have reaffirmed that it is far inferior in prognostic performance to other scores [35, 36]. Regarding the latter, the infarct size was measured in different ways: we chose the ASPECTS estimation on non-contrast CT, whereas the HeRS scored it in milliliters on magnetic resonance diffusion-weighted imaging (DWI MRI). Although both approaches are widely acceptable in hyperacute stroke settings, the ASPECTS is more suitable for non-contrast CT assessment, while the lesion volume can easily be quantified on DWI [37–39]. Furthermore, the ASPECTS, as well as the NIHSS, correlates strongly with the infarct volume (ASPECTS: Spearman ρ, −0.88; $p < 0.001$; NIHSS: Spearman ρ, 0.71; $p < 0.001$; VC, n = 248), but moderately with each other

Table 12 HTI ICR and ROC Analysis

	DC, n = 535	VC, n = 248
Ordinal α	0.82	0.83
Guttman bounds		
λ_2	0.83	0.85
λ_4	0.84	0.88
Raykov's ρ	0.81	0.81
McDonald's ω		
Categorical (95% BCa CI)	0.81 (0.77–0.84)	0.82 (0.76–0.86)
Hierarchical	0.83	0.87
Total	0.89	0.91
Greatest lower bound	0.84	0.89
ROC analysis (95% NB CI)		
AUC	0.85 (0.82–0.89)	0.83 (0.78–0.88)
Youden index	0.7 (0.63–0.78)	0.67 (0.57–0.77)
Cutpoint	2 (1–3)	2 (1–3)
Sensitivity	0.82 (0.73–0.9)	0.8 (0.66–0.94)
Specificity	0.89 (0.8–0.97)	0.87 (0.73–1.0)

(Spearman ρ, −0.66; $p < 0.001$; VC, n = 248). If the stroke volume variable had been added to our multivariate BLR equation, a multicollinearity issue would have occurred. We also suppose that a combination of clinical and imaging features is more reliable than the imaging data alone. To make our HTI score as much easy-to-use as possible, we have purposely refrained from MRI since CT is readily available in the most hospitals. Moreover, the HeRS score is computationally complicated; therefore, it seems less attractive from the practical point of view.

There are some important peculiarities between posterior and anterior circulation stroke. The differences include the value of screening instruments, optimum diagnostic modalities, clinical features, and outcomes [40, 41]. For instance, patients with vertebrobasilar infarction have lower NIHSS score and HT rates, less often AF, higher blood glucose level and rates of false-negative DWI findings, more WBC counts, and a better long-term outcome than those with carotid stroke [42–44]. However, all aforementioned tools predict HT regardless of the vascular basin (Table 13). Moreover, scores with imaging modalities, like the HAT and SEDAN, include CT signs of MCA stroke only. Meanwhile, a scoring system, the pc-ASPECTS, has been developed and validated for posterior circulation stroke [45]. Thus, the accuracy of predictive tools could be further improved by distinguishing the infarcted vascular basins; therefore, we have decided to restrict our study to the MCA territory.

There are a few limitations in our study. A relatively small, but sufficient for statistical inferences, sample size and lack of ethnic and racial diversity could be a source of potential bias. Almost all patients came from our local community, which was populated with Russian, Tatar, and Jewish ethnic groups; there were no patients of African, Asian or Hispanic origin. Furthermore, AIS patients following endovascular interventions were excluded

Table 13 Comparison of Different Composite Scores for Predicting HT in AIS Patients

Score	Predictors		Sample Size	Cerebral Vascular Territory	Predicted Outcome	IV rtPA Settings
Cucchiara [6]	Clinical	Age, NIHSS	1205	Any	Any HT	Yes
	Laboratory	Glucose, platelet count				
GRASPS [9]	Clinical	Age, ethnicity, NIHSS, sex, SBP	10,242	Any	SHT	Yes
	Laboratory	Glucose				
HAS-BLED [46]	Clinical	Age, alcohol abuse, bleeding history, drugs, SBP, stroke/TIA	3978	Any	Major Bleeding[a]	No
	Laboratory	Liver and renal function tests, INR				
HAT [5]	Clinical	Diabetes mellitus, NIHSS	400	Any	SHT	Yes
	Imaging	ASPECTS				
	Laboratory	Glucose				
HeRS [31]	Clinical	Age	345	Any	Any HT	Regardless
	Imaging	Infarct volume				
	Laboratory	Estimated glomerular filtration rate				
HTI	Clinical	NIHSS	783	MCA	Any HT	Regardless
	Imaging	ASPECTS, HMCA sign				
	Laboratory	AF on ECG				
iScore [32]	Clinical	AF, age, cancer, chronic heart failure, NIHSS, preadmission disability, renal dialysis, sex, stroke subtype	1696	Any	Any HT	Yes
	Laboratory	Glucose				
SEDAN [8]	Clinical	Age, NIHSS	1802	Any	SHT	Yes
	Imaging	ASPECTS, HMCA sign				
	Laboratory	Glucose				
SITS-SICH [7]	Clinical	Age, antiplatelet medication, hypertension, NIHSS, stroke onset to treatment time, SBP, weight	31,627	Any	SHT	Yes
	Laboratory	Glucose				
SPAN-100 [33]	Clinical	Age, NIHSS	624	Any	Any HT	Regardless

Note: [a]1-year risk for major bleeding (intracranial, hospitalization, hemoglobin decrease > 2 g/L, and/or transfusion) in a cohort of real-world patients with AF

Table 14 AUC Comparison Between the HTI and Alternative Scores (VC, *n* = 248)

Score	AUC (95% NB CI)	$\chi^2(1)$	*p*-Value
HTI	0.83 (0.78–0.88)	–	–
Cucchiara	0.72 (0.67–0.77)	31.6	<0.001
GRASPS	0.80 (0.75–0.84)	10.98	<0.001
HAS-BLED	0.53 (0.47–0.59)	86.47	<0.001
HAT	0.82 (0.77–0.88)	4.34	0.037
HeRS[a]	0.81 (0.75–0.86)	4.11	0.043
iScore	0.83 (0.79–0.87)	2.93	0.087
SEDAN	0.82 (0.76–0.87)	11.59	<0.001
SITS-SICH[b]	0.72 (0.66–0.78)	25.06	<0.001
SPAN-100	0.59 (0.53–0.65)	111.26	<0.001

Note: [a]Infarct volume was calculated on follow-up CT scans (≥12 h after the initial imaging) by using the ABC/2 formula. [b]For patients, who were not eligible for IV rtPA, stroke onset to treatment time was considered as stroke onset to admission time

from the analysis due to a small number of observations. Although some clinical and imaging data were collected prospectively, the research was retrospective in nature. As a result, we were not blinded to the outcome. The study was also confined to a single clinical center; to cope with that bias, we used bootstrapping. Finally, prospective multicenter external validation would be desirable.

Conclusions

The HTI is a four-item tool composed of ASPECTS, NIHSS, HMCA sign, and presence of AF on ECG at admission. The total score ranges from zero to eight. The higher the score, the more likely HT can occur. Knowing probability of any HT in advance could exert a significant influence on decision making to reinstitute anticoagulation in AIS patients with AF. It is a simple yet reliable instrument to predict any HT within 2 weeks after onset of AIS in the MCA territory regardless of the use of IV rtPA.

Abbreviations

AF: Atrial fibrillation; AHT: Asymptomatic hemorrhagic transformation; AIS: Acute ischemic stroke; ALT: Alanine transaminase; APTT: Activated partial thromboplastin time; ASPECTS: Alberta Stroke Program Early CT score; AST: Aspartate transaminase; AUC: Area under the ROC curve; BCa: Bias-corrected and accelerated (adjusted for ties); BLR: Binary logistic regression; CFA: Confirmatory factor analysis; CI: Confidence interval; CT: Computed tomography; DBP: Diastolic blood pressure; DC: Derivation cohort; DWI: Diffusion-weighted imaging; ECG: Electrocardiogram; EFA: Exploratory factor analysis; FMI: Fraction of missing information; HI-1: Hemorrhagic infarction type 1; HI-2: Hemorrhagic infarction type 2; HMCA: Hyperdense middle cerebral artery; HR: Heart rate; HT: Hemorrhagic transformation; HTI: Hemorrhagic transformation index; ICC: Intraclass correlation coefficient; ICR: Internal consistency reliability; INR: International normalized ratio; IQR: Interquartile range; IV rtPA: Intravenous recombinant tissue plasminogen activator; KDE: Kernel density estimate; LOWESS: Locally weighted scatterplot smoothing; LVEF: Left ventricular ejection fraction (echocardiography, Simpson method); MCA: Middle cerebral artery; MCMC: Markov chain Monte Carlo; MI: Multiple imputation; MRI: Magnetic resonance imaging; NB: Normal-based; NIHSS: National Institutes of Health Stroke Scale; OR: Odds ratio; PCF: Principal component factor; PF: Principal factor; PH-1: Parenchymal hematoma type 1; PH-2: Parenchymal hematoma type 2; PP: Predicted probability; PT: Prothrombin time; RBC: Red blood cells; RE: Relative efficiency; RIV: Relative increase in variance; ROC: Receiver operating characteristic; RRR: Relative risk ratio; SBP: Systolic blood pressure; SE: Standard error; SHT: Symptomatic hemorrhagic transformation; TIA: Transient ischemic attack; VC: Validation cohort; WBC: White blood cells

Acknowledgements

Not applicable.

Funding

No funding was received.

Authors' contributions

M.N.K. was involved in the design, data collection, analysis and interpretation, and reporting of this project. D.R.K. and M.M.I. helped with the design, data collection, data analysis, and revision of the manuscript. All authors have read and approved the final manuscript for publication.

Competing interests

The authors declare that they have no competing interests.

Author details

[1]Department of Neurology and Neurosurgery for Postgraduate Training, Kazan State Medical University, Kazan, Russia. [2]Department of Neurology, Interregional Clinical Diagnostic Center, 12A Karbyshev St, Kazan 420101, Russia. [3]Department of Radiology, Interregional Clinical Diagnostic Center, Kazan, Russia.

References

1. Lei C, Wu B, Liu M, Chen Y. Asymptomatic hemorrhagic transformation after acute ischemic stroke: is it clinically innocuous? J Stroke Cerebrovasc Dis. 2014;23:2767–72.
2. Sussman ES, Connolly ES Jr. Hemorrhagic transformation: a review of the rate of hemorrhage in the major clinical trials of acute ischemic stroke. Front Neurol. 2013;4:69.
3. Zhang J, Yang Y, Sun H, Xing Y. Hemorrhagic transformation after cerebral infarction: current concepts and challenges. Ann Transl Med. 2014;2:81.
4. Quain DA, Parsons MW, Loudfoot AR, Spratt NJ, Evans MK, Russell ML, et al. Improving access to acute stroke therapies: a controlled trial of organised pre-hospital and emergency care. Med J Aust. 2008;189:429–33.
5. Lou M, Safdar A, Mehdiratta M, Kumar S, Schlaug G, Caplan L, et al. The HAT score: a simple grading scale for predicting hemorrhage after thrombolysis. Neurology. 2008;71:1417–23.
6. Cucchiara B, Tanne D, Levine SR, Demchuk AM, Kasner S. A risk score to predict intracranial hemorrhage after recombinant tissue plasminogen activator for acute ischemic stroke. J Stroke Cerebrovasc Dis. 2008;17:331–3.
7. Mazya M, Egido JA, Ford GA, Lees KR, Mikulik R, Toni D, et al. Predicting the risk of symptomatic intracerebral hemorrhage in ischemic stroke treated with intravenous alteplase: Safe Implementation of Treatments in Stroke (SITS) symptomatic intracerebral hemorrhage risk score. Stroke 2012;43: 1524–31.
8. Strbian D, Engelter S, Michel P, Meretoja A, Sekoranja L, Ahlhelm FJ, et al. Symptomatic intracranial hemorrhage after stroke thrombolysis: the SEDAN score. Ann Neurol. 2012;71:634–41.
9. Menon BK, Saver JL, Prabhakaran S, Reeves M, Liang L, Olson DM, et al. Risk score for intracranial hemorrhage in patients with acute ischemic stroke treated with intravenous tissue-type plasminogen activator. Stroke. 2012;43:2293–9.
10. Heidbuchel H, Verhamme P, Alings M, Antz M, Diener HC, Hacke W, et al. Updated European Heart Rhythm Association Practical Guide on the use of non-vitamin K antagonist anticoagulants in patients with non-valvular atrial fibrillation. Europace. 2015;17:1467–507.
11. Koo CK, Teasdale E, Muir KW. What constitutes a true hyperdense middle cerebral artery sign? Cerebrovasc Dis. 2000;10:419–23.
12. National Institute of Neurological Disorders and Stroke rt-PA Stroke Study Group. Tissue plasminogen activator for acute ischemic stroke. N Engl J Med. 1995;333:1581–7.
13. Fiorelli M, Bastianello S, von Kummer R, del Zoppo GJ, Larrue V, Lesaffre E, et al. Hemorrhagic transformation within 36 hours of a cerebral infarct: relationships with early clinical deterioration and 3-month outcome in the European Cooperative Acute Stroke Study I (ECASS I) cohort. Stroke. 1999; 30:2280–4.
14. Gadermann AM, Guhn M, Bruno DZ. Estimating ordinal reliability for Likert-type and ordinal item response data: a conceptual, empirical, and practical guide. Practical Assessment, Research & Evaluation. 2012;17:3. http://pareonline.net/getvn.asp?v=17&n=3
15. Trizano-Hermosilla I, Alvarado JM. Best alternatives to Cronbach's alpha reliability in realistic conditions: congeneric and asymmetrical measurements. Front Psychol. 2016;7:769.
16. Green SB, Yang Y. Reliability of summed item scores using structural equation modeling: an alternative to coefficient alpha. Psychometrika. 2009;74:155–67.
17. DeLong ER, DeLong DM, Clarke-Pearson DL. Comparing the areas under two or more correlated receiver operating characteristic curves: a nonparametric approach. Biometrics. 1988;44:837–45.
18. Neumann-Haefelin T, Hoelig S, Berkefeld J, Fiehler J, Gass A, Humpich M, et al. Leukoaraiosis is a risk factor for symptomatic intracerebral hemorrhage after thrombolysis for acute stroke. Stroke. 2006;37:2463–6.
19. Marsh EB, Llinas RH, Schneider AL, Hillis AE, Lawrence E, Dziedzic P, et al. Predicting hemorrhagic transformation of acute ischemic stroke: prospective validation of the HeRS score. Medicine (Baltimore). 2016;95:e2430.
20. Tan S, Wang D, Liu M, Zhang S, Wu B, Liu B. Frequency and predictors of spontaneous hemorrhagic transformation in ischemic stroke and its association with prognosis. J Neurol. 2014;261:905–12.
21. Zou M, Churilov L, He A, Campbell B, Davis SM, Yan B. Hyperdense middle cerebral artery sign is associated with increased risk of hemorrhagic transformation after intravenous thrombolysis for patients with acute ischaemic stroke. J Clin Neurosci. 2013;20:984–7.
22. Terruso V, D'Amelio M, Di Benedetto N, Lupo I, Saia V, Famoso G, et al. Frequency and determinants for hemorrhagic transformation of cerebral infarction. Neuroepidemiology. 2009;33:261–5.
23. Paciaroni M, Agnelli G, Corea F, Ageno W, Alberti A, Lanari A, et al. Early hemorrhagic transformation of brain infarction: rate, predictive factors, and influence on clinical outcome: results of a prospective multicenter study. Stroke. 2008;39:2249–56.
24. Pundik S, McWilliams-Dunnigan L, Blackham KL, Kirchner HL, Sundararajan S, Sunshine JL, et al. Older age does not increase risk of hemorrhagic complications after intravenous and/or intra-arterial thrombolysis for acute stroke. J Stroke Cerebrovasc Dis. 2008;17:266–72.
25. Demchuk AM, Khan F, Hill MD, Barber PA, Silver B, Patel S, et al. Importance of leukoaraiosis on CT for tissue plasminogen activator decision making: evaluation of the NINDS rt-PA stroke study. Cerebrovasc Dis. 2008;26(2):120–5.

26. Nardi K, Leys D, Eusebi P, Cordonnier C, Gautier S, Hénon H, et al. Influence of lipid profiles on the risk of hemorrhagic transformation after ischemic stroke: systematic review. Cerebrovasc Dis Extra. 2011;1:130–41.
27. Kaesmacher J, Kaesmacher M, Maegerlein C, Zimmer C, Gersing AS, Wunderlich S, et al. Hemorrhagic transformations after thrombectomy: risk factors and clinical relevance. Cerebrovasc Dis. 2017;43:294–304.
28. Sandset EC, Berge E, Kjeldsen SE, Julius S, Holzhauer B, Krarup LH, et al. Heart rate as a predictor of stroke in high-risk, hypertensive patients with previous stroke or transient ischemic attack. J Stroke Cerebrovasc Dis. 2014; 23:2814–8.
29. Chen CH, Huang PW, Tang SC, Shieh JS, Lai DM, Wu AY, et al. Complexity of heart rate variability can predict stroke-in-evolution in acute ischemic stroke patients. Sci Rep. 2015;5:17552.
30. Tatlisumak T, Fisher M. Hematologic disorders associated with ischemic stroke. J Neurol Sci. 1996;140:1–11.
31. Marsh EB, Llinas RH, Hillis AE, Gottesman RF. Hemorrhagic transformation in patients with acute ischaemic stroke and an indication for anticoagulation. Eur J Neurol. 2013;20:962–7.
32. Saposnik G, Fang J, Kapral MK, Tu JV, Mamdani M, Austin P, et al. The iScore predicts effectiveness of thrombolytic therapy for acute ischemic stroke. Stroke. 2012;43:1315–22.
33. Saposnik G, Guzik AK, Reeves M, Ovbiagele B, Johnston SC. Stroke prognostication using age and NIH Stroke Scale: SPAN-100. Neurology. 2013;80:21–8.
34. Yong AG, Pearce S. A Beginner's guide to factor analysis: focusing on exploratory factor analysis. Tutor Quant Methods Psychol. 2013;9:79–94.
35. Asuzu D, Nystrom K, Amin H, Schindler J, Wira C, Greer D, et al. Comparison of 8 scores for predicting symptomatic intracerebral hemorrhage after IV thrombolysis. Neurocrit Care. 2015;22:229–33.
36. Sung SF, Chen SC, Lin HJ, Chen YW, Tseng MC, Chen CH. Comparison of risk-scoring systems in predicting symptomatic intracerebral hemorrhage after intravenous thrombolysis. Stroke. 2013;44:1561–6.
37. Demeestere J, Garcia-Esperon C, Garcia-Bermejo P, Ombelet F, McElduff P, Bivard A, et al. Evaluation of hyperacute infarct volume using ASPECTS and brain CT perfusion core volume. Neurology. 2017;88:2248–53.
38. González RG, Schaefer PW, Buonanno FS, Schwamm LH, Budzik RF, Rordorf G, et al. Diffusion-weighted MR imaging: diagnostic accuracy in patients imaged within 6 hours of stroke symptom onset. Radiology. 1999;210:155–62.
39. Schröder J, Cheng B, Ebinger M, Köhrmann M, Wu O, Kang DW, et al. Validity of acute stroke lesion volume estimation by diffusion-weighted imaging-Alberta Stroke Program Early Computed Tomographic Score depends on lesion location in 496 patients with middle cerebral artery stroke. Stroke. 2014;45:3583–8.
40. Merwick Á, Werring D. Posterior circulation ischaemic stroke. BMJ. 2014;348: g3175.
41. Sarikaya H, Arnold M, Engelter ST, Lyrer PA, Mattle HP, Georgiadis D, et al. Outcomes of intravenous thrombolysis in posterior versus anterior circulation stroke. Stroke. 2011;42:2498–502.
42. Libman RB, Kwiatkowski TG, Hansen MD, Clarke WR, Woolson RF, Adams HP. Differences between anterior and posterior circulation stroke in TOAST. Cerebrovasc Dis. 2001;11:311–6.
43. Tong X, Liao X, Pan Y, Cao Y, Wang C, Liu L, et al. Intravenous thrombolysis is more safe and effective for posterior circulation stroke: data from the Thrombolysis Implementation and Monitor of Acute Ischemic Stroke in China (TIMS-China). Medicine (Baltimore). 2016;95:e3848.
44. Oppenheim C, Stanescu R, Dormont D, Crozier S, Marro B, Samson Y, et al. False-negative diffusion-weighted MR findings in acute ischemic stroke. AJNR Am J Neuroradiol. 2000;21:1434–40.
45. Puetz V, Sylaja PN, Coutts SB, Hill MD, Dzialowski I, Mueller P, et al. Extent of hypoattenuation on CT angiography source images predicts functional outcome in patients with basilar artery occlusion. Stroke. 2008;39:2485–90.
46. Pisters R, Lane DA, Nieuwlaat R, de Vos CB, Crijns HJ, Lip GY. A novel user-friendly score (HAS-BLED) to assess 1-year risk of major bleeding in patients with atrial fibrillation: the Euro Heart Survey. Chest. 2010;138:1093–100.

Predictors of intensive care unit admission and mortality in patients with ischemic stroke: investigating the effects of a pulmonary rehabilitation program

Belma Doğan Güngen, Abdulkadir Tunç*, Yeşim Güzey Aras, Aslı Aksoy Gündoğdu, Adil Can Güngen and Serdar Bal

Abstract

Background: The aim of this study was to investigate the predictors of intensive care unit (ICU) admission and mortality among stroke patients and the effects of a pulmonary rehabilitation program on stroke patients.

Methods: This prospective study enrolled 181 acute ischemic stroke patients aged between 40 and 90 years. Demographical characteristics, laboratory tests, diffusion-weighed magnetic resonance imaging (DWI-MRI) time, nutritional status, vascular risk factors, National Institute of Health Stroke Scale (NIHSS) scores and modified Rankin scale (MRS) scores were recorded for all patients. One-hundred patients participated in the pulmonary rehabilitation program, 81 of whom served as a control group.

Results: Statistically, one- and three-month mortality was associated with NIHSS and MRS scores at admission and three months ($p<0.001$; $r=0.440$, $r=0.432$, $r=0.339$ and $r=0.410$, respectively). One and three months mortality- ICU admission had a statistically significant relationship with parenteral nutrition ($p<0.001$; $r=0.346$, $r=0.300$, respectively; $r=0.294$ and $r=0.294$, respectively). Similarly, there was also a statistically significant relationship between pneumonia onset and one- and three-month mortality- ICU admission ($p<0.05$; $r=0.217$, $r=0.127$, $r=0.185$ and $r=0.185$, respectively). A regression analysis showed that parenteral nutrition (odds ratio [OR] =13.434, 95% confidence interval [CI] =1.148–157.265, $p=0.038$) was a significant predictor of ICU admission. The relationship between pulmonary physiotherapy (PPT) and ICU admission- pneumonia onset at the end of three months was statistically significant ($p=0.04$ and $p=0.043$, respectively).

Conclusion: This study showed that PPT improved the prognosis of ischemic stroke patients. We believe that a pulmonary rehabilitation program, in addition to general stroke rehabilitation programs, can play a critical role in improving survival and functional outcomes.

Keywords: Stroke, Mortality, Intensive care unit, Pulmonary rehabilitation

* Correspondence: drkadirtunc@hotmail.com
Bezmialem Vakif Universitesi Tip Fakultesi Hastanesi, Istanbul, Turkey

Background

Severe stroke remains an important cause of mortality and morbidity, despite advances in disease management, acute treatment and secondary measures [1]. Predicting early mortality and disability after a stroke depends on many factors, such as age, the type of stroke, lesional location, level of consciousness, severity of neurological impairment, medical risk factors (hypertension and diabetes), premorbid conditions, fever and history of stroke [2]. Stroke patients may experience a reduction of up to 50% in respiratory function when compared to age- and gender-matched norms [3]. The reduction in respiratory function can lead to decreased endurance, dyspnoea and increased sedentary behaviour, as well as an elevated risk of stroke. The reduction in respiratory function may also cause aspiration, leading to pneumonia [4]. Previous research showed that pneumonia was an independent risk factor for mortality and a poor prognosis in stroke patients [1]. Research also showed that a reduction in respiratory muscle and abdominal muscle strength contributed to pulmonary and respiratory dysfunction following a stroke. Low respiratory muscle function decreases the efficacy of rehabilitation because it leads to exercise intolerance in stroke patients [5]. Thus, special exercise programs are needed to improve the pulmonary function and respiratory muscle strength of stroke patients.

The aim of pulmonary rehabilitation program is to enhance respiratory muscle resistance during breathing, thereby improving respiratory function. Previous studies demonstrated that pulmonary rehabilitation programs improved respiratory functions in cardiac disease and chronic obstructive pulmonary disease patients [6, 7]. There has been little research on the use of pulmonary rehabilitation programs in stroke patients. McCool and Tzelepis advised that respiratory muscle strength and endurance increased when initial stroke patients performed exercise at sufficient intensity to increase muscle strength, so that eventual improvement in respiratory functions could be expected [8]. In addition, pulmonary rehabilitation programs were considered to be capable of inducing positive effects on stroke patients' respiratory muscles through diaphragm breathing exercise and lip puckering breathing exercise in another study [9]. Another study showed that pulmonary physiotherapy (PPT) improved the quality of life of stroke patients [4].

The aims of the present study were to investigate the predictors of intensive care unit (ICU) admission and mortality among stroke patients and the effects of PPT on these stroke patients.

Methods

This prospective study enrolled 181 acute ischemic stroke patients aged between 40 and 90 years who were admitted to the neurology clinic stroke unit or the neurological ICU of the Sakarya University Training and Research Hospital between February 2015 and January 2016. The inclusion criteria were acute ischemic stroke confirmed by computed tomography (CT) or a diffusion-weighed magnetic resonance imaging (DWI-MRI) scan, aged > 40 years, ability to understand and follow simple verbal instructions, modified Rankin scale (MRS) score > 2, National Institute of Health Stroke Scale (NIHSS) score > 0, no unrestricted movement of the lips, no receptive aphasia and no history of thoracic or abdominal surgery. The exclusion criteria were as follows: blood pressure >180/100 mm Hg more than twice in 24 h; significant pulmonary disease, angina, myocardial infarction or acute heart failure within three months; neurological conditions other than stroke; presence of a severe visual disability and visual field defects; receiving medications that would influence the metabolic or cardiorespiratory responses to exercise; inability to perform the tests.

This study was approved by Sakarya University Human Ethics Committee (Reference number: 16214662/050.01.04/154). Prior to participation in the study, each individual completed a detailed written informed consent form.

Data collection

Demographical characteristics, laboratory tests, DWI-MRI time and nutritional status were recorded for all patients. Vascular risk factors, including hypertension, diabetes, smoking status and alcohol consumption, were evaluated. NIHSS and MRS scores were used at baseline and three months to assess stroke severity and functional disability [10, 11]. Infarct sizes and locations were recorded based on cranial MRI findings. Lesional areas were categorised according to the areas of the vessels: medial cerebral artery (MCA), anterior cerebral artery, posterior cerebral artery, basilar artery and cerebellar arteries. The MCA infarcts were further classified according to the dimensions of the lesions (MCA1: lacunar infarcts; MCA2: between lacunar infarcts and total MCA infarcts; and MCA3: total MCA infarcts).

The subtypes of ischemic stroke were classified according to the original Trial of Org 10172 Acute Stroke Treatment (TOAST) criteria [12]. The five major categories of the TOAST classification are: large artery atherosclerosis, including large artery thrombosis and artery-to-artery embolisms, cardioembolisms, small artery occlusions, stroke of other determined cause and stroke of undetermined cause. The definitions of the subtypes were made according to risk factor profiles, clinical features and results of diagnostic tests. CT, MRI, vascular imaging (carotid-vertebral artery Doppler ultrasound), electrocardiograms and echocardiography were performed, and pro-thrombotic syndromes were assessed.

Stroke management and three-month follow up

Stroke patients were transferred from the emergency unit to the stroke unit within 24 h. Stroke management was based on the guidelines of the American Heart Association/American Stroke Association [13]. Various measures were implemented. These included providing supportive treatment to ensure a patent airway, maintaining oxygen saturation above 92%, maintaining haemodynamic stability, providing fever and glycaemic control, providing hydration and nutrition and preventing pressure sores and deep venous thrombosis [2]. Antiplatelet agents (aspirin and clopidogrel) were used for the treatment of ischemic stroke [14]. Patients who required mechanical ventilation were admitted to the neurological ICU. The patients were followed up at the hospital or after discharge for a three-month period. Mortality and admission to the ICU were recorded at the end of the first and third months.

Pulmonary rehabilitation program

Patients were assigned randomly to either the PPT or control group by having each of the subjects take out 1 card from a box containing 2 types of cards representing both study groups. One-hundred patients participated in the pulmonary rehabilitation program (group 1), and 81 patients served as a control group (group 2). Both groups participated in a daily conventional rehabilitation program, which included joint mobility, eccentric contraction, muscle strengthening and walking exercises. Only the patients in group 1 participated in the PPT program. The program was conducted by physical therapists at our hospital for 30 min, three days/week. As part of the PPT, a physiotherapist monitored group 1 for 12 weeks. The same physiotherapist supervised all the exercises.

During the exercise program, all patients were clinically stable and all were receiving optimal medical therapy. Rehabilitation started with inspiratory diaphragm breathing exercises. The physiotherapist placed his hands on the superior rectus abdominis immediately below the anterior costal cartilage and induced inspiratory diaphragm breathing by instructing the patient to slowly and deeply inhale the air through the nose. Then the patient was instructed to perform expiratory pursed-lip breathing exercise by continuously exhale the air. During pursed-lip breathing exercise, the patient was instructed in sequence, to breathe in gently through the nose, purse his/ her lips as though whistling and then breathe out through the long pursed lips by not exerting power until she/ he is short of breath. The expiration time was set to be at least twice times longer than inspiration time [9, 15]. The patients took a rest when they complained about fatigue or dizziness during breathing exercise and conducted breathing exercise again.

The exercise intensity was based on the maximal heart rate and maximal effort of the patients. The exercise intensity was increased gradually over the course of the 12-week program. Each patient's performance during the exercise sessions was recorded and reported regularly to the patient's physician. NIHSS scores, MRS scores, pneumonia onset, admission to the ICU and mortality in groups 1 and 2 were recorded at the end of the first and third month.

Statistical analysis

Statistical analyses were carried out using SPSS/PC software (version 21.0). Descriptive statistics were presented as mean values, with standard deviations for numerical variables. Independent t tests were conducted to examine the difference between categorical variables in the two groups, and a one-way analysis of variance was used for examining the difference between the categorical variables in the two groups. A chi square test was used to determine the correlation between two categorical variables, and Pearson's correlation coefficients were used to examine the correlation between two numerical variables. The limit for statistical significance was accepted as $p<0.05$. To investigate the effect of the independent variables on the dependent variable (ICU admission), multiple linear regression analyses were used.

Results

As shown in Table 1, there were no significant differences in the baseline values of the two groups as regards their general characteristics, vascular risk factors, feeding type, NIHSS and MRS scores, and MRI findings and classification based on TOAST criteria ($p>0.05$). Group 1 had a mean age of 68.94±12.5 years, and 39 (21.5%) of the patients were males. In group 2, the mean age was 70.95±12.8 years, and 40 (22.7%) of the patients were males. The NIHSS score on admission was 6.53±5.038 in group 1, and it was 6.72±5.028 in group 2 ($p=0.805$).

ICU admission and mortality

Analysis of the effects of relevant determinants on one- and three-month mortality and ICU admission revealed no statistically significant effects of age, gender, hypertension, diabetes, nasogastric feeding, lesional areas on MRI and lesional subtypes according to TOAST criteria ($p>0.05$).

Statistically, one- and three-month mortality was associated with NIHSS and MRS scores at admission and three months ($p<0.001$; $r=0.440$, $r=0.432$, $r=0.339$ and $r=0.410$, respectively). No significant relationship was found between these parameters and ICU admission ($p>0.05$). One and three months mortality- ICU admission had a statistically significant relationship with parenteral nutrition ($p<0.001$; $r=0.346$, $r=0.300$, respectively; $r=0.294$ and $r=0.294$, respectively). Similarly, there was a statistically significant relationship between pneumonia onset and mortality- ICU admission at the end of one and three months ($p<0.05$; $r=0.217$, $r=0.127$, $r=0.185$ and $r=0.185$, respectively) (Table 2).

The multiple logistic regression using the potential variables (NIHSS scores, MRS scores, pneumonia, nasogastric feeding and parenteral nutrition) from the

Table 1 Demographic and clinical characteristics of the patients

		Stroke patients		*P* value*
		Pulmonary rehabilitation (+) Group 1 (n=100)	Pulmonary rehabilitation (-) Group 2 (n=81)	
Age (year)		68.94±12.505	70.95±12.875	0.290
Sex				
Male		39(21.5%) /	40(22.7%) /	0.161
Female		61(33.7%)	41(22.1%)	
Alcohol consumption		4(2.2%)	1(0.6%)	0.259
Smoking		27(14.9%)	17(9.4%)	0.201
Hypertension		69(38.1%)	59(32.6%)	0.421
Diabetes		39(21.5%)	26(14.4%)	0.336
WBC ($\times 10^9$/L)		7.54±2.199	8.16±3.312	0.068
Neutrophil count ($\times 10^9$)		4.54±1.957	4.24±1.714	0.292
Platelets		233.40±80.346	234.20±96.881	0.952
CRP (mg/L)		17.65 ±26.984	12.93±20.624	0.197
ESR(mm/hr)		31.30±23.6	28.51±20..81	0.410
Nasogastric feeding		13(7.2%)	16(8.8%)	0.218
Parenteral Nutrision		13(7.2%)	16(8.8%)	0.218
DWI time (hour)		9.96±5.151	10.34±4.069	0.595
NIHSS score at admission		6.53±5.038	6.72±5.028	0.805
Infarction size (cm)	0.5-1.5	31(17.1%)	23(12.7%)	0.914
	1.5-5	55(30.4%)	47(20.6%)	
	≥ 5	14(7.7%)	11(6.1%)	
MRS score	0	5(2.8%)	1(0.6%)	
	1	33(18.2%)	31(17.1%)	
	2	28(15.1%)	19(10.5%)	
	3	17(9.4%)	16(8.8%)	
	4	13(7.2%)	7(3.9%)	
	5	4(2.2%)	5(2.8%)	
	6	0	2(1.1%)	
Cranial magnetic resonance findings	MCA 1	24(13.3%)	18(9.9%)	0.511
	MCA 2	34(18.8%)	26(14.4%)	
	MCA 3	5(2.8%)	4(2.2%)	
	ACA	2(1.1%)	1(0.6%)	
	PCA	22(12.2%)	12(6.6%)	
	Basilary artery	8(4.4%)	10(5.5%)	
	Cerebellar artery	5(2.8%)	10(5.5%)	
TOAST criteria	large-artery atherosclerosis	30(16.6%)	25(13.8%)	0.751
	cardioembolism	31(17.1%)	23(12.7%)	
	small artery occlusion	24(13.3%)	24(13.3%)	
	other determined cause	4(2.2%)	4(2.2%)	
	undetermined cause	11(6.1%)	5(2.8%)	

Data are mean (SD) and frequency (%), unless stated otherwise. *WBC* white blood cells, *CRP* C-reactive protein (normal <0,9), *ESR* erythrocyte sedimentation rate (normal <20), *NIHHS* National Institute of Health Stroke Scale, *TOAST* Trial of Org 10172 in Acute Stroke Treatment, *DWI* diffusion-weighted MR imaging, *MCA* medial cerebral artery, *ACA* anterior cerebral artery, *PCA* posterior cerebral artery, *MRS* modified Rankin scale, *SD* standard deviation

* $p < 0.05$; statistical significance, with Student's t test

Table 2 The effects of relevant determinants on 1 and 3-months mortality and intensive care unit admission

	Stroke patients		1st month mortality	3th month mortality
	ICU admission at 1st month	ICU admission at 3th month		
Age	r:0.064	r:0.121	r:0.11	r:0.111
	p:0.389	p:0.104	p:0.135	p:0.135
Sex (Male)	r:0.028	r:0.066	r:0.056	r:0.056
	p:0.713	p:0.378	p:0.457	p:0.457
Hypertension	r:0.073	r:0.049	r:0.030	r:0.030
	p:0.329	p:0.511	p:0.690	p0.690
Diabetes	r:0.049	r:0.039	r:0.014	r:0.014
	p:0.513	p:0.331	p:0.848	p:0.848
Cranial magnetic resonance findings	r:0.138	r: 0.039	r:0.140	r:0.140
	p:0.065	p: 0.601	p:0.068	p:0.068
NIHSS score at admission	r:0.210	r:0.323	r:0.440	r:0.440
	p:0.005	p:0.001	p: <0.001	p: <0.001
NIHSS score at 3 months	r:0.276	r:0.355	r:0.432	r:0.432
	p:0.001	p:0.001	p: <0.001	p: <0.001
MRS score at admission	r:0.197	r:0.136	r:0.339	r:0.339
	p:0.008	p:0.069	p: <0.001	p: <0.001
MRS score at 3 months	r:0.195	r:0.169	r:0.410	r:0.410
	p:0.008	p:0.026	p: <0.001	p: <0.001
Nasogastric feeding	r:0.228	r:0.061	r:0.323	r:0.323
	p:0.002	p:0.415	p:0.001	p:0.001
Parenteral nutrition	r:0.346	r:0.300	r:0.294	r:0.294
	p:0.001	p:0.001	p:0.001	p:0.001
Pneumonia	r:0.217	r:0.127	r:0.185	r:0.185
	p:0.003	p:0.089	p:0.013	p:0.013
TOAST criteria	r:0.079	r:0.047	r:0.047	r:0.047
	p:0.292	p:0.530	p:0.530	p:0.530

ICU, intensive care unit; NIHHS, National Institute of Health Stroke Scale; MRS, modified Rankin scale; TOAST, Trial of Org 10172 in Acute Stroke Treatment
p < 0.05; r, correlation coefficient

bivariate analysis was adjusted to detect predictors of ICU admission. The regression analysis showed that parenteral nutrition (odds ratio [OR]: 13.434, 95% confidence interval [CI]: 1.148–157.265, *p*=0.038) was a significant predictor of ICU admission (Table 3).

Table 3 Multivariate logistic regression model for intensive care unit admission

	β	S.E. of β	*p* values*	OR (95% C.I.)
NIHSS score at admission	0.165	0.182	0.365	0.848 (0.593-1.212)
NIHSS score at 3 months	0.297	0.187	0.112	1.345 (0.933-1.943)
MRS score at admission	0.341	0.543	0.530	0.711 (0.245-2.060)
MRS score at 3 months	0.133	0.397	0.737	0.875 (0.402-1.905)
Pneumonia	0.648	1.085	0.550	1.912 (0.228-16.033)
Nasogastric feeding	0.211	1.309	0.872	0.810 (0.062-10.539)
Parenteral nutrition	2.598	1.255	0.038	13.434 (1.148-157.265)

Abbreviations: *NIHHS* National Institute of Health Stroke Scale, *MRS* Modified Rankin scale, *OR* Odds ratio, *CI* Confidence interval, *SE* Standart error
* *p* < 0.05

Effects of the pulmonary rehabilitation program

The three-month NIHSS scores were statistically significantly lower compared with the baseline scores in both groups (*p*<0.001). The three-month MRS scores were statistically significant in group 1 compared with the baseline scores (*p*<0.001). When the effect of the PPT program on one- and three- month mortality was examined, no significant difference was found in either group at the end of 1 month (0%). However, at the end of three months, the mortality in group 1 (*n* = 2, 2%) was slightly lower than that in group 2 (*n* = 3, 3.7%), as shown in Table 4.

The relationship between PPT and ICU admission and pneumonia onset at the end of three months was statistically significant (*p*=0.04 and *p*=0.043, respectively). In group 1, five (2.8%) patients had pneumonia, and one (1.0%) patient was admitted to the ICU. In group 2, 11 (6.1%) patients had pneumonia, and five (6.2%) patients were admitted to the ICU (Table 5).

Discussion

This study investigated the predictors of ICU admission and mortality and the effects of PPT on stroke patients. The results showed that the pulmonary rehabilitation program reduced ICU admission and pneumonia onset rates at the end of three months. They also revealed a statistically significant relationship between one- and three-month mortality and NIHSS and MRS scores at admission and three months and a statistically significant relationship between one- and three-month mortality and parenteral nutrition and pneumonia. Similarly, the relationship between parenteral nutrition, pneumonia onset and ICU admission was statistically significant. The regression analysis showed that parenteral nutrition was a significant predictor of ICU admission.

Based on a recent comparison of stroke results in different European regions, neurological impairment, a poor prognosis or mortality was recorded in 40% of patients at the end of the three months following the first episode of stroke [16]. In that study, age, stroke severity, comorbid factors and living pre-stroke dependency were determinants of post-stroke mortality and poor outcomes. Early post-stroke complications, such as pneumonia and increased intracranial pressure, were also reported to be independent risk factors for mortality and poor functional outcomes [17].

Table 4 Values of NIHSS- MRS scores at admission and 3 months and mortality- ICU admission at 1 and 3 months in both groups

PPT group				p^*
NIHSS score at admission	6.53 ±5.038	NIHSS score at 3 months	5.13 ±5.198	<0.001
MRS score at admission	3.2	MRS score at 3 months	2.5	<0.001
ICU admission at 1st month	3(3.0%)	ICU admission at 3 months	1(1.0%)	
1 month mortality	0(0%)	3 months mortality	2(2%)	
Control group				
NIHSS score at admission	6.72 ±5.028	NIHSS score at 3 months	5.86 ±5.239	0.002
MRS score at admission	2.3	MRS score at 3 months	2.04	0.507
ICU admission at 1st month	4(4.9%)	ICU admission at 3 months	5(6.2%)	
1 month mortality	0(0%)	3 months mortality	3(3.7%)	

Abbreviations: *PPT* Pulmonary physiotherapy, *ICU* Intensive care unit, *NIHHS* National Institute of Health Stroke Scale, *MRS* Modified Rankin scale
* $p < 0.05$

In stroke patients, the leading indications for ICU admission were reported to be deterioration of neurological status, thrombolytic treatment requirements, brain stem infractions and large hemispheric infarcts [18]. Other indications for ICU admission were a fluctuating clinical course, haemodynamic instability, multiple or septic emboli, significant cardiac dysrhythmia, respiratory and metabolic instability and the need for mechanical ventilation [18].

A previous study demonstrated that NIHSS and MRS scores were associated with the three-month prognosis in stroke patients [19]. In a study in Nepal, the NIHSS score at admission predicted seven-day mortality in ICUs, but the study did not evaluate long-term predictors of outcomes in acute stroke patients [20]. In the present study, the relationship between NIHSS and MRS scores at admission and three months and mortality rates at the end of one and three months were statistically significant, but there was no relationship between these scores and ICU admission. The relationship between NIHSS and MRS scores and mortality is concordant with that reported in previous studies [19, 20]. However, unlike the literature, these scores had no prognostic value as regards ICU admission. We attributed this finding to the limited number of patients and the effects of comorbid factors.

Table 5 Effects of pulmonary rehabilitation on mortality, pneumonia onset, ICU admission, NIHSS and MRS scores at 3 months

	PPT group	Control group	p^*
NIHSS score at 3 months	5.13 ±5.198	5.86 ±5.239	0.348
MRS score at 3 months	2.5	2.04	0.211
ICU admission at 3 months	1(1.0%)	5(6.2%)	0.04
3 months mortality	2(2%)	3(3.7%)	0.507
3 months pneumonia onset	5(2.8%)	11(6.1%)	0.043

PPT Pulmonary physiotherapy, *ICU* Intensive care unit, *NIHHS* National Institute of Health Stroke Scale; *MRS* Modified Rankin scale
* $p < 0.05$

In the present study, the relationship between parenteral nutrition and mortality and ICU admission was statistically significant, as was the relationship between pneumonia onset and mortality and ICU admission. Based on the multivariable analysis, parenteral nutrition increased the rates of ICU admission 13-fold. A stroke causes neurogenic oropharyngeal dysphagia, which limits food intake, considerably increasing the risk of malnutrition and tracheal aspiration, and triples the incidence of aspiration pneumonia. As reported in the literature, neurogenic oropharyngeal dysphagia occurred in about 25–90% of stroke patients, and swallowing disorders, frequently accompanied by tracheal aspiration, occurred in 45% of stroke patients [21]. Aspiration pneumonia was reported to develop in 50% of patients who suffered from tracheal aspiration [21]. The Berlin Stroke Register analysis demonstrated that pneumonia onset increased in-hospital death five-fold [22]. In the current study, the patients were received enteral feeding whenever possible. The patients with suspected aspiration or severe impaired consciousness were received parenteral nutrition, as patients receiving parenteral nutrition are expected to have a poor prognosis. In accordance with the previous studies [17, 22], pneumonia onset was also associated with a poor prognosis in the present study.

The cardiopulmonary functions of stroke patients are diminished due to damage of the hemi-thorax and deterioration of respiratory muscles [23]. As a result of the paralysis of the diaphragm and respiratory muscles following a stroke, the thorax cannot expand sufficiently, which can lead to shortening of the thoracic cells and muscle fibrosis. The expansion capacity of the thorax may consequently be reduced during breathing [24]. In addition, cardiorespiratory control and oxygen-transferring systems are impaired in stroke patients due to limited muscular movement. The latter has been associated with a lack of oxygen and increased metabolic demands [23]. The deterioration in cardiopulmonary function is a leading cause of morbidity in stroke patients [24].

Previous research reported that aerobic exercise decreased cardiovascular risk factors, in addition to improving cardiopulmonary functions and functionality in activities of daily life and enhancing motor-sensory functions, leading to improved walking abilities in stroke patients [25]. General stroke rehabilitation programs that focus only on physical and functional recovery may not adequately enhance cardiopulmonary function in stroke patients [23].

The present study demonstrated that PPT reduced ICU admission and pneumonia onset rates at the end of three months. The positive prognostic effect of the PPT program is in accordance with that found in previous studies [23–25]. The results suggest that a pulmonary rehabilitation program, in addition to general rehabilitation programs, would be beneficial for stroke patients.

This study has some potential limitations. First, the effects of the pulmonary rehabilitation program were monitored only at one and three months. A one-year follow-up would have been useful to shed light on the long-term effects of the PPT program on the prognosis. Second, the duration of PPT program was short and evaluation of pulmonary function tests before and after the PPT program were missing. A more effective PPT program considering its duration, intensity and frequency should be explored in the future. Third, the data were obtained from a single hospital setting and may not be generalizable to other settings. Finally, the effect of the infarct sizes, treatment regimens and information on patients' function before hospitalization on the prognoses were not studied.

The strengths of the study were that it included an examination of multiple factors that may affect the prognosis of stroke patients. In addition, the patients' disability scores were evaluated, and the same physician monitored all the patients.

Conclusions

This study showed that a PPT program was effective in improving the prognosis of ischemic stroke patients. We believe that pulmonary rehabilitation programs, in addition to general stroke rehabilitation programs, can play a critical role in improving the survival and functional outcomes of acute stroke patients.

Abbreviations

CI: Confidence interval; CT: Computed tomography; DWI-MRI: Diffusion-weighed magnetic resonance imaging; ICU: Intensive care unit; MCA: Medial cerebral artery; MRS: Modified Rankin scale; NIHSS: National Institute of Health Stroke Scale; OR: ODDS ratio; PPT: Pulmonary physiotherapy; TOAST: Trial of Org 10172 Acute Stroke Treatment

Acknowledgments

We gratefully acknowledge all participants for their help and willingness to participate this study.

Funding

No funding was obtained.

Authors' contributions

BDG, AT and YGA and contributed to the study design and concept. AAG, ACG and SB contributed to analysis and interpretation of data. BDG and AT were responsible for primary data analysis. BDG, AT, YGA, AAG, ACG and SB contributed to the writing and review. All authors read and approved the final manuscript.

Competing interests

The authors declare that they have no competing interests.

References

1. Ariza-Vega P, Lozano-Lozano M, Olmedo-Requena R, Martín-Martín L, Jiménez-Moleón JJ. Influence of cognitive impairment on mobility recovery of patients with hip fracture. Am J Phys Med Rehabil. 2016;8(9):e75719.
2. Nakibuuka J, Sajatovic M, Nankabirwa J, et al. Early mortality and functional outcome after acute stroke in Uganda: prospective study with 30 day follow-up. Spring. 2015;4:450.
3. Mackay-Lyons MJ, Makrides L. Exercise capacity early after stroke. Arch Phys Med Rehabil. 2002;83:1697–702.
4. Joo S, Shin D, Song C. The effects of game-based breathing exercise on pulmonary function in stroke patients: A Preliminary Study. Med Sci Monit. 2015;21:1806–11.
5. Teixeira-Salmela LF, Parreira VF, Britto RR, et al. Respiratory pressures and thoracoabdominal motion in community-dwelling chronic stroke survivors. Arch Phys Med Rehabil. 2005;86:1974–8.
6. Hill K, Jenkins SC, Philippe DL, et al. Comparison of incremental and constant load tests of inspiratory muscle endurance in COPD. Eur Respir J. 2007;30:479–86.
7. Mador MJ, Deniz O, Aggarwal A, et al. Effect of respiratory muscle endurance training in patients with COPD undergoing pulmonary rehabilitation. Chest. 2005;128:1216–24.
8. McCool FD, Tzelepis GE. Inspiratory muscle training in the patient with neuromuscular disease. Phys Ther. 1995;75:1006–14.
9. Seo K, Hwan PS, Park K. The effects of inspiratory diaphragm breathing exercise and expiratory pursed-lip breathing exercise on chronic stroke patients' respiratory muscle activation. J Phys Ther Sci. 2017;29(3):465–9.
10. Lan MY, Wu SJ, Chang YY, Chen WH, Lai SL, Liu JS. Neurologic and non-neurologic predictors of mortality in ischemic stroke patients admitted to the intensive care unit. J Formos Med Assoc. 2006;105(8):653–8.
11. Rankin J. Cerebral vascular accidents in patients over the age of 60. I General considerations Scott Med J. 1957;2:127–36.
12. Kolominsky-Rabas PL, Weber M, Gefeller O, et al. Epidemiology of ischemic stroke subtypes according to TOAST criteria: incidence, recurrence, and long-term survival in ischemic stroke subtypes: a population-based study. Stroke. 2001;32:2735–40.
13. Jauch EC, Saver JL, Adams HP Jr, et al. American Heart Association Stroke Council, Council on Cardiovascular Nursing; Council on Peripheral Vascular Disease; Council on Clinical Cardiology. Guidelines for the early management of patients with acute ischemic stroke: a guideline for healthcare professionals from the American Heart Association/American Stroke Association. Stroke. 2013; 44(3):870–947.
14. Li Z, Wang Y, Zhao X, et al. Treatment effect of clopidogrel plus aspirin within 12 hours of acute minor stroke or transient ischemic attack. J Am Heart Assoc. 2016;5(3):e003038.
15. Seo KC, Lee HM, Kim HA. The effects of combination of inspiratory diaphragm exercise and expiratory pursed-lip breathing exercise on pulmonary functions of stroke patients. J Phys Ther Sci. 2013;25:241–4.
16. Heuschmann PU, Wiedmann S, Wellwood I, et al. Three-month stroke outcome: the European Registers of Stroke (EROS) investigators. Neurology. 2011;76:159–65.
17. Grube MM, Koennecke HC, Walter G, et al. Berlin Stroke Register (BSR). Influence of acute complications on outcome 3 months after ischemic stroke. PLoS One. 2013;8(9):e75719.
18. Golestanian E, Liou JI, Smith MA. Long-term survival in older critically ill patients with acute ischemic stroke. Crit Care Med. 2009;37(12):3107–13.
19. Poudel RS, Thapa LJ, Shrestha S, et al. Efficacy of combined antithrombotic, statin and antihypertensive agents in acute ischemic stroke. J Nepal Med Assoc. 2015;53(197):5–11.

20. Dewan KR, Rana PV. A study of seven day mortality in acute ischemic stroke in a teaching hospital in Chitwan. J Nepal Health Res Counc. 2014;12(26):33–8.
21. Pinto G, Zétola V, Lange M, et al. Program to diagnose probability of aspiration pneumonia in patients with ischemic stroke. Int Arch Otorhinolaryngol. 2014;18(3):244–8.
22. Koennecke HC, Belz W, Berfelde D, et al. Factors influencing in-hospital mortality and morbidity in patients treated on a stroke unit. Neurology. 2011;77:965–72.
23. Kim J, Park JH, Yim J. Effects of respiratory muscle and endurance training using an individualized training device on the pulmonary function and exercise capacity in stroke patients. Med Sci Monit. 2014;20:2543–9.
24. Sutbeyaz ST, Koseoglu F, Inan L, et al. Respiratory muscle training improves cardiopulmonary function and exercise tolerance in subjects with subacute stroke: a randomized controlled trial. Clin Rehabil. 2010;24(3):240–50.
25. Katz-Leurer M, Shochina M, Carmeli E, et al. The influence of early aerobic training on the functional capacity in patients with cerebrovascular accident at the subacute stage. Arch Phys Med Rehabil. 2003;84(11):1609–14.

15

SCL20A2 mutation presenting with acute ischemic stroke

Xiaoyu Zhang†, Gaoting Ma†, Zhangning Zhao and Meijia Zhu*

Abstract

Background: Primary familial brain calcification (PFBC) is a rare disorder characterized by distinctive bilateral brain calcification and variable clinical presentations. However, cerebrovascular attack was rarely reported in PFBC patients. We here reported a *SLC20A2* mutation patient presenting with acute ischemic stroke.

Case presentation: A 56 years old man was transferred to our hospital because of 6 days of melena and 3 days of somnolence, agitation and mood changes. Computed tomography (CT) scan showed symmetrical calcifications in bilateral basal ganglia, caudate nucleus, thalami, subcortical white matter and cerebellum, which is consistent with PFBC. Brain magnetic resonance imaging (MRI) revealed acute ischemic stroke in bilateral basal ganglia and periventricular regions. Mutational analysis identified a *SLC20A2* gene mutation c.344C > T (p.Thr115Met) in exon 3. One of his daughters had also suffered from brain calcification. MR perfusion imaging revealed hypoperfusion in bilateral basal ganglia, prefrontal and temporal lobe. After treatment, he discharged with a favorable functional outcome but cognitive impairment.

Conclusions: Ischemic stroke can occur in PFBC patients, which may be associated with hypoperfusion and calcification of arteries. And hypoperfusion in frontotemporal lobar may be related with their cognitive impairment.

Keywords: Primary familial brain calcification, Stroke, *SLC20A2* mutation

Background

Primary Familial Brain Calcification (PFBC), also known as Fahr's disease (FD), is a rare disorder characterized by symmetrical calcification in the basal ganglia and other brain regions. The disorder was first described by Delacour in 1850 and the best-known case description was by Fahr in 1930 [1, 2]. Patients with PFBC mostly present with movement disorders, psychiatric symptoms or cognitive impairment. Although the exact mechanisms of PFBC remain unclear, recent discoveries of four causative genes namely *SCL20A2, PDGFB, PDGFRB*, and *XPR1* may offer important clues [3–6]. *SLC20A2* gene encodes for type III sodium-dependent phosphate transporter 2 (PiT2). *PDGFB* and *PDGFRB* genes are related with function of pericytes and integrity of blood brain barrier (BBB) [7]. It has been postulated that disturbance of neuronal calcium phosphorus metabolism and disruption of BBB in PFBC patients may contribute to metastatic deposition and cause intracranial calcification [8].

In pathological studies, calcium and other mineral deposits have been found in the walls of capillaries, arterioles and the perivascular spaces in patients with PFBC. Furthermore, small number of arteries may have severe calcification which could cause obstruction of the lumen [9]. It can be assumed that those brain regions with affected arteries may be easily attacked by ischemic stroke. However, ischemic stroke was rarely reported in PFBC patients. The relationship between PFBC and cerebrovascular disease is still confusing. Therefore, we here report a 55-year-old male with *SCL20A2* mutation presenting with acute ischemic stroke, and we further explore the relationship between PFBC and ischemic stroke.

Case presentation

A 56 years old man, with histories of lacunar stroke and gastric ulcer, came to our hospital because of 6 days of melena and 3 days of somnolence, agitation and mood changes. The patient was a farmer and did not take any antiplatelet and antacids drugs. He came to local community hospital for dizzy and melena on June 24th, 2017. Blood examination showed anemia with 73 g/L of hemoglobin. He was treated with proton pump inhibitors.

* Correspondence: zmjqfsyy@126.com
†Equal contributors
Department of Neurology, Qianfoshan Hospital, Shandong University, Jinan 250014, China

Two days later, he recovered from melena but presented with somnolence. Blood test was reexamined and showed aggravation of anemia with 58 g/L of hemoglobin. He was treated with red cell transfusions and then transferred to our hospital. On admission, vital signs were: blood pressure 96/48 mmHg, pulse 48 beats/min, respirations 12 breaths/min, body temperature 36.8 °C. The neurologic examination revealed somnolence, aphasia, bilateral decreased muscle power in grade 4 and bilateral babinski sign. He presented with agitation when he was awaken. The score of National Institutes of Health Stroke Scale (NIHSS) was 11 points. Computed tomography (CT) scan showed symmetrical calcifications in bilateral basal ganglia, caudate nucleus, thalami, subcortical white matter and cerebellum (Fig. 1). Brain magnetic resonance imaging (MRI) revealed acute ischemic stroke in bilateral basal ganglia and periventricular regions with hyperintense signal in diffusion weighted imaging (DWI) and hypointense signal in apparent diffusion coefficient (ADC) (Fig. 2). The patient was admitted to neurological department with the diagnosis of acute ischemic stroke.

At hospitalization, possible causes of intracranial calcification were investigated. The level of serum calcium was 2.08 mmol/L (normal range: 2.10–2.55 mmol/L). The level of serum phosphorus, copper, ceruloplasmin, thyroid hormone, parathyroid hormone and enzyme-linked immunosorbant assay for human immunodeficiency virus (HIV) were normal. Family history revealed that one of his three daughters (34 years old) had also suffered from brain calcification, but without neurological problems (Fig. 3). His parents and two brothers also have no neurological problems. His father died of cardiac disease 10 years ago and his mother died of cancer 13 years ago. Mutational analysis was performed with a sample of whole blood from the patient and showed a *SLC20A2* gene mutation c.344C > T (p.Thr115Met) in exon 3. Therefore, a diagnosis of PFBC was made.

In order to identify the possible mechanism of ischemic stroke, CT angiography of cervical and cerebral arteries were performed and showed arteriosclerosis (Fig. 1). Cerebral microbleeds were not observed in susceptibility weighted imaging (SWI) and cerebral veins were normal on magnetic resonance venography (MRV). Sinus rhythm was showed on electrocardiogram. Mural thrombus was not detected in ultrasound cardiogram. We hypothesized that ischemic stroke may be related with hypoperfusion. The level of low density lipoprotein was 2.78 mmol/L at admission. Risuvastatins were given according to the guideline of acute ischemic stroke. Antacids and volume expansion therapy were regularly administrated. Five days after admission, the patient presented with a normal state of consciousness and could speak simple words. However, his memory was not completely recovered. MR perfusion imaging was taken and revealed that there was hypoperfusion in bilateral basal ganglia, prefrontal and temporal lobe (Fig. 4). After treatment for 20 days, he discharged with a favorable functional outcome and could carry out daily activities independently. The score of NIHSS was one point (correctly answered one question when he was asked his age and the name of the current month) and modified Rankin Scale score was two points (unable to carry out all pre-stroke activities, such as working as a farmer). However, he still had cognitive impairment with the score of 18 by mini-mental state examination (MMSE). The level of hemoglobin was 90 g/L at discharge.

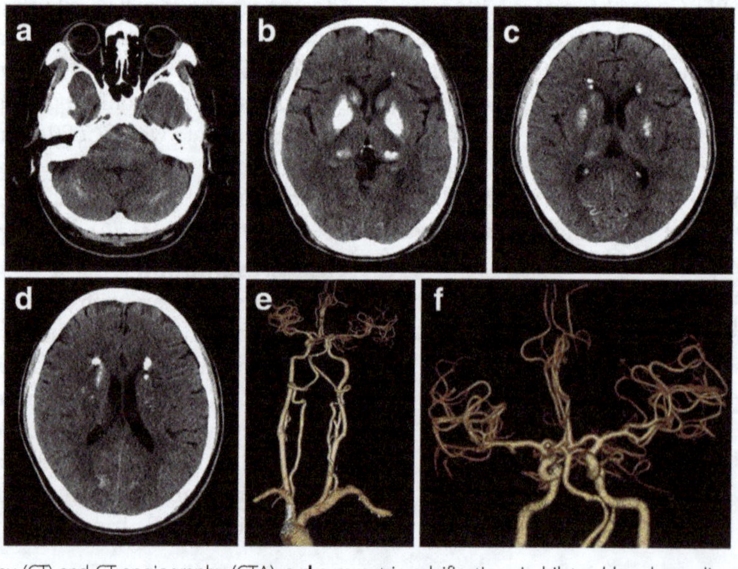

Fig. 1 Computed tomography (CT) and CT angiography (CTA). **a-d** symmetric calcifications in bilateral basal ganglia, caudate nucleus, thalami, subcortical white matter and cerebellum; **e-f** arteriosclerosis of cervical and cerebral arteries

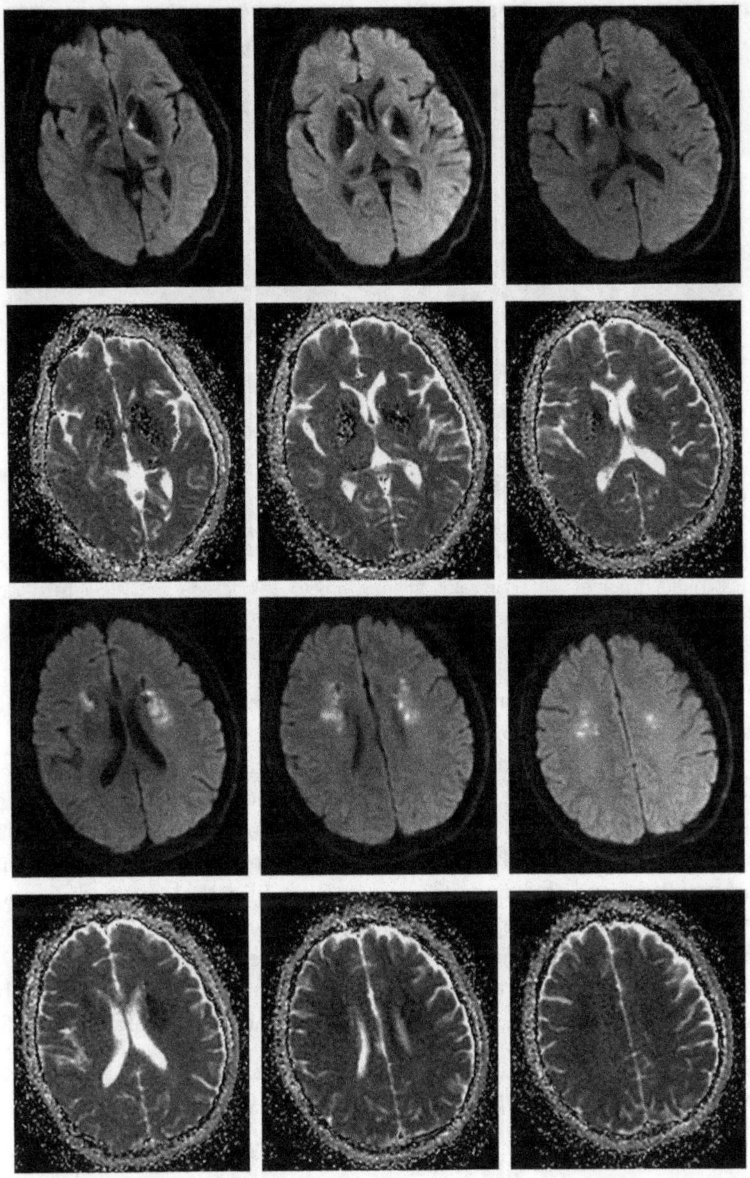

Fig. 2 Brain magnetic resonance imaging (MRI). Hyperintense signal in diffusion weighted imaging (DWI) and hypointense signal in apparent diffusion coefficient (ADC) in bilateral basal ganglia and periventricular regions

Discussion and conclusions

Primary familial brain calcification, or Fahr's disease, is a rare disorder characterized by distinctive bilateral brain calcification and variable clinical presentations. Four genes have been known to be associated with PFBC, including *SCL20A2, PDGFB, PDGFRB* and *XPR1*. *SLC20A2* is the most common gene involved with PFBC (55–66%), followed by *PDGFB* (31%) and *PDGFRB* (10%) [10]. It has also been reported that 14% patients with PFBC were sporadic cases. To date, about 40 variants in *SLC20A2* gene have been discovered [8]. In our patient, the mutation of c.344C > T (p.Thr115Met) in exon 3 has also been reported before [11].

The clinical presentations in PFBC patients are variable and almost a quarter of cases are asymptomatic. In previous studies, the most frequently described motor signs in PFBC patients were parkinsonism and dystonia [12]. Moreover, dysarthria, ataxia and chorea had also been described in published literatures [10]. Psychiatric features in PFBC patients include cognitive impairment, mood disorders, psychotic symptoms and obsessive-compulsive symptoms. In patients with *SLC20A2* mutations, the mostly described clinical presentations were parkinsonism, dystonia and cognitive impairment [12]. In our patient, parkinsonism was not observed. However, he may have cognitive impairment before stroke because

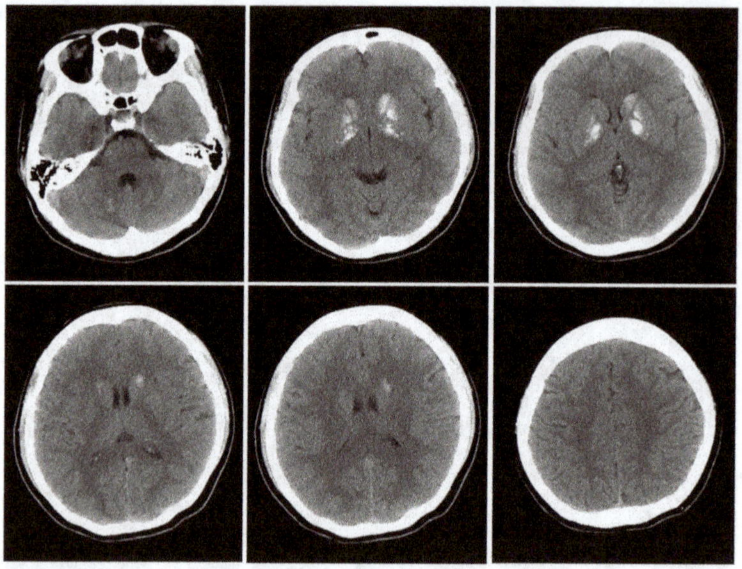

Fig. 3 Computed tomography (CT) of a daughter with brain calcification. Symmetric calcifications in bilateral basal ganglia, caudate nucleus, subcortical white matter and cerebellum

of forgetfulness provided by his daughters. And no clinical symptoms were observed in his daughter with brain calcification. In clinical practice, other causes of intracranial calcification should be distinguished from PFBC, including physiological calcification, disorders of calcium metabolism (hypoparathyroidism, pseudo-hypoparathyroidism, pseudo-pseudo-hypoparathyroidism and hyperparathyroidism), mitochondrial diseases, severe hypomagnesemia, HIV infection and other toxic conditions. Detailed medical histories and laboratory tests are helpful in determining the causes of intracranial calcification.

Cerebrovascular attack was rarely reported in PFBC patients. As far as we know, only two cases were reported in recent literatures, one patient with subarachnoid hemorrhage and the other with lacunar stroke in left genu of the internal capsule [13, 14]. The underlying mechanisms of ischemic stroke in PFBC patients are still unclear. In pathologic studies, calcium and other mineral deposits were found in the walls of capillaries, arterioles and in the perivascular spaces [9, 15]. A small number of these arteries even exhibited obstruction of the lumen because of severe calcification. Reactive astrocytes and

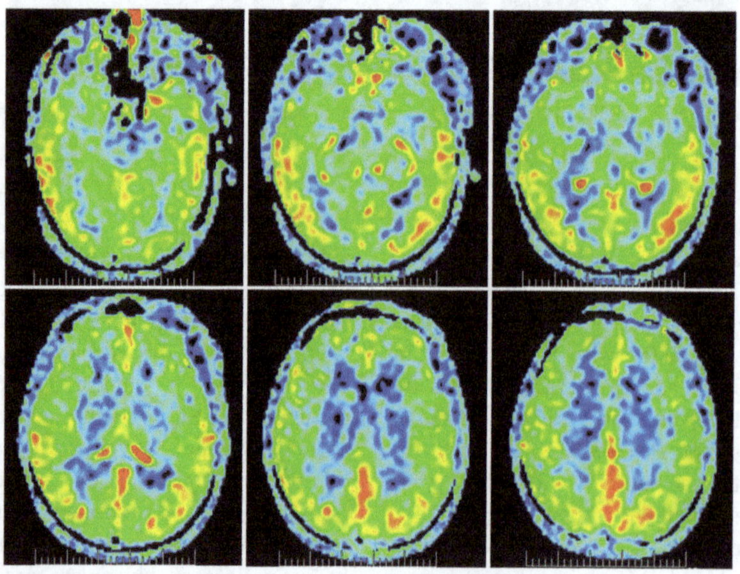

Fig. 4 MR perfusion imaging. Hypoperfusion in bilateral basal ganglia, prefrontal and temporal lobe

microglia accumulated around the calcified deposits, indicating a mild ongoing inflammatory process. Furthermore, microangiopathy was observed in skin biopsy of a patient with *PDGFB* mutation, showing thickened and fragmented areas in the basal lamina [16]. These changes may contribute to vascular stenosis and cause brain hypoperfusion. Evidences from neuroimagings also supported this assumption. Hypoperfusion were detected in basal ganglia region by single photon emission computed tomography (SPECT) and massive reduction of glucose metabolism were observed by position emission tomography (PET) [17, 18]. Therefore, it may be reasonable to postulate that vascular stenosis develop in affected vessels because of extensive calcium and mineral deposits, and ischemic stroke can occur once cerebral perfusion decreased. In our case, hypovolemia caused by gastrointestinal bleeding may result in hypoperfusion of brain and cause acute ischemic stroke in bilateral basal ganglia and periventricular regions. We also excluded other etiologies which may cause bilateral multiple ischemic stroke such as embolism, cerebral amyloid angiopathy and immunologically-mediated small vessel diseases.

Cognitive impairment is often observed in PFBC patients, while the underlying mechanisms are still largely unknown. In MR morphological evaluation, atrophy was detected in the left orbitofrontal gyrus and left hippocampus, which may affect their cognitive function [19]. In other studies, reduced perfusion by SPECT and decreased glucose metabolism by PET were found in frontal and temporal brain region, which is consistent with our MR perfusion results [17, 18]. Moreover, PFBC patients may presented with decreased resting state functional connectivity in executive control and working memory networks by functional MRI (fMRI) [19]. Therefore, both structural and functional network changes associated with frontotemporal lobar may contribute to cognitive impairment in PFBC patients. In our case, the patient presented with moderate dementia at discharge which may be related with decreased perfusion in frontotemporal lobar. However, it should be noted that many PFBC patients have no cognitive impairment, indicating that other factors may involve in the processes. More detailed studies are needed in the future.

In summary, we here presented acute ischemic stroke in a PFBC patient with *SLC20A2* gene mutation. The possible mechanism of ischemic stroke in PFBC patient may be associated with hypoperfusion and calcification of arteries. Furthermore, PFBC patient can present with cognitive impairment which may be attributed to structural and functional network changes of frontotemporal lobar.

Abbreviations

ADC: Apparent diffusion coefficient; BBB: Blood brain barrier; CT: Computed tomography; DWI: Diffusion weighted imaging; FD: Fahr's disease; FLAIR: Fluid attenuated inversion recovery; fMRI: functional MRI; HIV: Human immunodeficiency virus; MMSE: Mini-mental state examination; MRI: Magnetic resonance imaging; NIHSS: National Institutes of Health Stroke Scale; PET: Position emission tomography; PFBC: Primary familial brain calcification; PiT2: Sodium-dependent phosphate transporter 2; SPECT: Single photon emission computed tomography; SWI: Susceptibility weighted imaging

Acknowledgements

Xiaoyu Zhang and Gaoting Ma contributed equally to this manuscript.

Funding

None.

Authors' contributions

XYZ and GTM examined the patient and wrote the manuscript. XYZ and ZNZ analyzed neuroimagings. MJZ participated in the design of the case report and helped to draft the manuscript. All authors read and approved the final manuscript.

Competing interests

The authors declare that they have no competing interests.

References

1. Delacour A. Ossification des capillaires du cerveau. Ann Med Psychol (Paris). 1850;2:458–61.
2. Fahr T. Idiopathische Verkalkung der Hirngefäße. Zentralbl Allg Pathol. 1930;50:129–30.
3. Wang C, Li Y, Shi L, Ren J, Patti M, Wang T, et al. Mutations in SLC20A2 link familial idiopathic basal ganglia calcification with phosphate homeostasis. Nat Genet. 2012;44:254–6.
4. Keller A, Westenberger A, Sobrido MJ, Garcia-Murias M, Domingo A, Sears RL, et al. Mutations in the gene encoding PDGF-B cause brain calcifications in humans and mice. Nat Genet. 2013;45:1077–82.
5. Nicolas G, Pottier C, Maltete D, Coutant S, Rovelet-Lecrux A, Legallic S, et al. Mutation of the PDGFRB gene as a cause of idiopathic basal ganglia calcification. Neurology. 2013;80:181–7.
6. Legati A, Giovannini D, Nicolas G, Lopez-Sanchez U, Quintans B, Oliveira JR, et al. Mutations in XPR1 cause primary familial brain calcification associated with altered phosphate export. Nat Genet. 2015;47:579–81.
7. Betsholtz C, Keller A. PDGF, pericytes and the pathogenesis of idiopathic basal ganglia calcification (IBGC). Brain Pathol. 2014;24:387–95.
8. Taglia I, Bonifati V, Mignarri A, Dotti MT, Federico A. Primary familial brain calcification: update on molecular genetics. Neurol Sci. 2015;36:787–94.
9. Kimura T, Miura T, Aoki K, Saito S, Hondo H, Konno T, et al. Familial idiopathic basal ganglia calcification: Histopathologic features of an autopsied patient with an SLC20A2 mutation. Neuropathology. 2016;36:365–71.
10. Batla A, Tai XY, Schottlaender L, Erro R, Balint B, Bhatia KP. Deconstructing Fahr's disease/syndrome of brain calcification in the era of new genes. Parkinsonism Relat Disord. 2017;37:1–10.
11. Yamada M, Tanaka M, Takagi M, Kobayashi S, Taguchi Y, Takashima S, et al. Evaluation of SLC20A2 mutations that cause idiopathic basal ganglia calcification in Japan. Neurology. 2014;82:705–12.
12. Tadic V, Westenberger A, Domingo A, Alvarez-Fischer D, Klein C, Kasten M. Primary familial brain calcification with known gene mutations: a systematic review and challenges of phenotypic characterization. JAMA Neurol. 2015;72:460–7.
13. Al-Jehani H, Ajlan A, Sinclair D. Fahr's disease presenting with Aneurysmal subarachnoid hemorrhage. J Clin Imaging Sci. 2012;2:27.
14. Yang CS, Lo CP, Wu MC. Ischemic stroke in a young patient with Fahr's disease: a case report. BMC Neurol. 2016;16:33.
15. Miklossy J, Mackenzie IR, Dorovini-Zis K, Calne DB, Wszolek ZK, Klegeris A, et al. Severe vascular disturbance in a case of familial brain calcinosis. Acta Neuropathol. 2005;109:643–53.
16. Nicolas G, Marguet F, Laquerriere A, Mendes de Oliveira JR, Hannequin D. Microangiopathy in primary familial brain calcification: evidence from skin biopsies. Neurol Genet. 2017;3:e134.
17. Benke T, Karner E, Seppi K, Delazer M, Marksteiner J, Donnemiller E. Subacute dementia and imaging correlates in a case of Fahr's disease. J Neurol Neurosurg Psychiatry. 2004;75:1163–5.
18. Paschali A, Lakiotis V, Messinis L, Markaki E, Constantoyannis C, Ellul J, et al. Dopamine transporter SPECT/CT and perfusion brain SPECT imaging in idiopathic basal ganglia calcinosis. Clin Nucl Med. 2009;34:421–3.
19. Messina R, Rocca MA, Colombo B, Falini A, Comi G, Filippi M. Brain structural and functional abnormalities in Fahr's disease: a report of two cases. J Neurol. 2013;260:1927–30.

16

Feasibility and diagnostic accuracy of point-of-care handheld echocardiography in acute ischemic stroke patients

Peter Kraft[1,3*†], Anna Fleischer[2†], Silke Wiedmann[2,3], Viktoria Rücker[2], Daniel Mackenrodt[1,2,3], Caroline Morbach[3,5], Uwe Malzahn[2], Christoph Kleinschnitz[1,3,4], Stefan Störk[3,5] and Peter U. Heuschmann[2,3]

Abstract

Background: Standard echocardiography (SE) is an essential part of the routine diagnostic work-up after ischemic stroke (IS) and also serves for research purposes. However, access to SE is often limited. We aimed to assess feasibility and accuracy of point-of-care (POC) echocardiography in a stroke unit (SU) setting.

Methods: IS patients were recruited on the SU of the University Hospital Würzburg, Germany. Two SU team members were trained in POC echocardiography for a three-month period to assess a set of predefined cardiac parameters including left ventricular ejection fraction (LVEF). Diagnostic agreement was assessed by comparing POC with SE executed by an expert sonographer, and intraclass correlation coefficient (ICC) or kappa (κ) with 95% confidence intervals (95% CI) were calculated.

Results: In the 78 patients receiving both POC and SE agreement for cardiac parameters was good, with ICC varying from 0.82 (95% CI 0.71–0.89) to 0.93 (95% CI 0.87–0.96), and κ from 0.39 (−95% CI 0.14–0.92) to 0.79 (95% CI 0.67–0.91). Detection of systolic dysfunction with POC echocardiography compared to SE was very good, with an area under the curve of 0.99 (0.96–1.00). Interrater agreement for LVEF measured by POC echocardiography was good with κ 0.63 (95% CI 0.40–0.85).

Conclusions: POC echocardiography in a SU setting is feasible enabling reliable quantification of LVEF and preliminary assessment of selected cardiac parameters that might be used for research purposes. Its potential clinical utility in triaging stroke patients who should undergo or do not necessarily require SE needs to be investigated in larger prospective diagnostic studies.

Keywords: Ischemic stroke, Point-of-care echocardiography, Ejection fraction, Stroke unit, Systolic dysfunction, Feasibility, Accuracy

Background

About 30% of ischemic strokes are attributable to cardiac causes such as atrial fibrillation, patent foramen ovale, or other structural or rhythm abnormalities associated with systolic dysfunction [1]. In patients without known atrial fibrillation, echocardiography is considered essential to determine the underlying cause of stroke in research studies and for guiding secondary prevention in clinical routine; its use, therefore, is recommended by current clinical guidelines [2–4]. However, access of stroke patients to echocardiography that is executed by an ultrasound specialist is often limited, which may delay diagnosis, extend hospital stay and increase health-care costs [5]. Point-of-care (POC) echocardiography (so-called 'handheld echo') might be used in stroke patients as a screening tool for the detection of treatment

* Correspondence: kraft_p1@ukw.de
†Equal contributors
[1]Department of Neurology, University Hospital of Würzburg, Josef-Schneider-Str. 11, 97080 Würzburg, Germany
[3]Comprehensive Heart Failure Center, University of Würzburg, Würzburg, Germany
Full list of author information is available at the end of the article

relevant cardiac abnormalities, such as systolic dysfunction, aortic and mitral valve disease, left ventricular hypertrophy, atrial septal aneurysm, and pleural and pericardial effusion. In addition, POC echocardiography could contribute valuable information needed for research purposes, such as stroke etiology in diagnostic studies.

In this pilot study we investigated the diagnostic utility and accuracy of POC echocardiography in acute stroke patients performed by a non-expert examiner after a defined training phase on a stroke unit compared to a state-of-the-art transthoracic echocardiography performed by an expert sonographer under standardized cardiological conditions.

Methods

Population

Patients were recruited consecutively on the stroke unit of the University Hospital Würzburg between May and August 2014. The patient group is a sub-sample of the prospective SICFAIL (Stroke Induced Cardiac FAILure) cohort study evaluating the prevalence and time course of cardiac dysfunction in patients with ischemic stroke. Inclusion criteria were a diagnosis of acute ischemic stroke according to world health organization (WHO) definition [6], age ≥ 18 years, and written informed consent.

Echocardiography

POC echocardiography was performed using a portable cardiac ultrasound device (Vivid q, GE Healthcare) equipped with a M3S 1.5–4.0 MHz scanner (Additional file 1: Figure S1) in all study participants by a medical student (AF) specifically trained in this technique for the purpose of this study. A neurologist unfamiliar with echocardiography prior to study start (PK) received similar training to quantify inter-rater reliability. Training of the two non-cardiologist sonographers (AF, PK) was provided by expert sonographers of the Comprehensive Heart Failure Center Würzburg, spanned a period of about 3 months, included POC and standard echocardiography, and was completed via 3 certification scans 2 months prior to study initiation. For POC echocardiography measurements, patients were examined lying left-sided in their regular stroke unit beds, i.e. not on a dedicated echocardiography stretcher. The left arm had to be bended behind the head and the upper part of the bed was elevated by 20–30° to the horizontal plane. The patients had to follow the examiner's breathing instructions as far as possible. The examination started with the parasternal and continued with the apical and finally the subcostal insonation.

In addition, all patients underwent a reference transthoracic standard echocardiography according to current guidelines performed on a high-end ultrasound device (Vivid E9, GE Healthcare; GE M5S-D matrix single-crystal phased array transducer) by an expert sonographer of the Comprehensive Heart Failure Center [7].

In every patient 3 electrocardiography-triggered heart cycles were stored for both the POC and standard echocardiography. Basic cardiac parameters were assessed by standard scanning procedures including left ventricular ejection fraction (LVEF), left heart dimensions, wall thickness, major valve abnormalities, and pericardial or pleural effusion. LVEF was calculated according to the Simpson's biplane method or, in case of suboptimal imaging conditions, according to the Simpson's monoplane method. An LVEF <55% was defined as systolic dysfunction. Both scans, POC and standard echocardiography were performed within 48 h. In every case, the examiner performing the POC test vs. the standard echocardiography was blinded to the results of the respectively other examination.

Statistics and sample size calculation

For continuous variables the mean and standard deviation, for categorical variables the frequencies and proportions were reported. To assess the agreement between the POC and standard echocardiography for qualitative variables, Cohen's kappa with its respective 95% confidence interval (CI) was calculated. To assess the agreement between the POC and standard echocardiography for quantitative variables in the sense of conformity with standard echocardiography as reference, the intraclass correlation coefficient (ICC) for two raters (for continuous variables) with their respective 95% CI were calculated.

The sample size estimation was based on LVEF as the main read-out parameter as the SICFAIL study focused on echocardiographic measurement of cardiac function defined by ejection fraction. Area under the receiver operation curve (AUC), sensitivity and specificity were assessed for the detection of systolic dysfunction with POC echocardiography; 78 were required to detect an AUC of 0.95 with the power of 80% to the significance level of 5%. Analyses were performed with SPSS Software (SPSS 23, IBM Corp.).

Ethical approval

The study was approved from the University Hospital Würzburg Ethics Committee (AZ 176/13) and patients provided their written consent to participate in the study prior to any examination. The study was reported according to the Standards for Reporting Diagnostic accuracy studies (STARD) criteria.

Results

Eighty one patients with ischemic stroke were recruited for this study. Three subjects (3.7%) were excluded from analyses as they refused subsequent standard echocardiography. Hence, 78 patients provided two echocardiograms. In 76% of cases both echocardiographies were conducted within 24 h, in 24% within 48 h. In 56 patients (72%) standard echocardiography followed POC examination, in 22 patients (28%) POC echocardiography was conducted first. The demographic and clinical baseline characteristics are shown in Table 1.

In a first step we focused on the measurement of LVEF being the main read-out parameter in our study. Of the 78 patients with two echocardiograms, reliable LVEF assessment was achieved in 73 patients, since ultrasound quality of both POC and standard echocardiography was insufficient in 5 patients; in these subjects, LVEF was assessed by eyeballing (i.e. <55% or ≥55%). In a second step, we investigated a series of other potentially treatment-relevant cardiac structures. Table 2 summarizes the quality of ultrasound conditions and results of echocardiographic measurements in POC and standard echocardiography.

Interrater reliability was calculated between POC and standard echocardiography for all measured parameters. ICC ranged from 0.82 for LVEF to 0.93 for left ventricular end-systolic diameter (Table 2). Agreement coefficients for cardiac measurements ranged from 0.39 (pleural effusion) to 0.69 (atrial septum aneurysm), and for sonographic conditions from 0.65 (apical view) to 0.79 (subcostal view) (Table 2).

Given the study design and rationale as well as the LVEF-specific sample size estimation we restricted the calculation of further statistical values to LVEF as a marker for systolic function. Sensitivity of POC echocardiography for detecting systolic dysfunction was 100%, specificity 92.6%, and AUC 0.99 (95% CI, 0.96–1.00). Interrater reliability of the LVEF measurement by POC echocardiography between the two non-expert examiners was analyzed by an independent investigation of 18 patients. The ICC between the two raters for LVEF was 0.64 (95% CI 0.26–0.85).

Table 1 Demographical and baseline clinical data of patients

Age, years, mean (SD)	68.0 (13.5)
Male, n (%)	47 (61.0)
Hypertension, n (%)	44 (58.7)
Diabetes mellitus, n(%)	18 (24.0)
Hyperlipidemia, n (%)	21 (28.8)
Tobacco, n (%)	13 (17.1)
Atrial Fibrillation, n (%)	5 (6.8)
Angina Pectoris, n (%)	6 (8.1)
History of myocardial infarction, n (%)	4 (5.4)
History of heart failure, n (%)	3 (4.2)
Peripheral artery disease, n (%)	5 (6.8)
NIHSS at admission, median (IQR)	3 (1–4)
Systolic blood pressure, mmHg, mean (SD)	148.7 (22.0)
Diastolic blood pressure, mmHg, mean (SD)	77.4 (14.6)
Body mass index, kg/m^2, mean (SD)	27.5 (5.1)

SD standard deviation, *IQR* interquartile range *NIHSS* National Institutes of Health Stroke Scale score

Discussion

This pilot study showed that POC echocardiographic assessment performed in the ambitious setting of a stroke unit by stroke unit staff using a portable device is feasible and achieves reliable results regarding selected key characteristics of cardiac dimensions and function.

Feasibility and reliability of POC echocardiography have been assessed in different settings before. A recent report underscores the feasibility and usefulness to establish POC echocardiography even during the medical studies [8]. Our results are in line with previous investigations reporting good correlations between POC and standard echocardiography for the quantification of cardiac structures and functions in patients with suspected cardiac abnormalities (e.g. congestive heart failure) treated in cardiology departments [8, 9]. Of note, in most studies ultrasound examiners were experienced cardiologists and/or sonographers [4, 9–11], whereas in our study non-cardiologists performed the POC examinations. Another group found only moderate correlations between POC and standard echocardiography, and discordant findings (mainly regarding wall motion abnormalities) in 27% of adult out-patients even when performed and interpreted by experienced operators [11].

To the best of our knowledge, we present the first report evaluating portable echocardiography in patients with acute ischemic stroke in the setting of a stroke unit. The majority of patients had neurological deficits and POC echocardiography had to be performed in regular hospital beds which made the examination particularly challenging. Nevertheless, we were able to demonstrate high precision for the detection of systolic dysfunction and structural cardiac abnormalities compared to standard echocardiography performed by expert sonographers under routine conditions.

POC echocardiography might be a useful tool for documenting relevant cardiac abnormalities, used to inform research studies regarding the underlying cause of stroke. The role of POC echocardiography regarding intraventricular thrombus or other life threatening findings could not be assessed as they were not prevalent in our patient collective. Nevertheless, in this pilot study, atrial septal aneurysms could be detected with high precision. Further studies to evaluate the reliability of

Table 2 Point-of-care and standard echocardiographic data

	Point-of-care echocardiography	Standard echocardiography	Intraclass correlation coefficient (95% CI)	Agreement coefficient κ (95% CI)
Image quality, n (%)				
Parasternal				0.73 (0.61–0.86)
Good	35 (45.5)	40 (51.3)		
Moderate	22 (28.6)	20 (25.6)		
Poor	20 (26.0)	18 (23.1)		
Apical				0.65 (0.50–0.79)
Good	32 (42.1)	39 (50.0)		
Moderate	26 (34.2)	25 (32.1)		
Poor	18 (23.7)	14 (17.9)		
Subcostal				0.79 (0.67–0.91)
Good	38 (48.7)	41 (52.6)		
Moderate	28 (35.9)	24 (30.8)		
Poor	12 (15.4)	13 (16.7)		
Left ventricular ejection fraction, %, mean (SD)	60.8 (7.2)	62.3 (5.6)	0.82 (0.71–0.89)	
Left ventricular ejection fraction, n (%)				0.63 (0.40–0.85)
< 30%	0 (0.0)	0 (0.0)		
30–44%	3 (3.9)	1 (1.3)		
45–55%	10 (13.2)	7 (9.1)		
> 55%	63 (82.9)	69 (89.6)		
Not measurable, n	2	1		
Left ventricular end-diastolic wall thickness (septum), mm, mean (SD)	10.8 (1.7)	10.7 (1.7)	0.84 (0.76–0.90)	
Left ventricular end-diastolic wall thickness (posterior wall) mm, mean (SD)	10.5 (1.7)	10.0 (1.7)	0.85 (0.72–0.92)	
Left ventricular end-systolic diameter, mm, mean (SD)	33.7 (6.4)	32.9 (7.1)	0.93 (0.87–0.96)	
Left ventricular end-diastolic diameter, mm, mean (SD)	49.8 (5.5)	50.0 (5.5)	0.86 (0.79–0.91)	
Aortic valve maximal systolic flow velocity, m/s, mean (SD)	1.5 (0.4)	1.5 (0.4)	0.92 (0.88–0.95)	
Pericardial effusion, n (%)	0 (0.0)	0 (0.0)		0.00 (0.00–0.00)
Pleural effusion, n (%)	1 (1.3)	1 (1.3)		0.39 (−0.14–0.92)
Atrial septum aneurysm, n (%)	3 (3.9)	4 (5.1)		0.69 (0.39–0.98)
Heart rate during examination, 1/min, mean (SD)	69.8 (10.7)	69.7 (11.9)	0.67 (0.52–0.78)	

CI confidence interval, *SD* standard deviation

detection of persistent foramen ovale via transthoracic POC echocardiography applying right heart contrast agent seem promising and might make standard echocardiography unnecessary in certain patients.

Some limitations of the current pilot study need to be addressed. As it was mainly designed for measurement of LVEF in the SICFAIL study, we did not include all potentially treatment-relevant cardiac parameters into the echocardiography protocol (e.g. detailed description of regional LV dysfunction or mitral valve analysis). The sample size estimation was calculated for measurement of LVEF as a marker of systolic function only. Therefore, despite high accuracy of POC measurements, low patient numbers with peculiar cardiologic findings (pericardial effusion n = 0, pleural effusion n = 1, atrial septum aneurysm n = 4, intracardiac thrombus n = 0) impede reliable conclusions regarding these conditions. Due to the monocentric design, generalization of our results to conditions outside of our hospital is limited. The echocardiography device was of high quality and of the same brand as the reference device; this might have improved comparability and reliability of measurements. The stroke unit setting (e.g. type of hospital beds, illumination of patient rooms) may also vary amongst institutions. In addition, potential selection bias cannot be excluded as severely handicapped patients could not provide informed consent.

Conclusion

POC echocardiography is feasible in an acute stroke unit setting. Given the high accuracy for the detection of systolic dysfunction, it may be used for research purposes evaluating cardiac function after stroke. Its further clinical role as a screening tool for guiding individual patient treatment and management, such as fluid management in the acute situation, or for guiding secondary prevention, e.g. by detection of a cardiac source of embolism, which could render a standard echocardiogram unnecessary under certain conditions, needs to be established in larger prospective diagnostic studies with a sufficient number of patients with peculiar cardiologic findings.

Abbreviations

AUC: Area under curve; CI: Confidence interval; ICC: Intraclass correlation coefficient; IQR: Interquartile range; IS: Ischemic stroke; LVEF: Left ventricular ejection fraction; NIHSS: National Institutes of Health Stroke Scale score; POC: Point of care; SD: Standard deviation; SE: Standard echocardiography; SICFAIL: Stroke induced cardiac failure; SU: Stroke unit; WHO: World health organization

Acknowledgements

The authors thank Martina Bauer, Elisabeth Nau, and Jasmin Simon for providing training and echocardiography examinations.

Funding

This work was supported by the Federal Ministry of Education and Research within the Comprehensive Heart Failure Center Würzburg (grant 01EO1504). The funder did not influence the design of the study, the data collection, the analysis and interpretation of data and the writing of the manuscript.

Authors' contributions

PK and AF performed POC echocardiography examinations; PK, AF, SW, VR, CM, UM, SS and PUH statistically analyzed and interpreted data; PK, AF, SW, CM, SS and PUH drafted the manuscript; after that all authors (including DM and CK) contributed in revision of the manuscript for important intellectual content; all authors (including DM and CK) read and approved the final manuscript.

Authors' information

Not applicable

Competing interests

PK received honoraria for advisory boards and travel grants from Boehringer-Ingelheim, Bayer, Daiichi-Sankyo and Bristol-Myers Squibb. SW receives research support from the German Ministry of Research and Education and Deutsche Herzstiftung e.V.. PUH reports grants from German Ministry of Research and Education, European Union, Charité, Berlin Chamber of Physicians, German Parkinson Society, University Hospital Würzburg, Robert-Koch-Institute, German Heart Foundation, Charité–Universitätsmedizin Berlin (within Mondafis; supported by an unrestricted research grant to the Charité from Bayer), University Göttingen (within FIND-AF-randomized; supported by an unrestricted research grant to the University Göttingen from Boehringer-Ingelheim), University Hospital Heidelberg (within RASUNOA-prime; supported by an unrestricted research grant to the University Hospital Heidelberg from Bayer, BMS, Boehringer-Ingelheim, Daiichi Sankyo), outside the submitted work.

Author details

[1]Department of Neurology, University Hospital of Würzburg, Josef-Schneider-Str. 11, 97080 Würzburg, Germany. [2]Institute of Clinical Epidemiology and Biometry, University of Würzburg, Würzburg, Germany. [3]Comprehensive Heart Failure Center, University of Würzburg, Würzburg, Germany. [4]Department of Neurology, University Hospital Essen, Essen, Germany. [5]Department of Internal Medicine, University Hospital Würzburg, Würzburg, Germany.

References

1. Kolominsky-Rabas PL, Weber M, Gefeller O, Neundoerfer B, Heuschmann PU. Epidemiology of ischemic stroke subtypes according to TOAST criteria: incidence, recurrence, and long-term survival in ischemic stroke subtypes: a population-based study. Stroke. 2001;32:2735–40.
2. Herm J, Konieczny M, Jungehulsing GJ, et al. Should transesophageal echocardiography be performed in acute stroke patients with atrial fibrillation? J Clin Neurosci. 2013;20:554–9.
3. Kernan WN, Ovbiagele B, Black HR, et al. Guidelines for the prevention of stroke in patients with stroke and transient ischemic attack: a guideline for healthcare professionals from the American Heart Association/American Stroke Association. Stroke. 2014;45:2160–236.
4. Ringleb PA, Bousser MG, Ford G, Bath P, Brainin M, Caso V, et al. Guidelines for management of ischaemic stroke and transient ischaemic attack 2008. Cerebrovasc Dis. 2008;25:457–507.
5. Trambaiolo P, Papetti F, Posteraro A, et al. A hand-carried cardiac ultrasound device in the outpatient cardiology clinic reduces the need for standard echocardiography. Heart. 2007;93:470–5.
6. Aho K, Harmsen P, Hatano S, Marquardsen J, Smirnov VE, Strasser T. Cerebrovascular disease in the community: results of a WHO collaborative study. Bull World Health Organ. 1980;58:113–30.
7. Lang RM, Bierig M, Devereux RB, et al. Recommendations for chamber quantification. Eur J Echocardiogr. 2006;7:79–108.
8. Ho AM, Critchley LA, Leung JY, et al. Introducing final-year medical students to pocket-sized ultrasound imaging: teaching transthoracic echocardiography on a 2-week anesthesia rotation. Teach Learn Med. 2015;27:307–13.
9. Khan HA, Wineinger NE, Uddin PQ, Mehta HS, Rubenson DS, Topol EJ. Can hospital rounds with pocket ultrasound by cardiologists reduce standard echocardiography. Am J Med. 2014;127:669. e1-7
10. Andersen GN, Haugen BO, Graven T, Salvesen O, Mjolstad OC, Dalen H. Feasibility and reliability of point-of-care pocket-sized echocardiography. Eur J Echocardiogr. 2011;12:665–70.
11. Cullen MW, Blauwet LA, Vatury OM, et al. Diagnostic capability of comprehensive handheld vs transthoracic echocardiography. Mayo Clin Proc. 2014;89:790–8.

The clinical prognostic significance of hs-cTnT elevation in patients with acute ischemic stroke

Lanying He[1*†], Jian Wang[1*†] and Weiwei Dong[2]

Abstract

Background: Cardiac autonomic dysfunction caused by ischemic stroke might lead to an adverse outcome. Elevated high sensitivity cardiac troponin (hs-cTnT) is a marker of cardiac disease, it can elevate in acute stroke patients. The aim of the present study was to investigate association between serum hs-cTnT with prognosis among patients with acute ischemic stroke.

Methods: Five hundred and sixteen patients (mean age 66.19 ± 10.11) with acute ischemic stroke underwent a comprehensive clinical investigation and serum hs-cTnT activity test. All patients were followed up for 3 months. The prognosis was death or major disability (modified Rankin Scale score ≥ 3) at 3 months after acute ischemic stroke.

Results: 22.87% (118/516) of patients had serum hs-cTnT elevation (≥14 ng/l). Compared with normal hs-TnT group, the incidence of insular stroke (adjusted odds ratio, 2.84; 95% confidence interval, 1.48–4.17; $P = 0.001$) were more likely in patients with hs-cTnT elevation. In fully adjusted models, there was an association between serum hs-cTnT elevation and death (adjusted odds ratio, 3.14; 95% confidence interval, 1.16–8.49; $P = 0.02$) and major disability(adjusted odds ratio, 2.07; 95% confidence interval, 1.04–4.51; $P = 0.04$), and composite outcome(adjusted odds ratio,2.22;95% confidence interval,1.10–4.48; $P = 0.03$).

Conclusions: Higher levels of serum hs-cTnT were independently associated with increased risk of death or major disability after stroke onset, suggesting that serum hs-cTnT may have prognostic value in poor outcomes of ischemic stroke.

Keywords: Acute ischemic stroke, Heart damage, Hs-cTnT,electrocardiographic abnormality, Insular stroke

Background

Stroke is an important contributor to death and major disability. Ischemic stroke is the most common subtype of stroke. Autonomic dysfunction is a frequent in stroke patients. Studies showed that cardiac autonomic dysfunction caused by ischemic stroke might lead to an adverse outcome. Cardiac comorbidities account for almost 20% of deaths after ischemic stroke, appropriate preventive or therapeutic measures can be taken if the patient with acute stroke at risk of myocardial injury could be identified at the time of admission. High sensitivity cardiac troponin T (hs-cTnT) is the most sensitive marker of myocardial injury, however it can rise in several other conditions (e.g. renal failure, sepsis, heart failure, and pulmonary edema) [1, 2]. In the last decade, the importance of hs-cTnT elevated in acute stroke has attracted many scholars' interest. Previous studies have shown that serum hs-cTnT is elevated in 10–30% of acute stroke patients [3–5]. In addition, some studies have found that elevated serum hs-cTnT levels may be associated with specific areas of brain damage [6]. However, it still remains unclear the pathomechanism of hs-cTnT elevation during the acute stage of ischemic stroke, which may be developed by neurally mediated autonomic dysregulation after acute stroke. In the other hand, in published studies, there were small numbers of

* Correspondence: 531324679@qq.com; 383376877@qq.com
†Lanying He and Jian Wang contributed equally to this work.
[1]Department of Neurology, The Second People's Hospital of Chengdu, Chengdu 400010, People's Republic of China
Full list of author information is available at the end of the article

patients. To date, whether hs-cTnT levels is associated with death or poor outcome remain uncertain [7, 8].

To test the hypothesis that if serum hs-cTnT levels can help predict cardiac complications and poor outcome in acute ischaemic stroke(AIS), we studied the prognostic correlates of elevated hs-cTnT levels on admission in a cohort of consecutive patients.

Methods

Study population

The consecutive patients who were admitted to the Second People's Hospital of Chengdu due to AIS within 72 h of symptom onset between May 2012 and December 2017. Stroke patients were diagnosed as AIS if the brain computed tomography (CT) scan was normal or showed acute ischemic changes according to World Health Organization definition (sudden neurological deficit with a putative vascular cause). Acute ischemic stroke was confirmed by diffusion-weighted imaging (DWI) magnetic resonance imaging (MRI) using Siemens Magnetom Avanto 1.5 Tesla (Siemens Medical Solutions, Erlangen, Germany). The severity of stroke was assessed by National Institutes of Health Stroke Scale score(NIHSS). Eligible patients were all patients admitted to our stroke unit during the study period. This study was approved by ethics committee. Written informed consent was obtained from all study participants or their legal proxies.

Inclusion and exclusion criteria

Patients were included in the study only if they fulfilled all the following criteria:1. Admission for first-ever acute ischemic stroke.2. Evidence of a single acute hemispheric lesion consistent with clinical manifestations. 3. Cardiac(include acute myocardial infarction, congestive heart failure, a history of tachyarrhythmia/bradyarrhythmia or atrial fibrillation),pulmonary disease and impaired renal function (estimated glomerularfiltration rate < 60 mL/min per 1.73 m^2) were excluded.4. Any pharmacological treatment, including β-blockers, possibly affecting the autonomic function were excluded. 5.Cerebral hemorrhage, fever, hypoxia also were excluded. No patients received mechanical thrombectomy and thrombolytic therapy. All patients received standard therapy, which consisted of aspirin, lipid-lowering medications and so on. All patients were followed up for 3 months. The outcome was defined as death and major disability (scores 3–5 of modified Rankin Scale [mRS]) at 3 months after stroke onset.

Data collection

CT or MRI examination was conducted at the time of admission, and repeated examination was performed on 5 days after admission to confirm the location of the lesion. The presence of insular infarction was assessed by an experienced neuroradiologist blinded to clinical details.

Serum hs-cTnT was measured as part of routine laboratory testing on admission, which were measured by Elecsys and cobase analyzer (Roche diagnostics). Levels of serum hs-cTnT was considered abnormal if it was≥14 ng/l.

Standard 12-lead electrocardiogram (ECGs) examination was performed on admission and assessed by two inspectors, blinded for patients. The Data differences between observers were resolved by consensus.

After the heart investigation, if the patients were suspected to have acute coronary syndrome, the cardiologist would perform additional cardiac evaluations for the patients. The waveforms of 12-lead ECGs were uploaded in digitai form, and explained by a cardiologist. Two dimensional transthoracic echocardiography was performed on patients with suspected reversible cardiac ischemia, and then we excluded patients with reversible cardiac ischemia.

Statistical analysis

Firstly, patients were classified into normal and hs-cTnT elevation group according to the level of serum hs-cTnT on admission. Demographic characteristics, vascular risk factors, current smoke, and so on were compared between the 2 subgroups in univariate analysis, using Pearson χ 2 test, Fisher exact 2-sided test, or Student t test, mean values(±standard deviation) were calculated for continuous variables. Mann-Whitney U test was used to test differences between two groups. We then performed logistic regressions analyses to determine the association between serum hs-cTnT and outcome(death, major disability and death/major disability), adjusting for age, sex, hypertension, current Smoking, current alcohol drinking, diabetes, hyperlipidemia, insular stroke, family history of stroke and NIHSS score. Results were expressed as adjusted odds ratios (OR) with the corresponding 95% confidence interval (CI).The data were analyzed using SPSS software (SPASS 22.0). *P* values< 0.05 were considered as statistically significant.

Results

Characteristics of the study subjects

During the study period, 516 patients were identified, comprised 49.03%(253) men and 50.97%(263) women, and the mean age was 66.19 ± 10.11 years(38-96 years). In the study population, 367 patients had a history of hypertension, 154 had a history of diabetes, 274 had a history of hyperlipidemia, 149 patients smoke,153patients current alcohol drinking. Of these patients, 152were diagnosed as insular stroke. During the 3-month follow-up period, 49 out of 516(9.49%) patients had died.

Univariable models for predictors of elevated hs-cTnT

Serum hs-cTnT levels were normal in 398 (77.13%) patients, the elevated hs-cTnT level in 118 (22.87%). Baseline characteristics of patients in the normal hs-cTnT group(< 14 ng/L) and the elevated hs-cTnT group(≥14 ng/l) were compared (Table 1). Patients with elevated hs-cTnT showed significantly higher prevalence of older age, insular stroke and high NIHSS score than patients with normal hs-cTnT (both $P < 0.05$). In multivariate logistic regression, insular stroke associated with hs-cTnT elevation (adjusted odds ratio, 2.48; 95% confidence interval, 1.48–4.17; $P = 0.00$).

Multivariable models on the association between elevated hs-cTnT and prognosis

Mortality rates were 24.58%(29/118) in the elevated hs-cTnT group at 3 months, which was significantly higher than that in the normal hs-cTnT group(5.03%,20/398) ($P = 0.000$). In addition to 49 dead, the remaining 467 patients, major disability rates were 40.45%(36/89) in the elevated hs-cTnT group at 3 months, which was significantly higher than that in the normal hs-cTnT group(17.99%,68/378) ($P = 0.000$). After adjusting for age, sex, hypertension, current smoking, current alcohol drinking, diabetes, hyperlipidemia, insular stroke, family history of stroke and NIHSS score on admission,3-month mortality in the elevated hs-cTnT group was higher than in the normal hs-cTnT group (adjusted odds ratio, 3.14; 95% confidence interval, 1.16–8.49; $P = 0.02$), and 3-month major disability in the elevated hs-cTnT group was higher than in the normal hs-cTnT group (odds ratio, 2.17; 95% confidence interval, 1.04–4.51; $P = 0.04$). After adjusting for fully confounders, the combined prognosis of death/disability was significantly higher for the elevated hs-cTnT group at 3 months(adjusted odds ratio, 2.22; 95% confidence interval, 1.10–4.48; $P = 0.03$).(Table 2).

In this study, we also found that the concentration of hs-cTnT were significantly correlated with poor prognosis, the higher the hs-cTnT, the worse the prognosis. The levels of hs-cTnT in the death group and the survival group were respectively 18.67 ± 10.39, 10.26 ± 6.85 ($P = 0.00$), the levels of hs-cTnT in the mRS ≤ 2 group and the major disability group were respectively 9.14 ± 5.98, 14.14 ± 8.15(P = 0.00),and the levels of hs-cTnT in the mRS ≤ 2 group and the composite outcome group were respectively 9.14 ± 5.98, 15.59 ± 9.14(P = 0.00).

Discussion

Hs-cTnT is the most sensitive and specific biomarker of myocardial injury,which is widely used in the diagnosis of the patients with heart diseases, especially in patients with non-ST segment elevation acute coronary syndrome [9, 10]. Many studies have shown that serum Hs-cTnT of many patients with acute stroke increases significantly. The current treatment guidelines for acute ischemic stroke patients recommend troponin evaluation in acute stage [11]. It is still controversial whether the increase of troponin after AIS is related to the mortality and disability rate of stroke patients. Most studies suggest that there is a link between them, but a few studies that hold the opposite view. Some studies have shown that elevated troponin is related to poor functional prognosis, and high troponin levels is associated with increased mortality [12–15]. The potential pathophysiological mechanism of troponin elevation in the AIS is still unclear, leading to considerable uncertainty in the diagnosis and treatment for the clinician. In our study, 22.87%(118/516) of acute stroke patients had elevated serum hs-cTnT level which was congruent with

Table 1 Comparison of baseline characteristics between patients with normal and elevated hs-cTnT group

	hs-cTnT< 14 ng/L (398)	hs-cTnT≥14 ng/L (118)	OR(95%CI)	P*
Age, y(mean,SD)	65.36 ± 10.07	69.01 ± 9.77		*0.00*
Females,n(%)	205 (51.51)	58(49.15)	0.91 (0.60–1.37)	0.65
Men,n(%)	193(48.49)	60(50.85)	0.91(0.60–1.37)	0.65
Hypertension,patients,n(%)	287(72.11)	80(67.80)	0.81(0.52–1.27)	0.36
Current Smoking,n(%)	111(27.89)	38(32.20)	1.23(0.79–1.92)	0.36
Current alcohol drinking,n(%)	115(28.89)	38(32.20)	1.17(0.75–1.82)	0.49
Diabetes, n(%)	115(28.89)	39(33.05)	1.22(0.78–1.89)	0.39
Hyperlipidemia,n(%)	214(53.77)	60(50.85)	0.89(0.59–1.34)	0.58
ST/T change, n(%)	110 (27.64)	39(33.05)	1.293(0.83–2.01)	0.23
Insular stroke,n(%)	89(22.36)	63(53.39)	3.98(2.58–6.12)	*0.00*
Family history of stroke, n(%)	74(18,59)	27(22.88)	1.30(0.79–2.14)	0.30
NIHSS score(min-max)	2–25	2–30		
NIHSS score(mean,SD)	8.82 ± 4.39	11.80 ± 5.21		*0.00*

*Comparison between normal hs-cTnT group and elevated hs-cTnT group

Table 2 Multivariable Models Showing Association Between elevated hs-cTnT and Prognosis

	OR (95% CI)	P*
death	3.14(1.16–8.49)	0.02
Major disability(mRS 3–5)	2.17(1.04–4.51)	0.04
Major disability(mRS3–5) + death	2.22(1.10–4.48)	0.03

*Multivariable adjusted for age, sex, hypertension, current Smoking, current alcohol drinking, diabetes, hyperlipidemia, insular stroke, family history of stroke and NIHSS score

previous studies. Mortality rates and major disability rate in the elevated hs-cTnT group respectively were 24.58%,30.31% at 3 months, which was significantly higher than that in the normal hs-cTnT group. After adjusting for fully confounders, we found a significant association of elevated hs-cTnT level with risks of death or major disability within 3 months after acute ischemic stroke. These results suggested this association was independent of established risk factors, including age, and baseline NIHSS score, and increased serum hs-cTnT elevation could be an independent risk factor of poor outcomes and have prognostic value for death or major disability among patients with acute ischemic stroke.

The evidence on whether increased troponin is associated with stroke was inconsistent: some studies had shown that damage to the right or left insular is associated with higher baseline troponin levels [16, 17], while others had not found any association between insular stroke and troponin levels [18, 19].In our study, 152 were diagnosed as insular stroke, patients with elevated hs-cTnT levels showed significantly higher prevalence of insular stroke, after adjusting for fully confounders, we found a significant association of insular stroke with elevated hs-cTnT level. These results suggested insular damage might contribute to cardiac autonomic dysfunction, the underlying pathophysiological mechanism might be the downregulation of parasympathetic activity, hence the relative up-regulation of sympathetic effects on cardiac function. As a result, this may lead to myocardial injury by contraction zone necrosis or ischemia. In our study showed that the range of hs-cTnT activity was between 14.46~ 58.51 ng/L in patients with increased hs-cTnT levels, which was much lower than that in the myocardial infarction patients. So, hs-cTnT elevation during the acute stage of ischemic stroke, which may be developed by neurally mediated autonomic dysregulation after acute stroke.

Some limitations of this study merit consideration. Firstly, in this study, we relied on a single baseline blood sample and thus we could not account for variations in serum hs-cTnT levels that occur over time, serum hs-cTnT levels should be measured repeatedly to allow longitudinal analysis, which might provide additional information on the development and on its prognostic implications. Secondly, We did not study that association of elevated serum hs-cTnT level with recurrent stroke, which might have an effect on the experimental results. Thirdly, although we adjusted for NIHSS score, which has been show to correlate with infarction volume, we lacked data on infarction volume. Fourth, we lack data on the possible influence of the left and right insular stroke on hs-cTnT and prognosis, respectively, because left and right insular lesion have different influence on the cardiac autonomic function.. In future experiments, we will avoid the aboved limitation, in order to obtain more reliable result.

Conclusions

Routine serum hs-cTnT measurement in patients with ischemic stroke may provide important novel clinical use. In addition, some studies should be encouraged in regarding to correct cardiac autonomic dysfunction and whether lowering hs-cTnT could prevent the poor outcome of ischemic stroke.

In conclusion, our findings indicated that higher levels of serum hs-cTnT in acute ischemic stroke were associated with increased risk of death or major disability at 3 months. Serum hs-cTnT may have potential predictive value in risk stratification of ischemic stroke.

Abbreviations

CI: Confidence Interval; hs-cTnT: High sensitivity cardiac troponin; M: Mean; OR: Odds Ratio; SD: Standard Deviation

Acknowledgments

We thank all patients and their families for generously consenting to use of human tissues in this research.

Funding

This work was funded by the Health and Family Planning Commission of Chengdu (2015009), which is not involved in the database management (collection, analysis, interpretation of data) and has no access to patient information. The funding body did not participate in designing the study or writing the manuscript. The study protocol has undergone peer-review process by the funding body.

Authors' contributions

LYH was responsible for the concept and design of the study, data collection and analysis and the first draft of the paper and further manuscript. JW was responsible for concept and design of the study, the data analysis and interpretation. WWD was responsible for overseeing the concept and design of the study, the data analysis and interpretation, and writing the paper. All authors read and approved the final manuscript for publication.

Competing interests

The authors declare that they have no competing interests.

Author details

[1]Department of Neurology, The Second People's Hospital of Chengdu, Chengdu 400010, People's Republic of China. [2]Department of Neurology, First Affiliated Hospital, Chongqing Medical University, ChongqingChina, 400030, People's Republic of China.

References

1. Jeremias A, Gibson CM. Narrative review: alternative causes for elevated cardiac troponin levels when acute coronary syndromes are excluded. Ann Intern Med. 2005:142(9): 786–791. [Free full text] [Pubmed].
2. Kelley WE, Januzzi JL, Christenson RH. Increases of cardiac troponin in conditions other than acute coronary syndrome and heart failure. Clin Chem. 2009:55(12): 2098–2112. doi: https://doi.org/10.1373/clinchem.2009.130799. Epub 2009 Oct 8. [Free Article] [Pubmed].
3. Jensen JK, Kristensen SR, Bak S, Atar D, Hoilund-Carlsen PF, Mickley H. Frequency and significance of troponin T elevation in acute ischemic stroke. Am J Cardiol. 2007;99(1):108–12. https://doi.org/10.1016/j.amjcard.2006.10.052.
4. Liu J, Wang D, Xiong Y, et al. High-sensitivity cardiac troponin T levels and risk of cerebral microbleeds in acute ischemic strokepatients with atrial fibrillation and/or rheumatic heart disease. J Neurol Sci. 2016;369:15–8. https://doi.org/10.1016/j.jns.2016.08.003. Epub 2016 Aug 2
5. Suleiman HM, Aliyu IS, Abubakar SA, et al. Cardiac troponin T and creatine kinase MB fraction levels among patients with acute ischemic stroke in Nigeria. Niger J Clin Pract. 2017;20(12):1618–21. https://doi.org/10.4103/njcp.njcp_78_17.
6. Abdi S,Oveis-Gharan S, Sinaei F, Ghorbani A. Elevated troponin T after acute ischemic stroke: Association with severity and location of infarctin. Iran J Neurol., 2015,14(1):35–40. [Free PMC Article][Pubmed].
7. Jensen JK, Atar D, Mickley H. Mechanism of troponin elevations in patients with acute ischemic stroke. Am J Cardiol. 2007;99(6):867–70. https://doi.org/10.1016/j.amjcard.2006.10.052.
8. Freda BJ, Tang WH, Van LF, Peacock WF, Francis GS. Cardiac troponins in renal insufficiency: review and clinical implications. J Am Coll Cardiol. ,2002,40 (12): 2065–2071. [Free full text] [Pubmed].
9. Sayadnik M, Shafiee A, Jenab Y, Jalali A, Sadeghian S. Predictors of High-Sensitivity Cardiac Troponin T Elevation in Patients with Acute Paroxysmal Supraventricular Tachycardia and Ischemic Heart Disease. Tex Heart Inst J,2017,44(5):306–311. DOI:https://doi.org/10.14503/THIJ-15-5338
10. Abiko M, Inai K, Shimada E, Asagai S, Nakanishi T. The prognostic value of high sensitivity cardiac troponin T in patients with congenital heart disease. J Cardiol,2018,71(4):389–393. DOI:10.1016/j.jjcc.2017.09.012.
11. Jauch EC, Saver JL, Adams HP, et al. Guidelines for the early management of patients with acute ischemic stroke: a guideline for healthcare professionals from the American Heart Association. American Stroke Association Stroke. 2013;44:870–947. https://doi.org/10.1161/STR.0000000000000158 Epub 2018 Jan 24.
12. Ahn SH, Kim YH, Shin CH,et al. Cardiac Vulnerability to Cerebrogenic Stress as a Possible Cause of Troponin Elevation in Stroke. J Am Heart Assoc,2016,5(10):e004135. DOI:https://doi.org/10.1161/JAHA.116.004135[Free PMC Article][Pubmed].
13. Scheitz JF, Mochmann HC, Erdur H, et al. Prognostic relevance of cardiac troponin T levels and their dynamic changes measured with a high-sensitivity assay in acute ischaemic stroke: analyses from the TRELAS cohort. Int J Cardiol. 2014;177(3):886–93. https://doi.org/10.1016/j.ijcard.2012.01.055. Epub 2012 Feb 10
14. Faiz KW, Thommessen B, Einvik G, et al. Determinants of high sensitivity cardiac troponin T elevation in acute ischemic stroke.BMC Neurol 2014;14:96. DOI:https://doi.org/10.1186/1471-2377-14-96.[Free PMC Article][Pubmed].
15. Peddada K, Cruz-Flores S, Goldstein LB, et al. Ischemic stroke with troponin elevation: patient characteristics,resource utilization,and in-hospital outcomes. Cerebrovasc Dis,2016,42(2–3):213–223. DOI:https://doi.org/10.1159/000445526.Epub 2016 May 3.
16. Song HS,Back JH,Jin DK,et al.Cardiac troponin T elevation after stroke: relationships between elevated serum troponin T,stroke location, and prognosis. J Clin Neurol,2008,4:75–83. [Free PMC Article][Pubmed].
17. Scheitz JF, Endres M, Mochmann HC, et al. Frequency, determinants and outcome of elevated troponin in acute ischemic stroke patients. Int J Cardiol. 2012;157(2):239–42. https://doi.org/10.1016/j.ijcard.2012.01.055. Epub 2012 Feb 10
18. Christensen H, Johannesen HH, Christensen AF, et al. Serum cardiac troponin I in acute stroke is related to serum cortisol and TNF-alpha. Cerebrovasc Dis. 2004;18(3):194–9. https://doi.org/10.1159/000079941.
19. Barber M, Morton JJ, Macfarlane PW, et al. Elevated troponin levels are associated with sympathoadrenal activation in acute ischaemic stroke. Cerebrovasc Dis. 2007;23(4):260–6. https://doi.org/10.1159/000098325.

18

Plasma homocysteine levels and intracranial plaque characteristics: association and clinical relevance in ischemic stroke

Shan shan Lu[1], Jun Xie[1], Chun qiu Su[1], Song Ge[2], Hai bin Shi[1*] and Xun ning Hong[1*]

Abstract

Background: Elevated plasma homocysteine (Hcy) is an independent risk factor for ischemic stroke. This study aimed to evaluate the association between Hcy levels and intracranial plaque characteristics and to investigate their clinical relevance in ischemic stroke.

Methods: Ninety-four patients with intracranial atherosclerosis (ICAS) were enrolled. Plasma Hcy levels were measured. Intracranial plaque characteristics including plaque enhancement, stenosis ratio, T2 and T1 hyperintense components were assessed on high-resolution magnetic resonance imaging. Logistic regression model was constructed to analyze the association between high Hcy levels and plaque characteristics, and their synergistic effects to predict the likelihood for ischemic stroke, while adjusting for demographics and traditional atherosclerotic risk factors.

Results: Elevated Hcy level was associated with strong plaque enhancement independently of age, sex, serum creatinine levels and other atherosclerotic risk factors (($P < 0.001$, OR 6.00, 95% confidence interval [CI] 2.28–15.74). Both strong plaque enhancement ($P = 0.026$, OR 5.63, 95% CI 1.23–25.81) and high Hcy level ($P = 0.018$, OR 6.20, 95% CI 1.36–28.26) were correlated with acute ischemic stroke. The combination of them strengthened the ability to stratify the likelihood for ischemic stroke, with an improved area under the receiver operating characteristic curve (AUC) of 0.871, significantly higher than that of strong plaque enhancement (0.755) and high Hcy level (0.715) alone ($P < 0.05$ for both).

Conclusions: High Hcy level appears to have association with intracranial strong plaque enhancement. The combined assessment of plasma Hcy levels and plaque enhancement may improve ischemic stroke risk stratification.

Keywords: Homocysteine, Atherosclerosis, Magnetic resonance imaging, Ischemic stroke

Background

Acute ischemic stroke is the most common cerebrovascular disease and is one of the leading causes of death and long-term disability through the world [1]. Large artery atherosclerosis is a major cause of ischemic stroke and can be divided into intracranial atherosclerosis (ICAS) and extracranial atherosclerosis [2]. Recently, studies have reported that the prevalence of ICAS has racial and ethnic differences, with a greater incidence in Asian people [3]. A study by Cao et al. exhibited significantly greater plaque burden of middle cerebral artery (MCA) as compared to ipsilateral extracranial carotid artery and is more strongly associated with ischemia severity [4]. Bos et al. established ICAS as a major risk factor for stroke and suggested that its contribution to the proportion of all strokes may be greater than that of extracranial atherosclerosis [5]. Similarly, a retrospective study by Wong et al. also demonstrate that although extracranial atherosclerosis may be a more common lesion in whites in Europe and America, ICAS is more common in Asian patients [6].

* Correspondence: hbshi346@163.com; hongxunning@sina.com
[1]Department of Radiology, The First Affiliated Hospital of Nanjing Medical University, No.300 Guangzhou Road, Gulou district, Nanjing 210029, Jiangsu Province, China
Full list of author information is available at the end of the article

Elevated plasma homocysteine (Hcy) levels have been indicated as an independent risk factor for ischemic stroke [7, 8]. High Hcy levels may be associated with endothelial injury and vascular inflammation, leading to the development of atherogenesis [9]. Studies have revealed that high Hcy levels are associated with advanced carotid plaque and greater incidence of acute ischemic stroke in patients with carotid artery plaques [7, 10–13]. However, most of the previous findings were derived from carotid artery, presumably due to the technical limitation of imaging in the intracranial arteries. Although the plaque burden of intracranial artery is greater in Asian population, little data are available regarding the relationship between Hcy levels and intracranial plaque stability.

Currently, the application of high-resolution magnetic resonance imaging (HR-MRI) enables us to evaluate intracranial vasculopathy. Plaque characteristics on HR-MRI such as plaque enhancement and T1 hyperintensity can serve as markers of its stability and may associate with ischemic stroke [14–16]. In the present study, we aimed to evaluate the association between Hcy levels and intracranial plaque characteristics assessed on HR-MRI and investigated their clinical relevance in ischemic stroke events.

Methods

Subjects

This retrospective study was reviewed and approved by our institutional Review Board. The need for patient consent was waived by the same ethics committee. Between May 2016 and November 2017, we reviewed 146 consecutive patients with intracranial vasculopathy who had HR-MRI and, on luminal imaging, had intracranial arterial stenosis in our single institutional database. The detailed inclusion criteria were as follows: (1) plaque of MCA or basilar artery (BA) confirmed on HR-MRI; (2) absence of significant stenosis of extracranial carotid and vertebral artery (≥ 30%); (3) patients had one or more traditional atherosclerotic risk factors which included hypertension, vdiabetes mellitus, hypercholesterolemia and current cigarette smoking; and (4) the image quality of HR-MRI was adequate for evaluation. The exclusion criteria included: (1) non-atherosclerotic vasculopathies, such as vasculitis, dissection, or moyamoya disease; (2) patients had high risk factors for cardio-embolism, such as atrial fibrillation, valvular heart disease and infective endocarditis. Twelve patients with moyamoya diseases, 5 with arterial dissections, 2 with vasculitis, 10 with significant extracranial arterial stenosis, 7 with plaques only located in anterior cerebral artery or posterior cerebral artery, 7 with high-risk factors for cardio-embolism, and 9 with obvious motion artifacts on HR-MRI were excluded. Finally, 94 patients were recruited in the current study.

All the patients were divided into two groups based on the clinical information and diffusion-weighted imaging (DWI): 1) symptomatic group: patients who suffered from acute cerebral infarction or transient ischemic attack (TIA) in the distribution of MCA or BA territory within the recent 2 weeks; 2) asymptomatic group: patients with MCA or BA stenosis referred by luminal imaging before HR-MRI, yet had no history of stroke events.

Clinical profiles and laboratory measurement

Laboratory examination including plasma Hcy levels, serum creatinine levels, total cholesterol, low-density lipoprotein and blood glucose were measured within 24 h of admission. Blood samples were drawn from the patients after overnight fasting. Venous blood samples were collected in tubes containing EDTA, centrifuged within 30 min to avoid a false elevation in Hcy concentration. The plasma Hcy levels were determined by high-performance liquid chromatography. The physiological range of plasma Hcy are 5–15 μmol/L. Patients with Hcy levels above 15 μmol/L were defined as high Hcy (hyperhomocysteinemia) [7].

The traditional atherosclerotic risk factors were defined as follows: (1) hypertension: blood pressure > 140/90 mmHg on repeated measurements, or patients receiving antihypertensive medication; (2) hyperlipidemia: total cholesterol level ≥ 200 mg/dL, low-density lipoprotein ≥130 mg/dL, or use of lipid-lowering agent; (3) diabetes mellitus: fasting blood sugar ≥7.0 mmol/L, or 2-h post prandial blood sugar ≥11.1 mmol/L, or use of antidiabetic medication. Stress hyperglycaemia was carefully excluded according to the hemoglobin A1c levels; (4) current cigarette smoker.

MRI protocols

All the images were obtained with a 3.0 T MR imaging scanner (Magnetom skyra, Siemens Healthcare, Erlangen, Germany) equipped with a 20-channel head-neck coil. The HR-MRI protocols included a three-dimensional (3D) time-of-flight magnetic resonance angiography (TOF-MRA) and a 3D T1 weighted SPACE (Sampling Perfection with Application optimized Contrast using different angle Evolutions) sequence with fat-suppression before and after contrast administration. The detailed scan parameters used for T1 weighted SPACE were as follows: TR/TE, 900/4.2 ms; field-of-view, 240 × 216 mm; turbo-spin factor, 43 echos; echo spacing 4.2 ms. The acquired voxel size was $0.75 \times 0.75 \times 0.75\ mm^3$ and reconstructed to $0.4 \times 0.4 \times 0.75\ mm^3$. Contrast-enhanced T1 weighted SPACE was acquired with an approximately 5-min delay after administration of 0.1 mmol/kg contrast agent (gadodiamide, GE Healthcare, Ireland). Axial DWI was performed using a single-shot echo-planar spin-echo sequence with the following parameters: b-values, 0 and 1000 mm^2/s, FOV, 230 × 230 mm, section thickness, 5 mm, matrix, 192 × 192.

Image analysis

Two neuroradiologists (SSL and CQS, with 6 and 4 years of experience, respectively), who were provided each patient's clinical presentation, DWI and TOF-MRA results, analyzed the HR-MRI images independently. A plaque was identified as focal wall thickening when it was evident on both the short and long axis of the vessel compared to the normal vessel wall. A culprit plaque was defined as the only or a most stenotic lesion within the vascular territory of the ischemic stroke. Plaque characteristics evaluated in our study included the following: (1) strong enhancement, enhancement was greater than or equal to that of pituitary stalk [14]; (2) T2 hyperintense components: presence or absence of a T2 hyperintense band adjacent to the lumen, which may indicate the fibrous cap [17]. Lesion signal intensity on T2 was assessed relative to gray matter; (3) T1 hyperintense components: presence or absence of T1 hyperintense on unenhanced T1 images with fat-suppression, which may indicate the intraplaque hemorrhage [16]. Lesion signal intensity on T1 was assessed relative to normal-appearing white matter. For any discrepancy between the two readers, another senior neuroradiologist (XNH with 20 years of experience) re-evaluated the images and assisted in reaching a consensus agreement.

The degree of luminal stenosis was calculated using the following formula: stenosis ratio = (1- narrow lumen diameter/reference lumen diameter) × 100%. The reference lumen was defined as the neighboring segment of normal appearance proximal to the stenotic site. The measurement results of luminal stenosis ratio from the two neuroradiologists were averaged for subsequent analysis.

Statistical analysis

The inter-reader reproducibility for assessment of plaque characteristics was evaluated using Cohen's kappa statistics. The intraclass correlation coefficient were calculated for measurements of luminal stenosis ratio. In the univariate analyses comparing between the symptomatic and asymptomatic group, plaque characteristics, luminal stenosis ratio, Hcy and serum creatinine levels, patient demographics (age, sex) and atherosclerotic risk factors were compared using a Student's t test, or a Pearson's chi-square test, or a nonparametric Mann-Whitney U-test as appropriate. Correlation of Hcy levels (normal or high Hcy) with plaque characteristics were examined by Spearman correlation analysis. Multivariable logistic regression was constructed to evaluate the association between high Hcy levels and plaque characteristics reaching significance on univariate analysis (model 1), and their ability to stratify the likelihood of ischemic stroke after adjusting for demographics, serum creatinine levels and vascular risk factors (model 2). Odds ratio (OR) with 95% confidence interval (CI) was calculated for the covariate with statistical significance. Receiver operating characteristic (ROC) curves were constructed to assess the diagnostic performance of high Hcy levels, significant plaque characteristics and their combination (model 2) to determine the occurrence of ischemic stroke. The ROC analysis was performed using MedCalc (version 12.3.0, Mariakerke, Belgium). All other statistical analyses were performed using SPSS (version 16.0, Chicago, IL, USA). Statistical significance was set as $P < 0.05$.

Results

Patient demographics and plaque characteristics

A total of 94 patients with ICAS were enrolled in the study. They were divided into two groups, symptomatic group (males = 54; females = 21; average age = 59.7 ± 12.8; 71 with DWI-evidenced stroke and 4 with TIA) and asymptomatic group (males = 14; females = 5; average age = 62.3 ± 16.6). For 4 patients who had a matched clinical presentation of TIA, the vascular distributions were as follows: left MCA (aphasia and numbness and weakness of the right leg; aphasia and decreased sensation in right arm), right MCA (left face and arm numbness and weakness) and vertebrobasilar artery (transient dysphagia). For 19 asymptomatic patients, 11 patients had not any symptom, 3 with headache, 3 with memory decline, and 2 with dizziness.

The plasma Hcy levels were 16.78 ± 5.52 μmol/L in symptomatic group, significantly higher than that of asymptomatic group (13.63 ± 5.01 μmol/L) ($P = 0.026$). The inter-reader agreement was 0.820 for strong plaque enhancement, 0.745 for T2 hyperintense components, 0.724 for T1 hyperintense components and 0.965 for stenosis ratio. More plaques in symptomatic group showed strong enhancement and presence of T1 hyperintense compared to that of asymptomatic group ($P < 0.001$ and $P = 0.020$, respectively). No significant difference was found in other plaque features. The baseline patients' demographics and plaque characteristics are shown in Table 1.

Association between high Hcy levels and plaque characteristics

Table 2 shows the distribution of plaque characteristics in relation to plasma Hcy levels. Strong plaque enhancement was observed in 41 of 52 (78.8%) patients with high Hcy levels and significantly correlated with high Hcy ($r = 0.392$, $P < 0.001$). To further examine the association of strong plaque enhancement

Table 1 Patient demographics and plaque characteristics

Variables	Symptomatic group ($n = 75$)	Asymptomatic group ($n = 19$)	P value
Male, n (%)	54 (72.0%)	14 (73.7%)	0.883
Age, (Mean ± SD), y	59.7 ± 12.8	62.3 ± 16.6	0.454
Hypertension, n (%)	53 (70.7%)	16 (84.2%)	0.233
Diabetes mellitus, n (%)	28 (37.3%)	9 (47.4%)	0.424
Hyperlipidemia, n (%)	35 (46.7%)	10 (52.6%)	0.642
Current smoker, n (%)	24 (32.0%)	4 (21.1%)	0.351
Serum creatinine (μmol/L)	69.84 ± 16.31	71.32 ± 11.97	0.712
Homocysteine, (μmol/L)[a]	16.78 ± 5.52	13.63 ± 5.01	0.026
High Hcy, n (%)	48 (64.0%)	4 (21.1%)	0.001
Normal Hcy, n (%)	27 (36.0%)	15 (78.9%)	0.001
Plaque characteristics[b]			
Strong enhancement	54 (72.0%)	4 (21.1%)	< 0.001
Presence of T1 hyperintense	29 (38.7%)	2 (10.5%)	0.020
Presence of T2 hyperintense	38 (50.7%)	8 (42.1%)	0.505
Stenosis ratio (%)	61.7 ± 31.3	52.3 ± 30.0	0.303

Note: [a] The normal range of plasma Hcy is 5–15 μmol/L. High Hcy is defined as Hcy levels above 15 μmol/L. [b] Strong plaque enhancement, enhancement was greater than or equal to that of pituitary stalk; lesion T2 hyperintense components: presence or absence of T2 hyperintense band adjacent to the lumen; lesion T1 hyperintense components: presence or absence of T1 hyperintense on unenhanced T1 images with fat-suppression

with high Hcy, binary logistic regression analysis was performed (model 1). High Hcy was found to be associated with strong plaque enhancement independently of age, sex, serum creatinine levels and other traditional atherosclerotic risk factors ($P <$ 0.001, OR 6.00, 95% CI 2.28–15.74) (Table 3).

Ability of high Hcy and plaque characteristics to stratify ischemic stroke

In the multivariable logistic model (model 2), strong plaque enhancement ($P = 0.026$, OR 5.63, 95% CI 1.23–25.81) and high Hcy level ($P = 0.018$, OR 6.20, 95% CI 1.36–28.26) were associated with acute ischemic stroke independently of age, sex, serum creatinine levels and other traditional atherosclerotic risk factors (Table 4). The AUC (95% CI) for determining the occurrence of ischemic stroke were 0.755 (0.655–0.838) for strong plaque enhancement and 0.715 (0.612–0.803) for high Hcy level, respectively. The combination of high Hcy and strong plaque enhancement in model 2 improved the ability to stratify the likelihood for acute ischemic stroke, with improved AUC of 0.871 (0.786–0.931), significantly higher than that of strong plaque enhancement and high Hcy alone ($P < 0.05$ for both) (Fig. 1).

Table 2 Plasma homocysteine levels and intracranial plaque characteristics

Plaque characteristics[b]	High Hcy[a]	Normal Hcy	P value
Strong enhancement	41 (78.8%)	17 (40.5%)	< 0.001
Presence of T1 hyperintense	19 (36.5%)	12 (28.6%)	0.414
Presence of T2 hyperintense	24 (46.2%)	22 (52.4%)	0.548
Stenosis ratio (%)	61.3 ± 31.7	58.0 ± 30.6	0.684

Note: [a] High Hcy is defined as Hcy levels above 15 μmol/L. [b] Strong plaque enhancement, enhancement was greater than or equal to that of pituitary stalk; lesion T2 hyperintense components: presence or absence of T2 hyperintense band adjacent to the lumen; lesion T1 hyperintense components: presence or absence of T1 hyperintense on unenhanced T1 images with fat-suppression

Discussion

In the present study, we demonstrated a significant association between high plasma Hcy level and intracranial strong plaque enhancement independently of age, sex, serum creatinine levels and other traditional atherosclerotic risk factors in patients with large artery atherosclerosis. In addition, the combination of high Hcy and strong plaque enhancement improved the ability to stratify the likelihood for ischemic stroke in this group of patients.

Several plaque characteristics on HR-MRI were evaluated in our study. Plaque T1 hyperintensity is suggested as a possible indicator of recent intraplaque hemorrhage. The prevalence of T1 hyperintensity in our study was higher in plaques of symptomatic patients compared to those who were asymptomatic, which was consistent with previous study [16]. However, no correlation between high Hcy level and presence of T1 hyperintensity was found. Strong plaque enhancement may be the most promising imaging marker of intracranial plaque stability. In many previous reports, plaque enhancement has been documented as a very important predictor of plaque vulnerability in both extracranial and intracranial arteries [14, 15, 18–20]. A meta-analysis has shown that MRI-detected intracranial plaque enhancement is strongly associated with acute ischemic stroke [15]. In our study, plaques with strong enhancement was observed in 72% of plaques in symptomatic group, which is in accordance with previous findings. Pathologically, inflammation, neovascularity and increased endothelial permeability may contribute to the

Table 3 Determinants of strong plaque enhancement (model 1)

Variables	B	OR	95% CI	P value
High Hcy[a]	1.791	6.00	2.28–15.74	< 0.001
Sex (male = 1)	0.041	1.04	0.30–3.66	0.949
Age (/y)	−0.006	0.99	0.96–1.03	0.764
Hypertension	−0.430	0.65	0.21–1.98	0.448
Diabetes mellitus	−0.108	0.90	0.33–2.44	0.832
Hyperlipidemia	−0.565	0.57	0.21–1.54	0.266
Current smoker	−0.234	0.79	0.26–2.44	0.685
Serum creatinine	0.002	1.00	0.97–1.04	0.934

Note: *OR* indicates odds ratio, *CI* confidence interval. [a] High Hcy is defined as homocysteine level above 15 μmol/L

Table 4 Logistic regression analysis for predicting acute ischemic stroke (model 2)

Variables	B	OR	95% CI	*P* value
High Hcy[a]	1.824	6.20	1.36–28.26	0.018
Strong plaque enhancement	1.728	5.63	1.23–25.81	0.026
Presence of T1 hyperintense	1.748	5.74	0.81–40.77	0.080
Sex (male = 1)	0.381	1.46	0.26–8.37	0.668
Age (/y)	−0.015	0.99	0.94–1.04	0.559
Hypertension	−1.257	0.29	0.05–1.54	0.145
Diabetes mellitus	−1.069	0.34	0.08–1.50	0.155
Hyperlipidemia	0.287	1.33	0.32–5.52	0.692
Current smoker	0.799	2.22	0.45–10.90	0.324
Serum creatinine	−0.041	0.96	0.91–1.01	0.132

Note: *OR* indicates odds ratio, *CI* confidence interval. [a] High Hcy is defined as homocysteine level above 15 μmol/L

contrast enhancement of vulnerable plaques [21]. Plaques with strong enhancement reflects active inflammatory response and may lead to the occurrence of downstream cerebral infarction.

High plasma Hcy levels appeared to have association with intracranial strong plaque enhancement in our study. Previous studies have revealed that high Hcy may represent a sensitive risk factor for the development of advanced and unstable carotid plaques [7, 13]. Higher level of plasma Hcy were correlated with increased intima-media thickness in carotid artery [10, 22]. Our finding extends this association from carotid artery atherosclerosis to ICAS, further strengthening the existing evidence that elevated plasma Hcy level is a modifiable risk factor for vascular atherosclerosis. Hcy may impact the development of atherosclerosis through its involvement in complex pathways of inflammation and calcification [23]. It is postulated that high plasma Hcy levels may cause the impairment of vascular smooth muscle cell migration and endothelial cell function via the activation of methylation-sensitive transcription factors. It may also cause abnormalities in the function of fibrinogen and thrombin generation, leading to the formation of atherosclerotic plaques [24].

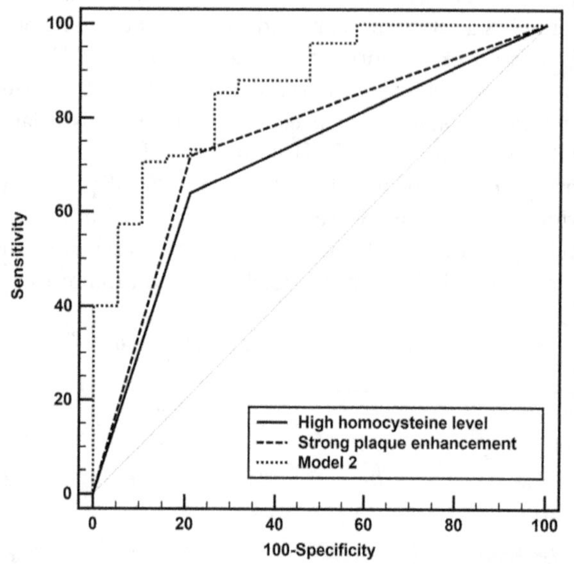

Fig. 1 ROC curves for the ability of strong plaque enhancement and high homocysteine (Hcy) level to determine ischemic stroke. The AUC was 0.755 and 0.715 for strong plaque enhancement and high Hcy level, respectively. The combination of them after adjusting for sex, age, serum creatinine levels and other traditional atherosclerotic risk factors (hypertension, diabetes mellitus, hyperlipidemia, current smoker) in model 2 significantly improved the AUC to 0.871

Elevated plasma Hcy level has been proved as an independent cardiovascular risk factor for ischemic stroke. Wu et al. found a significant correlation between elevated plasma Hcy and a greater incidence of acute cerebral infarction in patients with carotid artery plaques [7]. A prospective cohort study of Ji et al. supported the atherogenic role of Hcy. An elevated Hcy level can represent a sensitive predictor for severe neurological impairment, a poor functional outcome, and stroke recurrence in large artery atherosclerosis stroke subtype [25]. Several previous cohort studies such as the Northern Manhattan cohort study, the Framingham Study and the British Regional Heart Study also demonstrate elevated plasma Hcy was associated with an increased risk of ischemic stroke [26–28]. Our findings support this association. Both high Hcy levels and strongly enhanced plaques were significantly associated with symptomatic ischemic stroke. Importantly, the combined measurements of them were found to increase the ability to predict ischemic stroke events independently of sex, age, serum creatinine levels and other atherosclerotic risk factors. Such finding was consistent with a previous published study that the combination of carotid intima-media thickness and plasma Hcy levels could improve the prediction of ischemic stroke events [22]. High plasma Hcy is linked to mechanisms involved in the development of atherosclerosis, which may explain the synergism.

Our present study has certain limitations. First, homocysteine level is influenced by several factors which were not considered in this study, such as dietary habits (alcohol, coffee consumption, et al), folate and vitamin B_{12} levels, and therefore may potentially cause the bias. Second, this was a retrospective study, the selection bias cannot be discounted. The sample size was from a single Chinese center and relatively small, which may not be an accurate representation for all stroke patients, particularly in Western populations. Third, plaque characteristics in the present study were visually assessed. Quantitative analysis of plaque features, such as plaque burden and volume may provide incremental information on vulnerable lesions. Nevertheless, we consider that plaque enhancement is a non-invasive, sensitive and simple imaging marker in clinical practice. Finally, a longer period of following-up would probably allow us to examine the impact of plaque characteristics and/or Hcy levels on functional status (e.g., hospitalization duration and modified Rankin Scale), which is not discussed in the present study, but is clinically significant and deserve further investigation.

Conclusions

Our data revealed a significant association between high plasma Hcy levels and strong plaque enhancement on HR-MRI. The combined assessment of plasma Hcy levels and plaque enhancement may improve ischemic stroke risk stratification.

Abbreviations

Hcy: Plasma homocysteine; HR-MRI: High-resolution magnetic resonance imaging; ICAS: Intracranial atherosclerosis; MCA: Middle cerebral artery; BA, basilar artery

Acknowledgements

We sincerely thank Dr. Yan Zhou for her help in collecting the clinical information for all the patients.

Funding

No funding was received from any organization or individuals.

Authors' contributions

LSS, HXN and SHB were responsible for the concept and design of the study. LSS, XJ and SCQ were responsible for collecting and analyzing the data. LSS was responsible for drafting the manuscript. GS was responsible for the study coordination and interpretation of data. All authors participated in review and revision of the manuscript. All authors read and approval the final manuscript.

Competing interests

The authors declare that they have no competing interests.

Author details

[1]Department of Radiology, The First Affiliated Hospital of Nanjing Medical University, No.300 Guangzhou Road, Gulou district, Nanjing 210029, Jiangsu Province, China. [2]Department of Neurology, The First Affiliated Hospital of Nanjing Medical University, Nanjing 210029, Jiangsu Province, China.

References

1. Towfighi A, Saver JL. Stroke declines from third to fourth leading cause of death in the United States: historical perspective and challenges ahead. Stroke. 2011;42:2351–5.
2. Adams HP Jr, Bendixen BH, Kappelle LJ, Biller J, Love BB, Gordon DL, et al. Classification of subtype of acute ischemic stroke. Definitions for use in a multicenter clinical trial. TOAST. Trial of org 10172 in acute stroke treatment. Stroke. 1993;24:35–41.
3. Holmstedt CA, Turan TN, Chimowitz MI. Atherosclerotic intracranial arterial stenosis: risk factors, diagnosis, and treatment. Lancet Neurol. 2013;12:1106–14.
4. Cao Y, Sun Y, Zhou B, Zhao H, Zhu Y, Xu J, et al. Atherosclerotic plaque burden of middle cerebral artery and extracranial carotid artery characterized by MRI in patients with acute ischemic stroke in China: association and clinical relevance. Neurol Res. 2017;39:344–50.
5. Bos D, Portegies ML, van der Lugt A, Bos MJ, Koudstaal PJ, Hofman A, et al. Intracranial carotid artery atherosclerosis and the risk of stroke in whites: the Rotterdam study. JAMA Neurol. 2014;71:405–11.
6. Wong LK. Global burden of intracranial atherosclerosis. Int J Stroke. 2006;1: 158–9.
7. Wu W, Guan Y, Xu K, Fu XJ, Lei XF, Lei LJ, et al. Plasma homocysteine levels predict the risk of acute cerebral infarction in patients with carotid artery lesions. Mol Neurobiol. 2016;53:2510–7.
8. Boysen G, Brander T, Christensen H, Gideon R, Truelsen T. Homocysteine and risk of recurrent stroke. Stroke. 2003;34:1258–61.
9. Wang H, Fan D, Zhang H, Fu Y, Zhang J, Shen Y. Serum level of homocysteine is correlated to carotid artery atherosclerosis in Chinese with ischemic stroke. Neurol Res. 2006;28:25–30.
10. Dietrich M, Jacques PF, Polak JF, Keyes MJ, Pencina MJ, Evans JC, et al. Segment-specific association between plasma homocysteine level and carotid artery intima-media thickness in the Framingham offspring study. J Stroke Cerebrovasc Dis. 2011;20:155–61.
11. Sasaki T, Watanabe M, Nagai Y, Hoshi T, Takasawa M, Nukata M, et al. Association of plasma homocysteine concentration with atherosclerotic carotid plaques and lacunar infarction. Stroke. 2002;33:1493–6.
12. Alsulaimani S, Gardener H, Elkind MS, Cheung K, Sacco RL, Rundek T. Elevated homocysteine and carotid plaque area and densitometry in the Northern Manhattan study. Stroke. 2013;44:457–61.
13. Yang X, Zhou Y, Liu C, Gao X, Wang A, Guo Y, et al. Homocysteine and carotid plaque stability: a cross-sectional study in Chinese adults. PLoS One. 2014;9:e94935.
14. Qiao Y, Zeiler SR, Mirbagheri S, Leigh R, Urrutia V, Wityk R, et al. Intracranial plaque enhancement in patients with cerebrovascular events on high-spatial-resolution MR images. Radiology. 2014;271:534–42.
15. Gupta A, Baradaran H, Al-Dasuqi K, Knight-Greenfield A, Giambrone AE, Delgado D, et al. Gadolinium enhancement in intracranial atherosclerotic plaque and ischemic stroke: a systematic review and meta-analysis. J Am Heart Assoc. 2016;5(8):e003816.
16. Xu WH, Li ML, Gao S, Ni J, Yao M, Zhou LX, et al. Middle cerebral artery intraplaque hemorrhage: prevalence and clinical relevance. Ann Neurol. 2012;71:195–8.
17. Xu WH, Li ML, Gao S, Ni J, Zhou LX, Yao M, et al. In vivo high-resolution MR imaging of symptomatic and asymptomatic middle cerebral artery atherosclerotic stenosis. Atherosclerosis. 2010;212:507–11.
18. Chung GH, Kwak HS, Hwang SB, Jin GY. High resolution MR imaging in patients with symptomatic middle cerebral artery stenosis. Eur J Radiol. 2012;81:4069–74.
19. Qiao Y, Etesami M, Astor BC, Zeiler SR, Trout HH 3rd, Wasserman BA. Carotid plaque neovascularization and hemorrhage detected by MR imaging are associated with recent cerebrovascular ischemic events. AJNR Am J Neuroradiol. 2012;33:755–60.
20. Skarpathiotakis M, Mandell DM, Swartz RH, Tomlinson G, Mikulis DJ. Intracranial atherosclerotic plaque enhancement in patients with ischemic stroke. AJNR Am J Neuroradiol. 2013;34:299–304.
21. Millon A, Boussel L, Brevet M, Mathevet JL, Canet-Soulas E, Mory C, et al. Clinical and histological significance of gadolinium enhancement in carotid atherosclerotic plaque. Stroke. 2012;43:3023–8.
22. Jung JM, Kwon DY, Han C, Jo I, Jo SA, Park MH. Increased carotid intima-media thickness and plasma homocysteine levels predict cardiovascular and all-cause death: a population-based cohort study. Eur Neurol. 2013;70:1–5.
23. Held C, Sumner G, Sheridan P, McQueen M, Smith S, Dagenais G, et al. Correlations between plasma homocysteine and folate concentrations and carotid atherosclerosis in high-risk individuals: baseline data from the homocysteine and atherosclerosis reduction trial (HART). Vasc Med. 2008;13:245–53.
24. Zhang D, Wen X, Wu W, Xu E, Zhang Y, Cui W. Homocysteine-related hTERT DNA demethylation contributes to shortened leukocyte telomere length in atherosclerosis. Atherosclerosis. 2013;231:173–9.
25. Ji Y, Song B, Xu Y, Fang H, Wu J, Sun S, et al. Prognostic significance of homocysteine levels in acute ischemic stroke: a prospective cohort study. Curr Neurovasc Res. 2015;12:334–40.
26. Sacco RL, Anand K, Lee HS, Boden-Albala B, Stabler S, Allen R, et al. Homocysteine and the risk of ischemic stroke in a triethnic cohort: the NOrthern MAnhattan study. Stroke. 2004;35:2263–9.
27. Bostom AG, Rosenberg IH, Silbershatz H, Jacques PF, Selhub J, D'Agostino RB, et al. Nonfasting plasma total homocysteine levels and stroke incidence in elderly persons: the Framingham study. Ann Intern Med. 1999;131:352–5.

19

Pragmatic trial of multifaceted intervention (STROKE-CARD care) to reduce cardiovascular risk and improve quality-of-life after ischaemic stroke and transient ischaemic attack

Thomas Toell[1], Christian Boehme[1], Lukas Mayer[1], Stefan Krebs[2], Clemens Lang[2], Karin Willeit[1,3], Barbara Prantl[1], Michael Knoflach[1], Gerhard Rumpold[4], Gudrun Schoenherr[1], Andrea Griesmacher[5], Peter Willeit[1], Julia Ferrari[2], Wilfried Lang[2,6], Stefan Kiechl[1*] and Johann Willeit[1*]

Abstract

Background: Patients with ischaemic stroke or transient ischaemic attack (TIA) are at high risk of future cardiovascular events. Despite compelling evidence about the efficacy of secondary prevention, a substantial gap exists between risk factor management in real life and that recommended by international guidelines. Moreover, stroke is a leading cause of disability and morbidity which partly emerges from post-stroke complications.

Methods/design: We designed a block-randomised (2:1 ratio) open pragmatic trial [NCT02156778] with blinded outcome assessment comparing STROKE-CARD to usual post-stroke-patient care. STROKE-CARD is a multifaceted post-stroke disease management program with the objective of reducing recurrent cardiovascular events and improving quality of life in ischaemic stroke and TIA-patients. It combines intensified multi-domain secondary prevention, systematic detection and treatment of post-stroke complications, and patient self-empowerment. Enrolment of 2160 patients with acute ischaemic stroke or TIA (ABCD2-Score ≥ 3) is planned at two study centres in Austria. The co-primary efficacy endpoints are (i) the composite of major recurrent cardiovascular events (nonfatal stroke, nonfatal myocardial infarction, and vascular death) occurring within 12 months after the index event and (ii) one-year health-related quality-of-life measured with the European Quality of Life-5 Dimensions (EQ-5D-3 L) questionaire. Secondary endpoints include all-cause mortality, functional outcome, and target-level achievement in risk factor management.

Discussion: This trial will provide evidence on whether the pragmatic post-stroke intervention program STROKE-CARD can help prevent cardiovascular events and improve quality-of-life within the setting of a high-quality acute stroke care system. In case of success, STROKE-CARD may be implemented in daily clinical routine and serve as a model for other disease management initiatives.

Keywords: Stroke, Transient ischemic attack, Secondary prevention, Disease management

* Correspondence: stefan.kiechl@i-med.ac.at; johann.willeit@i-med.ac.at
[1]Department of Neurology, Medical University of Innsbruck, Anichstraße 35, A-6020 Innsbruck, Austria
Full list of author information is available at the end of the article

Background

Stroke is the second leading cause of death and one of the leading contributors to disability worldwide [1, 2]. While the age-standardised incidence of stroke is decreasing in high-income countries due to improved health care services and primary prevention, the absolute number of stroke patients is still on the rise, mainly based on continuous population aging and growth [3]. Stroke survivors represent a population-segment particularly vulnerable to further cerebro- and cardiovascular events. Apart from persistent deficits, potentially avoidable medium- and long-term post-stroke complications are significant contributors to functional impairment and an appealing target for concerted interventions.

The risk of stroke recurrence is high at up to 10% within one year and more than 25% within 5 years [4]. Recurrent strokes account for about one fifth of all strokes in state-wide registries [5], have a worse clinical outcome, have a higher fatality rate, and cause higher healthcare costs than first-ever strokes [6].

More than 90% of the global stroke burden is attributable to modifiable risk factors, including behavioural and metabolic factors [7, 8] and most patients with acute ischaemic stroke have one or more un- or insufficiently controlled risk factors - a condition recently termed "preventable stroke" [9]. Vice versa, current evidence-based secondary prevention strategies combining behavioural and pharmacological interventions were estimated to reduce the risk for recurrent vascular events by more than 80% [10]. In real life, however, prevention goals and target levels of risk factors are rarely achieved [11, 12]. Furthermore, discontinuation of prescribed medications represents a major challenge in patient management, occurring in roughly one-third of ischaemic stroke patients within the first year of hospital discharge [13].

Multimodal and multi-disciplinary interventions within the framework of structured disease-management programs have been shown to improve quality of care and outcomes in patients with various chronic diseases other than stroke [14, 15]. Also, digital health care interventions are a promising novel tool to improve individualised risk factor management [16].

To address the substantial gap between risk factor management in real life and that recommended by international guidelines, we designed the STROKE-CARD program, which is a multifaceted pragmatic post-stroke disease management program combining intensified multi-domain secondary prevention, detection and treatment of post-stroke complications, and patient self-empowerment. In a pragmatic trial, we compare STROKE-CARD to usual care in its ability to reduce rates of recurrent cardiovascular events and improve quality-of-life in ischaemic stroke and TIA-patients.

Methods/design

Trial objectives

In this trial, we test the hypothesis that the pragmatic disease-management program STROKE-CARD designed for ischaemic stroke and TIA patients is capable of (a) preventing recurrent cardiovascular events by optimised guideline-compliant secondary prevention and target level achievement and (b) ameliorating health-related quality of life (QoL) and patient-wellbeing by early detection and consequent treatment of post-stroke complications.

Study design and centres

STROKE-CARD is a randomised, controlled, open interventional phase III trial with blinded outcome assessment [ClinicalTrials.gov NCT02156778] conducted in Austria. It initially started as a single-centre study in January 2014 and was extended to a second centre in December 2014. It compares two standards of post-stroke patient care, both complying with the current state-of-the-art. The trial does not involve experimental interventions but compares usual with intensified care as specified below. Primary outcome events are adjudicated based on pre-specified diagnostic criteria blinded to treatment allocation.

The two trial centres are located at the Departments of Neurology at the Innsbruck University Hospital (IUH) and the Hospital St. John of God in Vienna. IUH serves as the comprehensive stroke unit for the entire federal state of Tyrol (catchment area ≈ 1 Mio) and as a primary stroke unit for the city of Innsbruck and 65 surrounding suburban communities with approximately 0.3 Mio inhabitants. Patients from this exclusive catchment area represent an unselected cohort of ischaemic stroke and TIA patients [5]. The Hospital St. John of God Vienna houses one of the four comprehensive stroke units in Vienna. The Viennese stroke network includes additional six primary stroke units and serves the city of Vienna with a catchment area of more than 1.8 Mio inhabitants.

Study population

The study population comprises consecutive patients with acute ischaemic stroke or TIA (ABCD2-Score ≥ 3) [17] admitted to the two study centres. Patients are eligible for inclusion irrespective of whether the index event was a first or recurrent event. Ischaemic stroke is ascertained using the American Heart Association criteria based on clinical and imaging features [18].

All patients with ischaemic stroke or TIA admitted to the study centres are screened for potential inclusion in the STROKE-CARD trial during the first days of their hospital stay and in most instances included before discharge after signing an informed consent. Further details on the inclusion and exclusion criteria are provided in Table 1.

Table 1 STROKE-CARD inclusion and exclusion criteria

Inclusion criteria	Exclusion criteria
Patients with acute ischaemic stroke or TIA (ABCD2 Score ≥ 3 points) Age ≥ 18 years Signed informed consent	Patients living outside the catchment area Malignancy or other severe disease with life-expectancy less than the expected duration of the trial Drug addiction or severe alcohol abuse Patients with permanent severe disability and low perspectives for successful rehabilitation (mRS [19] = 5 at discharge)

TIA transient ischaemic attack, *mRS* modified Rankin Scale [19]

Randomisation and follow-up

We block-randomise patients in a 2:1 ratio to receive the STROKE-CARD program or standard care on the basis of the exact date and time of the qualifying event, with the durations of the blocks ranging from 4 to 8 weeks. The target sample size is 2160 patients overall, 1440 patients in the STROKE-CARD group, and 720 in the control group (Fig. 1). We strive for inclusion of about 500 patients per year. Patients are followed-up for 12 months, but we also obtain consent from the patients to contact them later on and extend follow-up for future research projects. Patients who do not adhere to the extended standard care program, especially do not attend the 3-month assessment, are followed in the same way as adherent patients for primary and secondary outcome events.

Intervention

Standard care

In the control arm, patients are managed according to the usual stroke care protocol [5] of the study centres which includes: (a) detailed patient counselling and education about stroke pathophysiology, risk factor management, life style improvement and medication compliance by a stroke specialist (involving the next of kin and caregivers if appropriate); (b) provision of the complimentary book "After a stroke" [20] dealing with all aspects of stroke care; (c) individual in-hospital advice by a dietitian for patients with diabetes, severe dyslipidaemia, and obesity, and smoking cessation support for heavy smokers; (d) provision of standardised information materials (e.g. for oral anticoagulation therapy); and (e) provision at discharge of detailed medical reports for the general practitioner as well as the patient containing target levels for risk factor management. Post-discharge risk-factor-management is performed by the patient's general practitioner. Only selected high-risk patients are seen in the centres' outpatient clinics. A standardised 3-month telephone interview by a study nurse for assessment of functional outcome (mRS, Barthel Index, nursing allowance, life situation, support services, medication) is part of the country-wide quality program but has no interventional character [5]. As part of the STROKE-CARD protocol, all patients undergo a comprehensive standardised clinical visit 12 months after recruitment.

Stroke-CARD

In addition to the procedures listed above, the intervention-arm includes two additional interventions:

(a) a three-month outpatient appointment with standardised re-assessment of all risk factors and re-evaluation of stroke aetiology, screening for post-stroke complications (e.g. spasticity, foot-drop, fatigue, pain, incontinence, communication problems, depression and anxiety, impaired cognition, seizures, fatigue, syncope, falls, fractures etc.), other health problems and residual deficits, estimation of the patient's demand for nursing services and the patient's adherence to drug prescriptions. All this information is used to optimise secondary prevention [21–23] with best possible achievement of target levels, to refine rehabilitation and treatment goals, and to manage post-stroke complications. Further details on the target levels are listed in Table 2. Patient assessment and counselling is done by a multidisciplinary team of physicians, nurses, physiotherapists, occupational and speech therapists. Treatment decisions are determined by experienced stroke neurologists. The overall visit takes about 3–4 h. The general practitioner receives a detailed medical report with precise instructions and treatment goals. Additional 6-month and 9-month visits are performed exceptionally (target < 5% of cases) at the discretion of the study team in case of medical need, complications requiring follow-up, or very poor risk factor control.

(b) Patients are offered access to an interactive password-protected web-based patient portal called "**My Strokecard**" [https://ches.tirol-kliniken.at/cms/]. If patients are unable to use a computer, caregivers are asked to assist with the usage of "My Strokecard". The patient-portal has been designed building on existing software for electronic patient-reported outcome monitoring [24] and contains three components: (i) An adapted version of the 'post-stroke checklist' for ascertainment of post-stroke complications is available for screening purposes at any time and pop up automatically three weeks before the three- and twelve-month

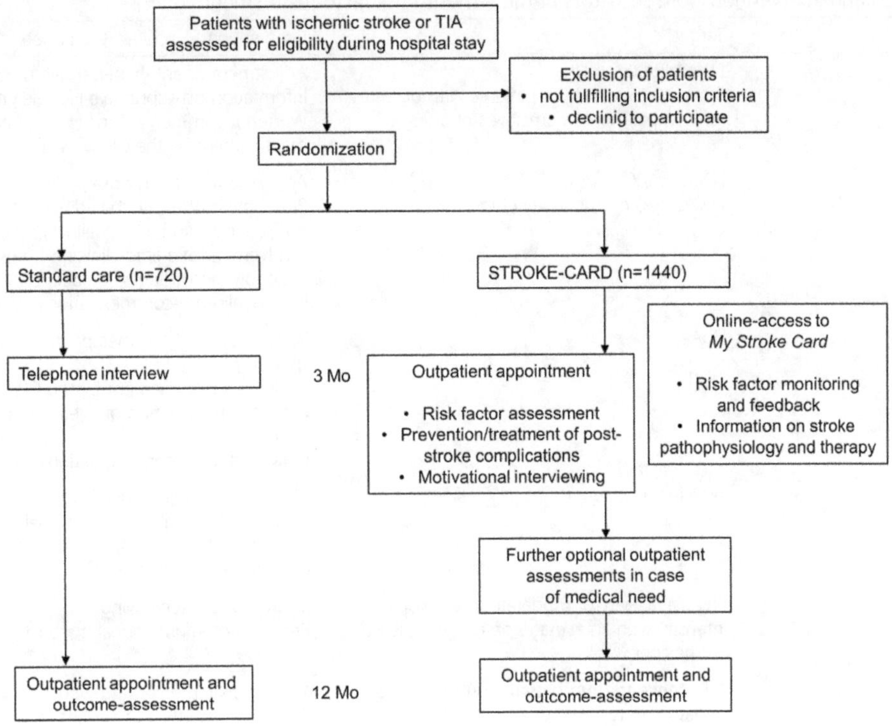

Fig. 1 Patient flow and allocation

outpatient appointment, so that the readout of the questionnaires is already available before the medical visit. (ii) A self-administered internet-based tool for risk factor monitoring and patient self-empowerment (i.e. blood pressure, body weight, nicotine consumption, physical activity, LDL-C and HbA1c in case of diabetes) automatically generates feedback on target level achievement [tabular protocols and simple graphs visualising the current stage and time trends for the patient and GP, ***see*** Additional file 1]. (iii) Extensive information and educational materials on stroke pathophysiology, symptoms and risk factor management are provided.

During the in-hospital phase, clinical care does not differ between the two groups, with the exception of the training for the use of "My Stroke Card" in the extended care group before discharge.

There will be (i) a continuous monitoring of different benchmarks, including the duration of hospital stay and access to rehabilitation facilities to ensure that the two groups do not receive differential attention and to minimise surveillance biases, and (ii) a monitoring of trial progress by a data monitoring board.

Outcome

Primary outcomes (Co-primary endpoint)

- Incidence of major cardiovascular events defined as nonfatal stroke (ischaemic or haemorrhagic), nonfatal myocardial infarction (including acute coronary syndrome requiring emergency vascularisation), and vascular death (i.e. sudden cardiac death and death from acute myocardial infarction, ischaemic or haemorrhagic stroke, heart failure, cardiovascular procedures, pulmonary embolism, or peripheral artery disease) within one year of the index event.
- Health-related QoL assessed by the European Quality of Life-5 Dimensions (EQ-5D-3 L) overall health utility score one year after the index event.

Secondary outcomes

- Recurrent ischaemic or haemorrhagic stroke and TIA (defined as transient neurological deficit < 24 h and absence of DWI positive lesions on MRI) within one year of the index-event.
- All-cause mortality at 12 months.
- Favorable functional outcome (mRS ≤2 and change in mRS) at one year and at three months.

Table 2 Target levels and interventions for risk factors at the 3-month risk factor assessment

Condition	Target	Intervention to achieve the targets
Hypertension	BP < 140/90 mmHg BP < 130/85 mmHg in patients with diabetes, renal impairment or small-vessel disease	Adjustment of anti-hypertensive medication Information on supportive lifestyle changes Written recommendations to and intensified management by the GP
Dyslipidaemia	LDL-C < 100 mg/dL LDL-C < 70 mg/dL in very high-risk patients	Adjustment of statin dosage Prescription of ezetimibe additionally to high-dose statins (according to guidelines) Involvement of a lipid-clinic and prescription of PCSK9 inhibitors (according to guidelines) Individualised recommendations by a dietitian
Diabetes	HbA_{1c} < 7%	Re-evaluation of the therapeutic regime by a diabetes-specialist Additional management by the GP, re-instruction in correct administration of injectable pharmacological agents Individualised recommendations by a dietitian
Smoking	Nicotine abstinence	Motivational interviewing and counselling Provision of informational material Involvement of a psychiatric specialist for behavioural or pharmacological therapy
Physical inactivity	Physical activity of moderate to vigorous intensity with an average of 40 min at least 3 times per week	Motivational interviewing Provision of informational material
Non-adherence to drug prescriptions	Adherence to drug prescription (proportion of days covered ≥90%)	Motivational interviewing with information on indication & therapeutic effect of current medication Simplification of drug-regimes Home support by nurses and/or relatives
Poor "stroke-knowledge" of patients & family-members or caregivers		Information on stroke pathophysiology & individual stroke mechanism Provision of a book and standardised information material
Post-stroke complications[a] & poor functional outcome	Improvement of QoL	Individualised treatment & prevention of post-stroke complications Provision of further outpatient or inpatient rehabilitation Re-assessment on nursing demands, social integration & outpatient care Involvement of a social worker

BP blood pressure, *GP* general practitioner, *LDL-C* low-density lipoprotein cholesterol, *PCSK9* proprotein convertase subtilisin/kexin type 9, HbA_{1c} glycated haemoglobin, *QoL* quality of life
[a]spasticity, pain, risk of falling, post stroke-depression (PSD), fatigue, anxiety, dysphagia, social deprivation, post-stroke dementia

- Individual components of the EQ-5D-3 L questionnaire, i.e. mobility, self-care, usual activities, pain and discomfort, anxiety and depression after one year.
- Achievement of predefined target levels in secondary prevention 12 months after the index event: BP < 140/90 mmHg [< 130/85 mmHg in selected patients], target HbA_{1c} in patients with diabetes [mainly < 7.0%, less stringent targets in elderly], nicotine abstinence, LDL-C < 100 mg/dL [LDL-C < 70 mg/dL in high-risk patients] [23], physical activity with an average of 40 min at least 3 times per week, platelet inhibitor or anticoagulation according to ischaemic stroke aetiology [in case of oral anticoagulation with vitamin K antagonists: INR 2–3, time in therapeutic range (TTR) > 70%], statins except for patients with ischaemic strokes of non-atherosclerotic origin and no evidence of atherosclerosis (e.g. vessel dissection), medication adherence [proportion of days covered (PDC) ≥ 90%] [25]. The latter criterion focuses on statins, platelet inhibitors other than aspirin (which is typically purchased over the counter), antihypertensive medication, oral anti-diabetic drugs, and anticoagulation.

Clinical assessments and study protocols

The protocol uses validated and field-proven forms, scales and questionnaires. All the study team members are highly experienced and NIHSS- and mRS-certified.

The clinical baseline-assessment (entire study population) and the outpatient appointment (3-month intervention [intervention arm only] and 12-month outcome assessment [entire study population]) will be performed by trained health care professionals of the multidisciplinary study team composed of experienced stroke neurologists, PhD-students, physiotherapists, and stroke nurses. Data are collected prospectively according to pre-specified

Table 3 Trials on multimodal secondary prevention strategies in ischaemic stroke or TIA-patients

Study, Country	Y	Inclusion criteria	n	Age	M (%)	Intervention type/model	FU (Mo)	Outcome measures	Significant results
PRAISE, USA [42]	2014	Ischaemic stroke, TIA < 5 years, age > 40 y	600	63 ± 11	40	Education & self-management (peer-led), 6 weekly workshops	6	Cholesterol, BP, antithrombotics use	BP-lowering
ICARUSS, Australia [43]	2009	Ischaemic stroke, haemorrhagic stroke, TIA, age > 20 y	233	66 ± 13	54	Education & pre-arranged visits at the GP's at 2 weeks, 3, 6, 9, 12 Mo. Telephone assessment prior to each visit	12	RF-modification, disability, QoL, cognitive function, ADLs	Cholesterol-, BP-lowering, exercise, disability, QoL
Hornnes et al., Denmark [44]	2011	Ischaemic stroke or TIA, all age-groups	349	69 ± 12	45	Pre-discharge or outpatient appointment, nurse-led home visits at 1, 4, 7, 10 Mo	12	BP after one year	BP-lowering
INSPiRE-TMS, Germany [51]	2013	TIA, minor stroke, age > 18 y	Target = 2082	N/A	N/A	RF-management & support program, up to 8 assessments	24	Stroke, ACS, cardiovascular death, RF-control, mortality, hospital admissions	ongoing
SMART study, China [45]	2014	Ischaemic stroke, TIA related to atherosclerosis	3821	61 ± 12	68	Medication & lifestyle advice, education (computer software)	12	Adherence to drugs, stroke, ACS, all-cause death	better adherence to statins
STANDFIRM, Australia [46]	2017	Ischaemic stroke, haemorrhagic stroke, TIA, age > 18 y	563	70	N/A	Community-based intervention, evidence-based care plan, 3 education sessions, 2 telephone assessments	24	Targets for cardiometabolic factors	cholesterol levels
COMPASS, USA [52]	2017	Ischaemic stroke, haemorrhagic stroke, TIA, age > 18 y	Target = 6000	N/A	N/A	holistic approach integrating medical & community resources, clinical visit after 14 days, 4 telephone assessments	3	Functional status, Qol, cognitive function, hospitalisations, caregiver measures	ongoing
SUCCEED, USA [53]	2017	Ischaemic stroke, TIA, haemorrhagic stroke, hypertension, age > 40 y	Target = 516	N/A	N/A	3 clinic visits, 3 home visits, & telephone coordination by community health worker, self-coordination program	36	BP, RF-control, medication adherence, cost-effectivness	ongoing
NAILED, Sweden [47]	2015	Ischaemic stroke, haemorrhagic stroke, TIA, all age-groups	537	71 ± 11	57	Nurse-led, telephone-based follow-up, medication adjustment	12	BP, LDL-C, RF-control	cholesterol-, BP-lowering
Kono et al., Japan [48]	2013	Ischaemic stroke (mRS 0–1), non-cardio-embolic origin	70	64	68	Lifestyle intervention program with counselling at BL, 3, 6 Mo, exercise training (2x/week) for 24 weeks	36	Stroke or cardiac death, hospitalisation due to stroke recurrence, MI, AP or pAD, RF-control	vascular events, physical activity BP-lowering, salt intake.
McAlister et al., Canada [49]	2014	Ischemic stroke, TIA, slight or no disability	275	68	63	Pharmacist-led or a nurse-led case manager intervention with 6 monthly visits	12	BP and lipid control, FRS and CDLEM	cholesterol-, BP-lowering, global vascular risk
STROKE-CARD, Austria	2017	Ischaemic stroke (mRS 0–4), TIA (ABCD2-Score ≥ 3); age > 18 y	Target = 2170	N/A	N/A	3 Mo clinical visit with RF-assessment, online RF-monitoring	12	Major cardiovascular event, vascular death, QoL	ongoing

ACS acute coronary syndrome, *ADLs* activities of daily living, *AP* angina pectoris, *BL* baseline, *BP* blood pressure, *CDLEM* Cardiovascular Disease Life Expectancy Model, *FRS* Framingham Risk Score, *FU* follow up, *GP* general practitioner, *M* percentage of male participants, *Mo* month, *MI* myocardial infarction, *N/A* not available, *pAD* peripheral artery disease, *QoL* quality-of-life, *RF* risk factor, *SBP* systolic blood pressure, *TIA* transient ischaemic attack protocols and questionnaires with electronic data entry and storage and undergo subsequent quality checks and validation (e.g. by hospital records and feedback from the GP). All hospitals in the survey area dispose of electronic records, to which study investigators were granted access via protected data links according to the patients' informed consent.

The **baseline assessment** includes detailed documentation of the following components: ischaemic stroke aetiology [TOAST-criteria [26], Causative Classification of Stroke [27]], stroke severity [NIHSS [28] on admission and discharge], clinical syndrome [stroke/TIA symptoms, vessel territories], acute stroke therapy and recanalization procedures, pre-stroke disability and disability on admission [mRS], prior cardiovascular events and comorbidities, cardiovascular risk factors (hypertension, dyslipidaemia, smoking-status [current, former, never] and burden [pack-years, Fagerstroem questionnaire [29]], alcohol consumption [quantity, patterns, type of beverages], diabetes [ADA criteria] [30], atrial fibrillation, physical activity [Baecke Physical Activity Questionnaire] [31]), family history of cardiovascular disease, previous and current medication, cognitive function [Mini-Mental State Examination [32] and Montreal Cognitive Assessment [33]], depression [Beck Depression Inventar, anxiety [Hospital Anxiety and Depression Scale [34]], fatigue [Fatigue Severity Scale [35]], health related quality of life [European Quality of Life-5 Dimensions EQ5D-3 L [36]], anthropometric measures [body mass index, waist–to hip ratio], repeated blood pressure recordings [acute setting and before discharge], ankle-brachial index, atherosclerosis of the carotid arteries [intima-media thickness, plaque burden], [37] pulse wave velocity [Complior® system], and routine laboratory measures [including lipid profile, renal function, liver function, thyroid function, cardiac markers, differential blood count, coagulation diagnostics, and inflammation markers].

The **3- and 12-month visits** involve a neurological evaluation with documentation of clinical deficits and functional outcome [NIHSS, mRS, and Barthel Index [38]], routine laboratory examination and assessment of recurrent cardiovascular events, hospital stays and procedures [interventional and surgical], falls and fractures, all incident diseases and morbidities [including bleeding events], current medication, adherence to prescribed drugs, and risk factor control. Cognitive function, depression, anxiety, fatigue, and QoL all are re-evaluated [see baseline assessment]. Carotid ultrasound [see baseline protocol] is obligatorily repeated during the 12-month visit and, if clinically indicated, also after three months.

Blood and urine samples are drawn after an overnight fast and at least 12-h abstinence from smoking [during the hospital stay and 3 and 12 months thereafter], immediately processed, used for routine testing, and stored in a biobank [plasma, serum, whole blood, and urine]. Samples are stored at – 80 °C in compliance with the OECD guidelines and Austrian Bioethics Commission recommendations [39].

Sample size

Sample size calculations for this trial were based on the primary composite cardiovascular disease endpoint. Assuming a 1-year cumulative risk of 15% in the usual care group, 2045 subjects are required to detect a 5% absolute risk reduction ($\alpha = 0.05$) with a 90% power.

Expecting an attrition rate of 15% (7.5% dropout rate [withdrawal of consent] and a loss-to-follow-up of 7.5%), we aimed to include a total of 2400 patients. Between January 2014 and June 2017, 1866 patients were recruited, with an attrition rate substantially lower than expected (< 5.0% as opposed to the anticipated 15%). Accordingly, the data monitoring board recommended revision of the recruitment goal from 2400 to 2160 patients. A sample size of 2160 patients provides the trial with a 90% power to detect a difference of 0.03 points on the EQ-5D-3 L overall health utility score (co-primary efficacy endpoint) assuming a standard deviation of 0.2.

Statistical analyses

The primary efficacy analysis is based on time from hospital discharge to first occurrence of primary composite end-point as defined above. It is an unadjusted survival analysis according to the intention-to-treat principle with use of the log-rank test. Hazard ratios and 95% confidence intervals will be estimated using Cox models with the assumption of proportional hazards checked by means of Schoenfeld residuals. Prespecified sensitivity analyses include adjusted models and a per-protocol analysis. Consistency of intervention effects in four prespecified subgroups (men and women, age groups, type of index event, and patients with or without regular use of My StrokeCard) will be assessed by means of test for interaction. The continuous efficacy endpoint QoL will be analysed with linear regression models.

Owing to the fact that our study attempts to encourage patients to adhere to current evidence-based prevention guidelines and does not include experimental treatment concepts, we do not perform a formal safety analysis. We however analyze whether there are any differences in the occurrence of potential side effects, risks and consequences of intensified secondary prevention in both study arms including (a) major bleeding [40], (b), syncopes and fractures, (c) laboratory abnormalities (ALT, CK, GFR), and (d) muscle-related outcomes. No formal interim analysis will be performed. All reported P values are two-sided.

Discussion

The risk of stroke recurrence within one year after ischaemic stroke or TIA is high and can effectively be reduced by effective guideline-compliant secondary prevention. Vice versa, poor adherence to guidelines leads to preventable recurrent events, worse outcome and higher health care costs. Post-stroke complications are frequent, often remain unrecognised and contribute to stroke disability and poor QoL.

The STROKE-CARD concept

STROKE-CARD is the first comprehensive pragmatic post-stroke disease management in Austria and, to our knowledge, one of the largest interventions of its kind worldwide. STROKE-CARD is addressing a real-life-cohort of ischaemic stroke- and TIA-patients with the primary objectives of enhancing adherence to prevention guidelines and thereby lowering rates of recurrent vascular events and post-stroke complications, and improving functional outcome and QoL. Whereas disease management programs traditionally rely on expert opinion, our initiative strives for a rigorous scientific evaluation involving outcome and health economy analyses. It pursues the concept that optimal acute stroke care extends to a thorough three-month assessment and individualised counselling. We employ a multidisciplinary but lean and cheap intervention leveraging contemporary e-technology and encouraging patient self-empowerment with the prospect of a widespread implementation in case of success. Access to Internet and social media is now broadly available and STROKE-CARD offers web-based educational patient-operated tools for risk factor to record and manage risk factors combined with linkage of patient data to medical caregivers. The STROKE-CARD concept was presented as an abstract at the European Stroke Organisation Conference 2018 [41].

Other post-stroke disease management programs

Previous trials on multimodal secondary prevention strategies in ischaemic stroke or TIA-patients have shown variable improvements in risk factor control or medication adherence but most were not designed and powered to analyse potential effects recurrent cardiovascular disease and stroke events. An overview on trials focusing on multimodal secondary stroke prevention is provided in Table 3. Limitations shared by these trials include the usually limited sample size (443 median, IQR 347.3) [42–50] and the common focus on TIA or minor stroke patients only [48, 49, 51].

Only one large-scale study has been completed so far [45] and enrolled more than 3800 ischaemic stroke and TIA-patients in 47 hospitals in China. In spite of a better adherence to statin-medications no difference in the hard clinical end points after one year of follow-up could be demonstrated.

Two ongoing studies deserve special consideration: (i) The Comprehensive Post-Acute Stroke Service (COMPASS) study, [52] a cluster-randomised trial involving 40 hospitals in North Carolina, plans enrolment of 6000 ischaemic and haemorrhagic stroke patients and investigates potential effects of the COMPASS care model (telephone follow-up, one clinic visit within two weeks after discharge, and an individualised patient electronic care plan) on the patient-reported 90-day functional outcome (primary endpoint), hospital re-admission rates, and 90-day mortality. (ii) The Intensified Secondary Prevention intending a Reduction of Recurrent Events in TIA and Minor Stroke patients (INSPiRE-TMS) study, [51] from Germany intends to recruit 2082 patients with minor stroke or TIA, provides up to eight appointments in outpatient clinics and focuses on two-year recurrent vascular events or vascular death.

Type and intensity of intervention vary widely among the different trials. Several programs envisage nurse-led home visits or telephone-based assessments for risk factor control [44, 47, 50]. The ICARUSS-strategy [43] in Australia trusts on several pre-arranged GP visits whereas the STANDFIRM-trial ($n = 500$), [46] a community-based intervention, consists of educational sessions, multiple follow-up assessments, and as telephone interviews conducted by study nurses and general practices. A recent intervention [49] has achieved a substantial and sustained (six months) reduction in global vascular risk (Framingham Risk Score, Cardiovascular Disease Life Expectancy Model) by non-physician provider case management. Digital health interventions (e.g. telemedicine, web-based strategies, email and- mobile phone-reminders) improved risk factor control in vascular diseases other than stroke [16].

Strengths and limitations

Key and in part unique features of STROKE-CARD are its comprehensive focus on both recurrent vascular events (risk factor control and compliance) and post-stroke complications and QoL, its lean and easily applicable intervention, and the inclusion of moderate and severe ischaemic stroke patients (all except those with permanent severe disability).

The primary analysis may be viewed as conservative in two respects: [1] It relies on a short one-year follow-up whereas potential effects are expected to increase over time. Extension of follow-up is a decided goal and fund raising is in progress [2]. Our program is realised within the framework of a highly developed stroke care setting and bears the challenge of a strong comparator group with high-quality management of ischaemic stroke/TIA patients. Although findings of our trial are not easily extrapolated to less developed stroke systems, the potential benefit of the intervention is presumably even higher on the low-quality stroke care background.

Our program is focused on ischaemic stroke but may serve as a model for other diseases sensitive to post-discharge management.

In case of success, the next steps would be a refinement of STROKE-CARD components and identification of subgroups with a health benefit and cost effectiveness in order to end up with a practicable tool for broad clinical implementation in the whole of Tyrol, Austria and beyond.

Abbreviations

ACS: Acute coronary syndrome; ADLs: Activities of daily living; ALT: Alanine aminotransferase; AP: Angina pectoris; BL: Baseline; BP: Blood pressure; CDLEM: Cardiovascular Disease Life Expectancy Model; CK: Creatine kinase; DWI: Diffusion weighted imaging; EQ-5D-3L: European Quality of Life-5 Dimensions; FRS: Framingham Risk Score; FU: Follow up; GFR: Glomerular filtration rate; GP: General practitioner; HbA1c: Glycated haemoglobin; IUH: Innsbruck University Hospital; LDL-C: low-density lipoprotein cholesterol; MI: Myocardial infarction; Mo: Month; MRI: Magnet resonance imaging; mRS: Modified Rankin Scale; N/A: Not available; NIHSS: National institute of health stroke scale; pAD: Peripheral artery disease; PCSK9: proprotein convertase subtilisin/kexin type 9; PDS: Post stroke-depression; QoL: Quality of life; RF: Risk factor; SBP: Systolic blood pressure; TIA: Transient ischaemic attack; TOAST: Trial of Org 10,172 in Acute Stroke Treatment

Acknowledgements

Not applicable.

Funding

The Medical University of Innsbruck served as the sponsor of this study and received financial support from the university hospital (Tirol Kliniken), Tyrolean Health Insurance Company (TGKK), the Tyrol Health Care Funds (TGF), and unrestricted research grants from Boehringer Ingelheim, Otto Bock and Sanofi Aventis. The study centre in Vienna additionally received a grant from Bayer Healthcare. The sponsor and partners had no influence on the study design and clinical decisions, and no role in data analysis, interpretation, and publication.

Authors' contributions

TT, JW, SK, WL, and MK designed the study protocol and gained ethical approval. TT, CB, LM, SK, CL, KW, BP, GR, GS, AG, JF are involved in patient recruitment or data acquisition. PW coordinates data management and analysis. TT and CB performed the systematic review. TT wrote the first version of the manuscript. All authors reviewed and edited the manuscript and approved the final version of the manuscript.

Competing interests

The author(s) declared no potential conflicts of interest with respect to the research, authorship, and/or publication of this article.

Author details

[1]Department of Neurology, Medical University of Innsbruck, Anichstraße 35, A-6020 Innsbruck, Austria. [2]Department of Neurology, Hospital St. John of God, Johannes von Gott Platz 1, A-1020 Vienna, Austria. [3]Department of Neurology, Inselspital Bern, University Hospital, Freiburgstrasse, CH-3010 Bern, Switzerland. [4]Department of Medical Psychology, Medical University of Innsbruck, Schöpfstraße 23a, A-6020 Innsbruck, Austria. [5]Central Institute of Medical and Chemical Laboratory Diagnostics, University Hospital of Innsbruck, Anichstraße 35, A-6020 Innsbruck, Austria. [6]Sigmund Freud Private University, Medical Faculty, Campus Prater Freudplatz 1, A-1020 Vienna, Austria.

References

1. Hay SI. Global, regional, and national incidence, prevalence, and years lived with disability for 328 diseases and injuries for 195 countries, 1990–2016: a systematic analysis for the global burden of disease study 2016. Lancet. 2017;390:1211–59.
2. Steel N. Global, regional, and national age-sex specific mortality for 264 causes of death, 1980–2016: a systematic analysis for the global burden of disease study 2016. Lancet. 2017;390(10100):1151–210.
3. Feigin VL, Forouzanfar MH, Krishnamurthi R, Mensah GA, Connor M, Bennett DA, et al. Global and regional burden of stroke during 1990–2010: findings from the global burden of disease study 2010. Lancet. 2014;383(9913): 245–55.
4. Mohan KM, Wolfe CDA, Rudd AG, Heuschmann PU, Kolominsky-Rabas PL, Grieve AP. Risk and cumulative risk of stroke recurrence: a systematic review and meta-analysis. Stroke. 2011;42(5):1489–94.
5. Willeit J, Geley T, Schöch J, Rinner H, Tür A, Kreuzer H, et al. Thrombolysis and clinical outcome in patients with stroke after implementation of the Tyrol stroke pathway: a retrospective observational study. Lancet Neurol. 2015;14(1):48–56.
6. Samsa GP, Bian J, Lipscomb J, Matchar DB. Epidemiology of recurrent cerebral infarction a Medicare claims–based comparison of first and recurrent strokes on 2-year survival and cost. Stroke. 1999;30(2):338–49.
7. Feigin VL, Roth GA, Naghavi M, Parmar P, Krishnamurthi R, Chugh S, et al.. Global burden of stroke and risk factors in 188 countries, during 1990–2013: a systematic analysis for the Global Burden of Disease Study 2013. Lancet Neurol [Internet]. 2016 [cited 2016 Nov 16]; Available from: https://doi.org/10.1016/S1474-4422(16)30073-4.
8. O'Donnell MJ, Chin SL, Rangarajan S, Xavier D, Liu L, Zhang H, et al. Global and regional effects of potentially modifiable risk factors associated with acute stroke in 32 countries (INTERSTROKE): a case-control study. Lancet. 2016;388(10046):761–75.
9. Fisher M, Moores L, Alsharif MN, Paganini-Hill A. Definition and implications of the preventable stroke. JAMA Neurol. 2016;73(2):186.
10. Hackam DG, Spence JD. Combining multiple approaches for the secondary prevention of vascular events after stroke: a quantitative modeling study. Stroke. 2007;38(6):1881–5.
11. Heuschmann PU, Kircher J, Nowe T, Dittrich R, Reiner Z, Cifkova R, et al. Control of main risk factors after ischaemic stroke across Europe: data from the stroke-specific module of the EUROASPIRE III survey. Eur J Prev Cardiol. 2015;22(10):1354–62.
12. on behalf of the ASPIRE-S Study Group, Brewer L, Mellon L, Hall P, Dolan E, Horgan F, et al.. Secondary prevention after ischaemic stroke: the ASPIRE-S study. BMC Neurol [Internet]. 2015 Dec [cited 2016 Nov 16];15(1). from: https://doi.org/10.1186/s12883-015-0466-2
13. Bushnell CD, Olson DM, Zhao X, Pan W, Zimmer LO, Goldstein LB, et al. Secondary preventive medication persistence and adherence 1 year after stroke. Neurology. 2011;77(12):1182–90.
14. Gonseth J, Guallar-Castillón P, Banegas JR, Rodríguez-Artalejo F. The effectiveness of disease management programmes in reducing hospital re-admission in older patients with heart failure: a systematic review and meta-analysis of published reports. Eur Heart J. 2004;25(18):1570–95.
15. Riedl R, Robausch M, Berghold A. The Evaluation of the Effectiveness of Austrians Disease Management Program in Patients with Type 2 Diabetes Mellitus - A Population-Based Retrospective Cohort Study. Reboldi G. PLOS ONE. 2016;11(8):e0161429.
16. Widmer RJ, Collins NM, Collins CS, West CP, Lerman LO, Lerman A. Digital health interventions for the prevention of cardiovascular disease: a systematic review and meta-analysis. Mayo Clin Proc. 2015;90(4):469–80.
17. DeLange T, Frech G, Kelen G. Validation and refinement of scores to predict very early stroke risk after transient ischaemic attack. Lancet. 2007;369:283–92.
18. Sacco RL, Kasner SE, Broderick JP, Caplan LR, Connors JJ, Culebras A, et al. An updated definition of stroke for the 21st century: a statement for healthcare professionals from the American Heart Association/American Stroke Association. Stroke. 2013;44(7):2064–89.
19. Van Swieten JC, Koudstaal PJ, Visser MC, Schouten HJ, Van Gijn J. Interobserver agreement for the assessment of handicap in stroke patients. Stroke. 1988; 19(5):604–7.
20. Kiechl S, Lalouschek W, Lang W. NACH EINEM SCHLAGANFALL. 2nd ed. Holzhausen Verlag; 2014. 152 p.

21. Kernan WN, Ovbiagele B, Black HR, Bravata DM, Chimowitz MI, Ezekowitz MD, et al. Guidelines for the prevention of stroke in patients with stroke and transient ischemic attack. Stroke. 2014;45(7):2160–236.
22. Van Horn L, Carson JAS, Appel LJ, Burke LE, Economos C, Karmally W, et al.. Recommended Dietary Pattern to Achieve Adherence to the American Heart Association/American College of Cardiology (AHA/ACC) Guidelines: A Scientific Statement From the American Heart Association. Circulation. 2016; CIR.0000000000000462.
23. Catapano AL, Graham I, De Backer G, Wiklund O, Chapman MJ, Drexel H, et al. 2016 ESC/EAS guidelines for the Management of Dyslipidaemias. Eur Heart J. 2016;37(39):2999–3058.
24. Holzner B, Giesinger JM, Pinggera J, Zugal S, Schöpf F, Oberguggenberger AS, et al. The computer-based health evaluation software (CHES): a software for electronic patient-reported outcome monitoring. BMC Med Inform Decis Mak. 2012;12(1):126.
25. Choudhry NK, Shrank WH, Levin RL, Lee JL, Jan SA, Brookhart MA, et al. Measuring concurrent adherence to multiple related medications. Am J Manag Care. 2009;15(7):457–64.
26. Adams HP, Bendixen BH, Kappelle LJ, Biller J, Love BB, Gordon DL, et al. Classification of subtype of acute ischemic stroke. Definitions for use in a multicenter clinical trial. TOAST. Trial of org 10172 in acute stroke treatment. Stroke. 1993;24(1):35–41.
27. Ay H, Benner T, Murat Arsava E, Furie KL, Singhal AB, Jensen MB, et al. A computerized algorithm for etiologic classification of ischemic stroke: the causative classification of stroke system. Stroke. 2007;38(11):2979–84.
28. Lyden P, Brott T, Tilley B, Welch KM, Mascha EJ, Levine S, et al. Improved reliability of the NIH stroke scale using video training. NINDS TPA Stroke Study Group Stroke. 1994;25(11):2220–6.
29. Heatherton TF, Kozlowski LT, Frecker RC, K-O F. The Fagerström test for nicotine dependence: a revision of the Fagerstrom tolerance questionnaire. Br J Addict. 1991;86(9):1119–27.
30. American Diabetes Association. Diagnosis and Classification of Diabetes Mellitus. Diabetes Care. 2010;33(Supplement_1):S62–9.
31. Baecke JA, Burema J, Frijters JE. A short questionnaire for the measurement of habitual physical activity in epidemiological studies. Am J Clin Nutr. 1982; 36(5):936–42.
32. Folstein MF, Folstein SE, McHugh PR. "Mini-mental state": a practical method for grading the cognitive state of patients for the clinician. J Psychiatr Res. 1975;12(3):189–98.
33. Nasreddine ZS, Phillips NA, Bédirian V, Charbonneau S, Whitehead V, Collin I, et al. The Montreal cognitive assessment, MoCA: a brief screening tool for mild cognitive impairment. J Am Geriatr Soc. 2005;53(4):695–9.
34. Zigmond AS, Snaith RP. The hospital anxiety and depression scale. Acta Psychiatr Scand. 1983;67(6):361–70.
35. Krupp LB, LaRocca NG, Muir-Nash J, Steinberg AD. The fatigue severity scale: application to patients with multiple sclerosis and systemic lupus erythematosus. Arch Neurol. 1989;46(10):1121–3.
36. Brooks R, Group E. EuroQol: the current state of play. Health Policy. 1996; 37(1):53–72.
37. Willeit K, Pechlaner R, Egger G, Weger S, Oberhollenzer M, Willeit J, et al. Carotid atherosclerosis and incident atrial fibrillation. Arterioscler Thromb Vasc Biol. 2013;33(11):2660.
38. Collin C, Wade DT, Davies S, Horne V. The Barthel ADL index: a reliability study. Int Disabil Stud. 1988;10(2):61–3.
39. OECD Organization for Economic Cooperation and Development. Eur J Health Law. 2010;17(2):191–204.
40. Schulman S, Kearon C, The subcommittee on control of anticoagulation of the scientific and standardization committee of the international society on thrombosis and haemostasis. Definition of major bleeding in clinical investigations of antihemostatic medicinal products in non-surgical patients. J Thromb Haemost. 2005;3(4):692–4.
41. European Stroke Organisation Conference. Late Breaking Abstracts. Eur Stroke J. 2018;3(1_suppl):587–620.
42. Kronish IM, Goldfinger JZ, Negron R, Fei K, Tuhrim S, Arniella G, et al. The effect of peer education on stroke prevention: the prevent recurrence of all Inner-City strokes through education (PRAISE) randomized controlled trial. Stroke J Cereb Circ. 2014;45(11):3330–6.
43. Joubert J, Reid C, Barton D, Cumming T, McLean A, Joubert L, et al. Integrated care improves risk-factor modification after stroke: initial results of the integrated Care for the Reduction of secondary stroke model. J Neurol Neurosurg Amp Psychiatry. 2009;80(3):279.
44. Hornnes N, Larsen K, Boysen G. Blood pressure 1 year after stroke: the need to optimize secondary prevention. J Stroke Cerebrovasc Dis. 2011;20(1):16–23.
45. Peng B, Ni J, Anderson CS, Zhu Y, Wang Y, Pu C, et al. Implementation of a structured guideline–based program for the secondary prevention of ischemic stroke in China. Stroke. 2014;45(2):515–9.
46. Olaiya MT, Cadilhac DA, Kim J, Nelson MR, Srikanth VK, Gerraty RP, et al. Community-based intervention to improve Cardiometabolic targets in patients with stroke. Stroke. 2017;48(9):2504.
47. Irewall A-L, Ögren J, Bergström L, Laurell K, Söderström L, Mooe T. Nurse-Led, Telephone-Based, Secondary Preventive Follow-Up after Stroke or Transient Ischemic Attack Improves Blood Pressure and LDL Cholesterol: Results from the First 12 Months of the Randomized, Controlled NAILED Stroke Risk Factor Trial. Pizzi C, editor. PLOS ONE. 2015;10(10):e0139997.
48. Kono Y, Yamada S, Yamaguchi J, Hagiwara Y, Iritani N, Ishida S, et al. Secondary prevention of new vascular events with lifestyle intervention in patients with Noncardioembolic mild ischemic stroke: a single-center randomized controlled trial. Cerebrovasc Dis. 2013;36(2):88–97.
49. McAlister FA, Grover S, Padwal RS, Youngson E, Fradette M, Thompson A, et al. Case management reduces global vascular risk after stroke: secondary results from the the preventing recurrent vascular events and neurological worsening through intensive organized case-management randomized controlled trial. Am Heart J. 2014;168(6):924–30.
50. Rochette A, Korner-Bitensky N, Bishop D, Teasell R, White CL, Bravo G, et al. The YOU CALL-WE CALL randomized clinical trial: impact of a multimodal support intervention after a mild stroke. Circ Cardiovasc Qual Outcomes. 2013;6(6):674–9.
51. Leistner S, Michelson G, Laumeier I, Ahmadi M, Smyth M, Nieweler G, et al. Intensified secondary prevention intending a reduction of recurrent events in TIA and minor stroke patients (INSPiRE-TMS): a protocol for a randomised controlled trial. BMC Neurol. 2013;13(1):11.
52. Duncan PW, Bushnell CD, Rosamond WD, Jones Berkeley SB, Gesell SB, D'Agostino RB, et al. The comprehensive post-acute stroke services (COMPASS) study: design and methods for a cluster-randomized pragmatic trial. BMC Neurol. 2017;17:133.
53. Towfighi A, Cheng EM, Ayala-Rivera M, McCreath H, Sanossian N, Dutta T, et al. Randomized controlled trial of a coordinated care intervention to improve risk factor control after stroke or transient ischemic attack in the safety net: secondary stroke prevention by uniting community and chronic care model teams early to end disparities (SUCCEED). BMC Neurol. 2017;17:24.

20

Increased serum exosomal miR-134 expression in the acute ischemic stroke patients

Jingxia Zhou[†], Lin Chen[†], Bocan Chen, Shaozhu Huang, Chaosheng Zeng, Hairong Wu, Cong Chen and Faqing Long[*]

Abstract

Background: The exosomal miRNAs have been emerged as biomarkers and therapeutic targets for various diseases, however, the function of exosomal miRNAs in stroke remains largely unknown.

Methods: The blood samples from acute ischemic stroke (AIS) patients and normal controls were collected. The exosomes were isolated from the blood samples, which were confirmed by electron microscopy and western blot with the specific exosomes biomarker CD9, CD63 and Tsg101.

Results: RT-qPCR analysis showed that exosomal miR-134 was significantly increased in AIS patients within 24 h after stroke onset compared with that of control group. Highly expressed exosomal miR-134 was correlated with the National Institutes of Health Stroke Scale (NIHSS) scores, infarct volume and positively associated with the worse prognosis of the stroke patients. Additionally, the exosomal miR-134 was strong positively correlated with the expression of serum interleukin 6 (IL-6) and plasma high-sensitivity C relative protein (hs-CRP). The receiver operating characteristic (ROC) curve suggested that miR-134 might be a potential factor to discriminate AIS patients from non-stroke controls.

Conclusions: The exosomal miR-134 as a possible novel biomarker for the diagnosis and prognosis of stroke.

Keywords: Acute ischemic stroke, Exosome, miR-134, National Institutes of Health stroke scale scores, Infarct volume

Background

Stroke is the main cause of neurological dysfunction, which has been considered as the second most common cause of death worldwide and brings heavy burden to the society and family [1–6]. Although remarkable progress has been made in the treatment of stroke, the diagnosis of stroke is still difficult as determining the cause of stroke remains complicated in up to 25% of the patients. Currently, there are no blood-based biomarkers with clinical utility for acute ischemic stroke. Therefore, exploring novel biomarkers involved in the pathogenesis of stroke still remains a challenge.

Tissue responding to the injury caused by stroke and the neuron remodeling after ischemia have been considered as a promising strategy for stroke treatment [7–10]. This process requires the alternation of gene expression in neurons. MicroRNAs (miRNAs) are characterized as non-coding RNAs that inhibit the gene expression via post- transcriptionally regulating the targets via binding the 3′-untranslational region [11–14]. MiRNAs are key regulators of the cell proliferation, differentiation and migration [15]. Aberrant expression of miRNAs has been found in a variety of human diseases. Recent studies showed that circulating miRNAs are highly stable and detectable in the serum of patients with ischemic stroke [16–19]. Up-regulated or down-regulated circulating miRNAs has been identified in stroke patients, which suggested that circulating miRNAs might be a potential biomarkers and therapy targets in stroke.

It has been reported that miRNA can be secreted from cells into the body fluids via exosomes [20–23]. Exosomes

* Correspondence: drctorlong@aliyun.com
[†]Jingxia Zhou and Lin Chen contributed equally to this work.
Department of Neurology, The Second Affiliated Hospital of Hainan Medical University, Haikou 570311, Hainan Province, People's Republic of China

are identified as 30–100 nm vesicles that are released into the extracellular space, which deliver protein, mRNA, miRNA or lipid from parent cells to recipient cells [24]. Exosomal miRNAs establish the communication between cell-to-cell and are involved in regulating different biological processes via modulating the expression of target genes. Notably, the critical role of exosomal miRNAs in the development of stroke is emerging [17, 19, 25]. Recent study showed that the plasma exosomal miR-422a and miR-125b-2-3p were potential blood-base biomarkers for monitoring and diagnosing of IS patients [26]. Additionally, the exosome mediated delivery of miR-124 promoted the cortical neurogenesis after stroke [27]. On the other hand, aberrant release of exosomal miRNAs leads to the alternation of gene expression that may induce the initiation and development of cerebral ischemia reperfusion injury. Among these miRNAs, miR-134 was a brain-specific miRNA that was associated with the development of dendritic and synaptic spine [28]. It has been reported that miR-134 was differentially expressed in brain tissues with ischemic injury [29, 30]. In rat model, miR-134 was down-regulated by electroacupuncture and promoted the expression of LIM domain kinase to enhance the synaptic-dendritic plasticity after ischemic stroke [31]. It was also found that overexpression of miR-134 significantly promoted neuron death induced by oxygen-glucose deprivation/reoxygenation by in vitro study [29]. These reports suggested the potential critical roles of miR-134 in regulating cerebral ischemic injury, however, the expression and correlation between miR-134 with the clinical parameters of acute ischemic stroke patients remains largely unknown.

Here, in this study, we detected the expression level of miR-134 in the serum exosomes from the patients with stroke and non-stroke subjects. To determine the clinical significance of miR-134 in stroke, the correlation between the expression of exosomal miR-134 with the National Institutes of Health Stroke Scale (NIHSS) scores, infarct volume, and prognosis of stroke patients were analyzed. The potential application of exosomal miR-134 as a novel biomarker for the diagnosis and therapy of stroke was also discussed.

Methods

Clinical sample collection

The 50 stroke patients were recruited between April 2015 and December 2016 in The Second Affiliated Hospital of Hainan Medical University. The ischemic stroke of these patients was confirmed by magnetic resonance imaging (MRI). The severity of stroke was evaluated with the NIHSS score by experienced neurologists. These AIS patients were divided into different Trial of Org 10,172 in Acute Stroke Treatment (TOAST) subtypes including cardioembolism, large artery atherosclerotic stroke and small artery stroke (Table 1). Control group were enrolled from those who underwent an annual medical examination and denied history of stroke attack at The Second Affiliated Hospital of Hainan Medical University. The cell-free serum samples were collected from the peripheral blood via centrifugation and stored at − 80 °C. This study was approved by The Second Affiliated Hospital of Hainan Medical University. Written consent was obtained from each participant. The clinical characteristics of the stroke patients and controls were described in Table 2.

Serum collection and exosomes isolation

Five milliliters of fresh whole blood from stroke patients within 24 h of stroke onset or control groups was collected into the promoting coagulating tubes and incubated at 37 °C for 20 min. And then the blood was centrifuged at 1600 *g* for 10 min. The serum was transferred into a new tube and centrifuged at 20,000 g at 4 °C for 15 min. The supernatant was collected and kept at − 80 °C until use. The serum exosomes were extracted with the ExoQuick exosome precipitation solution (System Biosciences, CA, USA). Briefly, the serum sample was centrifuged at 3000 g for 15 min at 4 °C. The supernatant was transferred into a fresh tube and one-fourth volume of ExoQuick Solution was added. The samples were mixed well and incubated at 4 °C for 2 h. And then the mixture was centrifuged at 1500 g for 30 min. The supernatant was discarded and the pellet was re-centrifuged for another 5 min at 4 °C. The exosome-containing pellet was resuspended with nuclease-free water. The size and morphology of exosomes were detected by transmission electron microscopy (TEM, Phillip CM120, 60 kV).

RT-qPCR analysis

Total RNA extraction from the serum exosomes was performed with the Exosome RNA Purification Kit (System Biosciences Inc., Mountain View, CA, USA) according to the manufacturer's instructions. The concentration and quality of the RNA was determined using the NanoDrop ND-2000 spectrophotometer (Thermo Scientific Rockford, IL, USA). Single strand cDNA was synthesized with the First Strand cDNA Synthesis Kit (Ferments, Vilnius, Lithuania). The expression of miR-134 was detected by real time PCR using the SYBR Green Master Mix (Applied Biosystems) on the Applied Biosystems 7900 real-time

Table 1 Stroke patients with different TOAST subtypes

Subtypes	Number
Cardioembolism	23
Large artery atherosclerotic stoke	10
Small artery stroke	17
Total	50

Table 2 Baseline clinical characteristics of the AIS patients and normal controls

Parameter	AIS patients (n = 50)	Control (n = 50)	*P* value
Mean age	65.42 ± 10.25	63.33 ± 14.32	> 0.05
Gender (Male/Female)	26/24	22/28	> 0.05
Race (Asian, %)	100%	100%	> 0.05
Ethnicity (Han, %)	100%	100%	> 0.05
Stroke risk factors			
Hypertension	30 (60.0%)	27 (54.0%)	> 0.05
Diabetes mellitus	24 (48.0%)	8 (16.0%)	< 0.01
Atrial Fibrillation	15 (30.0%)	12 (24.0%)	> 0.05
Hyperlipidemia	30 (60.0%)	13 (26.0%)	< 0.01
NIHSS score	7.82 ± 1.36	NA	NA
mRS ≤2	32 (64.0%)	NA	NA
> 2	18 (36.0%)	NA	NA

PCR machine. All the reactions were performed in triplicate. The PCR condition was set as the follows: 95 °C for 10 min, and then 42 cycles of 95 °C for 10s and 60 °C for 1 min. The relative expression abundance of miR-134 was calculated with the $2^{-\Delta\Delta Ct}$ method.

Western blot

Exosomal protein was extracted with the RIPA lysis buffer (Thermo Fisher Scientific, IL, USA). The protein concentration was determined by the Pierce BCA protein assay kit (Thermo Fisher Scientific, IL, USA). 20 μg of protein was loaded and separated by the 12% SDS-PAGE followed by transferred to polyvinylidene fluoride membranes. Afterwards, the membrane was blocked with 5% non-fat milk for 1 h at room temperature (RT) and then incubated with the indicated primary antibodies for 2 h at RT. The bands were detected by incubating the membrane with horse radish peroxidase (HRP)-conjugated secondary antibody for 1 h at RT and visualized using the ECL detection kit (Thermo Fisher Scientific, IL, USA).

Antibody characterization

The antibodies against CD9 (1:1000, sc-13,118, Santa Cruz Biotechnology), CD63 (1:1000, sc-365,604, Santa Cruz Biotechnology), β-actin (1:2000, sc-47,778, Santa Cruz Biotechnology) and Tsg101 (1:2000, ab30875, Abcam) were purchased from the company.

Statistical analysis

The statistical analysis was performed with the SPSS software (version 13.0, Chicago, IL, USA). Difference between two groups was compared by the Student's *t* test and multiple comparisons between more than two groups were determined by the one-way analysis of variance (ANOVA) followed by the Bonferroni test. The Chi-squared test was used to assess the correlation between the expression of miR-134 and clinicopathological factors. The exosomal miR-134 expression with the conventional risk factors of stroke was analyzed by the multivariable logistic regression. The correlation between the expression level of miR-134 and the NIHSS score of the stroke patients was determined with the Pearson's correlation test. $P < 0.05$ was considered as statistically significant.

Results

Identification of the serum exosomes isolated from the AIS patients

To isolate exosomes from the blood, ExoQuick kit was used to precipitate the microvesicles. Electron microscopy and western blot analysis have been the gold standard for exosome confirmation. The vesicles isolated in the study displayed a spherical structure with 30–100 nm nano-size (Fig. 1a), which is consistent with the diameter of exosomes. To further confirm this, the expression of CD9, CD63 and Tsg101, the commonly used exosomal markers, was detected by western blot. As shown in Fig. 1b, the protein bands of CD9, CD63, Tsg101 and β-actin were all observed with the indicated antibodies respectively. These data suggested that the isolation method we used was suitable for exosome purification.

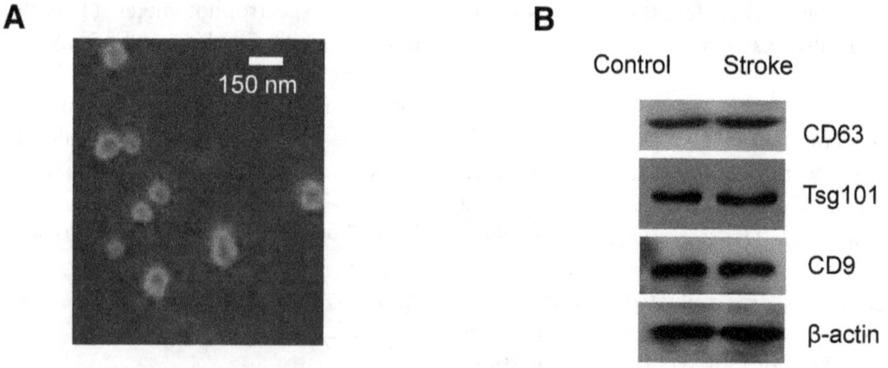

Fig. 1 The isolation of exosomes from the serum of AIS patients and controls. **a** The transmission electron microscope of the exosomes purified from the serum. Scale bar, 150 nm. **b** Western blot analysis of the exosomal markers with the indicated antibodies

The level of exosomal miR-134 was significantly elevated in stroke patients

To compare the expression abundance of exosomal miR-134 in stroke patients and normal controls, RT-qPCR analysis was performed with exosomes isolated from patients and the control group. As shown in Fig. 2a, compared with the control group, the expression of exosomal miR-134 was significantly increased in stroke patients within 24 h of the stroke onset. To detect whether the increased expression of miR-134 was a dynamic process after stroke, the expression level of miR-134 in the circulating exosome was examined at 24-, 48- and 72 h after stroke occurred. The data showed that there was no significant difference for the expression of exosomal miR-134 between different time points of the stroke (Fig. 2b).

Exosomal miR-134 was a possible biomarker for the diagnosis of AIS

The high expression of exosomal miR-134 in stroke patients led us to determine whether exosomal miR-134 was an independent risk factor in AIS. To this end, logistic regression analysis was performed to evaluate the impact of diabetes mellitus and hyperlipidemia on the expression of exosomal miR-134 between the stroke patients and normal controls. The data suggested that exosomal miR-134 has the possibility to be an independent risk factor of AIS (Table 3). To determine whether the serum exosomal miR-134 can be considered as a biomarker for the diagnosis of AIS, the receiver operating characteristic (ROC) curve was generated with the expression level of miR-134 in the serum exosomes. As shown in Fig. 3, the area under the curve (AUC) of miR-134 was 0.834 (95% confidence interval, 0.88–0.97), with a sensitivity of 75.3%, a specificity of 72.8%, a positive of 94.0%, and a negative predictive value of 88.0%. This data suggested that miR-134 is a possible potential biomarker to discriminate AIS patients from non-stroke controls.

Table 3 Expression of serum exosomal miR-134 and the risk of stroke

Characteristics	*P* value	OR	95% CI
miR-134	0.003	2.668	1.183–6.441
Diabetes mellitus	0.001	2.842	1.514–5.333
Hyperlipidemia	0.047	1.617	1.128–3.038

The relationship between the expression of exosomal miR-134 and the NIHSS score, infarct volume of the stroke patients

To determine the clinical significance of exosomal miR-134 in the diagnosis of acute ischemic stroke, the correlation between the expression of miR-134 and NIHSS scores, infarct volume was examined by the Pearson correlation test. As presented in Fig. 4a, significant correlation between the level of miR-134 and the NIHSS score was observed. Consistent with this data, the expression abundance of exosomal miR-134 was also significantly correlated with the infarct volume of the acute ischemic stroke patients (Fig. 4b). Additionally, to detect the relationship between the expression of circulating exosomal miR-134 with the 3-month prognosis of the stroke patients, the expression level of miR-134 in patients with good or poor outcome was compared. As shown in Fig. 4c, higher abundance of the exosomal miR-134 was found in stroke patients with poor prognosis. These findings suggested the potential clinical application of exosomal miR-134 in stroke.

The level of serum exosomal miR-134 was positively correlated with the serum level of IL-6 and plasma hs-CRP

Increasing evidence suggested that inflammation plays critical roles in the development of cardiovascular diseases [32–34]. The pro-inflammatory cytokine IL-6 and

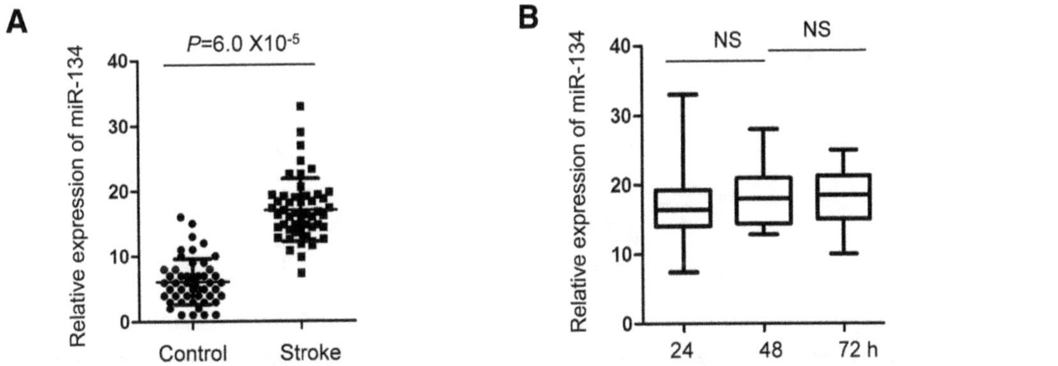

Fig. 2 The level of exosomal miR-134 was significantly elevated in stroke patients. **a** RT-qPCR analysis was performed to detect the expression of serum exosomal miR-134 in both the AIS patients and healthy controls. Student's *t* test, *n* = 50 in stroke group and n = 50 in control group. **b** The expression level of serum exosomal miR-134 of the AIS patients at different time points after the stroke occurred. *N* = 50. Ns, no significance. One-way ANOVA

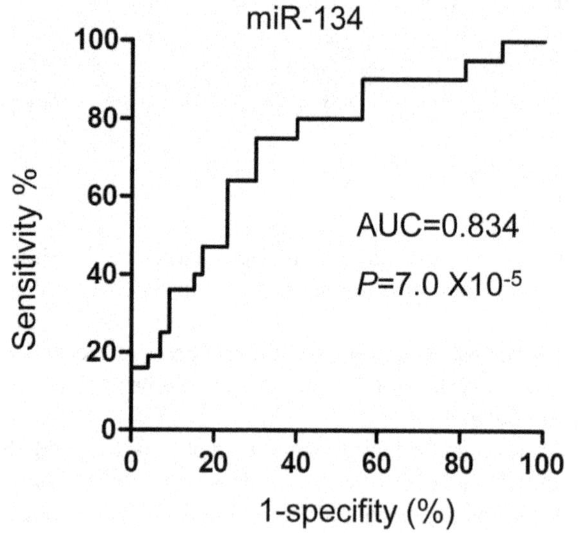

Fig. 3 Diagnostic value of serum exosomal miR-134 in AIS. ROC curve was generated based on the level of serum exosomal miR-134 to distinguish AIS patients (n = 50) from normal controls (n = 50). The area under the cure was 0.834 (95% confidence interval, 0.88–0.97)

hs-CRP was reported to reflect the degree of brain ischemic damage and stroke [35–41]. In this study, the levels of plasma hs-CRP and serum IL-6 were measured in AIS patients and control participants. The results showed that both plasma hs-CRP and serum IL-6 was significantly increased in the AIS patients in comparison with that of the control group (Fig. 5a and b). To further characterize the relationship between exosomal miR-134 and stroke, the correlation between the expressions of exosoma miR-134 and hs-CRP, IL-6 was analyzed, respectively. As shown in Fig. 5c and d, the level of miR-134 presented positive correlations with plasma hs-CRP and serum IL-6.

Discussion

Aberrant expression of miRNAs is associated with the initiation and development of human diseases. Notably, the plasma exosomal miRNAs have been found as diagnosis biomarkers and potential therapeutic targets in some diseases, however, the expression of exosomal miRNAs in acute ischemic stroke and its correlation with the clinical characteristics of the stroke patients remain largely unknown. In this study, we isolated the exosomes from blood of AIS patients and found that exosomal miR-134 was highly expressed in the stroke patients compared with that of the control group. Additionally, miR-134 was

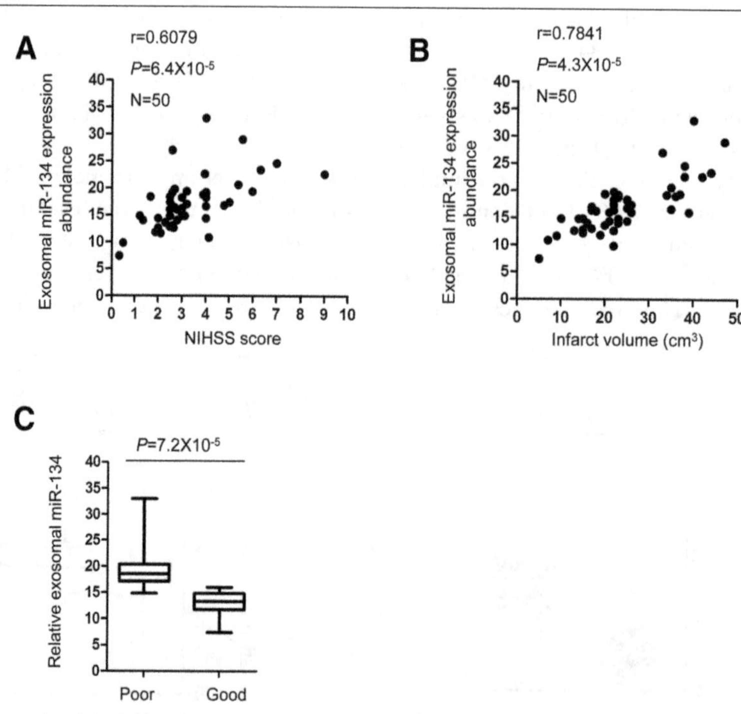

Fig. 4 The correlation between the abundance of serum exosomal miR-134 with the NIHSS, infraction volume of AIS patients. **a** The correlation between exosomal level of miR-134 with the NIHSS score of the stroke patients was analyzed by the Person correlation test. N = 50. **b** The correlation between exosomal level of miR-134 with the infarction volume of the stroke patients was analyzed by the Person correlation test. N = 50. **c** The correlation between serum exosomal miR-134 with the outcome of AIS patients. The expression level of miR-134 in AIS patients with good prognosis (modified Rankin Scale (mRS) ≤ 2, $n = 32$) and poor prognosis ((mRS > 2, $n = 18$) was analyzed by the Student's t test

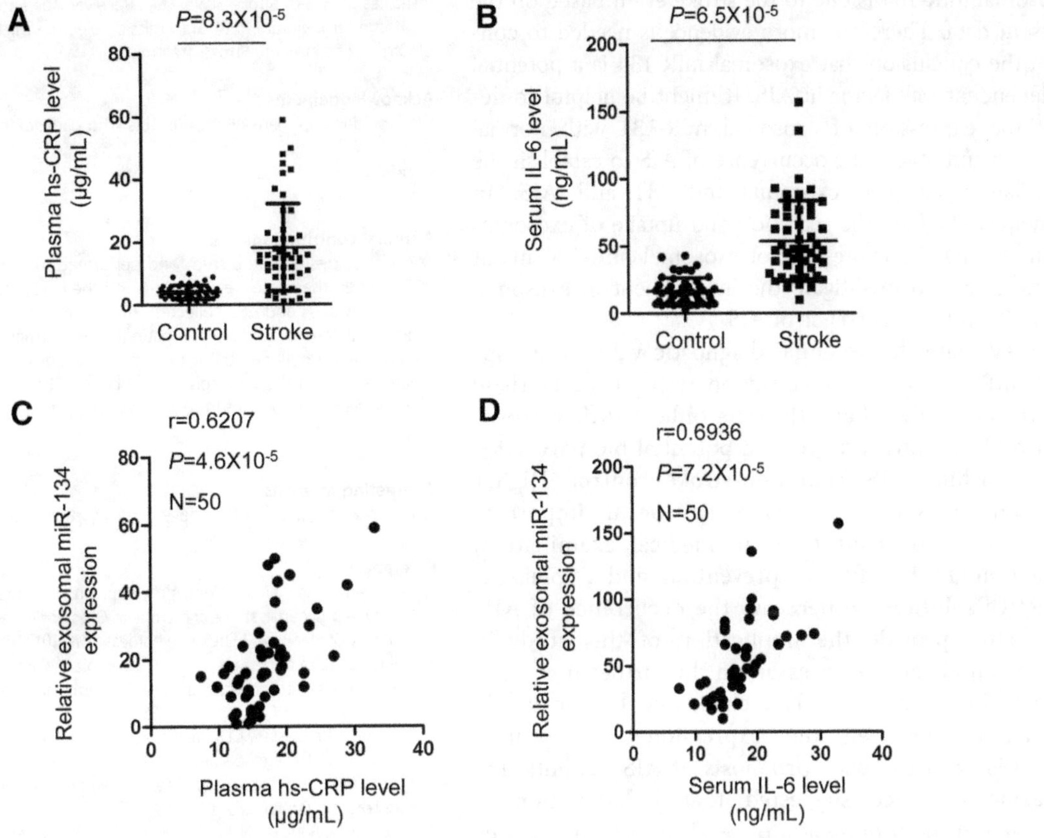

Fig. 5 The level of serum exosomal miR-134 was positively correlated with the serum level of IL-6 and plasma hs-CRP. **a, b** The levels of plasma hs-CRP and serum IL-6 were detected in AIS patients and control participants. Student's *t* test. **c, d** The exosomal miR-134 was positively correlated with the concentration of plasma hs-CRP and serum IL-6 in AIS patients

positively correlated with the NIHSS score and poor prognosis of these patients. These findings suggested that potential involvement of exosomal miR-134 in AIS.

The intercellular communication is an essential process under both physiological and pathological conditions. It has been well documented that extracellular vesicles and exosomes are important platform to change the genetic information between cells [42]. The extraordinary value of exosomes in the diagnosis and treatment of stroke has drawn wide attention during recent years. The function of exosome in brain injury and neurondegenerative diseases has been demonstrated [43–48]. It has been reported that exosomes protected the brain tissues from ischemia-reperfusion injury after hypoxia precondition [49]. The protection role of exosomes secreted by the mesenchymal stem cells was achieved by delivering functional proteins or RNAs to neurons or astrocytes after ischemic injury [24, 50]. Previous study has showed that increased plasma microvesicles during cerebral ischemia [51, 52]. The number of microvesicles derived from endothelial cells was positively correlated with the occurrence of ischemic stroke [53, 54]. In the present study, increased exosomal miR-134 might indicate the enhanced production of exosomes in stroke patients, which responds to the intercellular brain injury. Further investigation is needed to explore the specific cell type or brain tissue where the exosome derived from.

MiRNAs have emerged as important regulators of cardiovascular physiological processes [55]. It has been documented that miR-21, miR-223 and miR-146b served as biomarkers for acute ischemic stroke [17, 56, 57]. Additionally, elevated serum expression of miR-15a, miR-16 and miR-17-5p was also found to be strongly associated with the AIS [58]. Recent findings showed that miR-134 regulated the ischemia injury-induced neuronal cell death [29]. In the present study, the exosomal miR-134 was significantly increased in AIS samples after stroke in comparison with that of the control group. No remarkable difference was observed for the level of exosomal miR-134 at the time point of 24-, 48- and 72 h after the stroke event. Further study is necessary to explore the alternation of exosomal miR-134 expression with relatively earlier time frame. In the present study, as blood samples of AIS patients were collected within 24 h after the stroke onset, we couldn't rule out the possibility that the increase of exosomal miR-134 is due to the stroke event based on the present data. Therefore, more evidence is needed to confirm the conclusion that exosomal miR-134 is a potential independent risk factor in AIS. It might be helpful to detect the expression of exosomal miR-134 with normal subjects and follow the occurrence of AIS to establish the correlation between exosomal miR-134 and AIS. In principle, blocking the secretion and uptake of exosomes or inhibiting the expression of exosomal miR-134 might be necessary to investigate the involvement of exosomal miR-134 in the occurrence of AIS.

To evaluate the potential diagnostic value of exosomal miR-134 in AIS, receiver operating characteristic curve was analyzed and the data indicated that exosomal miR-134 might serve as a potential biomarker for distinguishing AIS from non-stroke control. Higher exosomal miR-134 expression may be an important indicator to be considered in medical examination, which might benefit the prevention and implement effective solutions to decrease the occurrence of AIS. To better provide the implication of this study, a larger sample size is necessary in the further investigation. Additionally, our data elucidated the positively correlation between the expression of exosomal miR-134 with the poor prognosis of AIS patients. Increasing evidence suggested that inflammation is involved in the progression of cerebrovascular diseases [59–62]. The plasma hs-CRP and serum IL-6 are important markers of inflammation and associated with the development of stroke. Consistently, our results found that serum exosomal miR-134 was significantly correlated with the increased expression of hs-CRP and IL-6 in AIS patients, which supported the conclusion that exosomal miR-134 was potential candidate for AIS prediction. As the function of miRNAs is achieved via modulating the expression of downstream target genes, further studies will be designed to explore the underlying molecular mechanism by which exosomal miR-134 in response to the ischemic stroke.

Conclusions

Our study demonstrated that the expression of exosomal miR-134 in AIS patients was significantly increased. Enhanced abundance of the exosomal miR-134 was significantly correlated with the poor prognosis of AIS. Due to the relative small sample sizes in this study, further large-scale prospective data and longer follow-up studies were quite necessary to confirm the specificity and accuracy of exosomal miR-134 as a biomarker in the diagnosis of AIS.

Abbreviations

AIS: Acute ischemic stroke; ANOVA: One-way analysis of variance; HRP: Horse radish peroxidase; hs-CRP: High-sensitivity C relative protein; IL-6: Interleukin 6; miRNAs: microRNAs; MRI: Magnetic resonance imaging; NIHSS: National Institutes of Health Stroke Scale; ROC: Receiver operating characteristic; RT: Room temperature; TEM: Transmission electron microscopy; TOAST: Trial of Org 10,172 in Acute Stroke Treatment

Acknowledgements

We would like to thank all the subjects who participate in this study.

Funding

None.

Authors' contributions

JXZ and LC designed the study and performed most of the experiments. BCC purified the exosomes and detected the exosomes with the electron microscopy. SZH and CSZ collected the samples and analyzed the baseline clinical characteristics of the AIS patients and normal controls, as well as the correlation between the expression of exosomal miR-134 and the risk of stroke. HRW and CC interpreted the data. FQL wrote the manuscript. All authors read and approved the final manuscript.

Competing interests

The authors declare that they have no competing interests.

References

1. Fargeot G, Stefanizzi S, Depuydt S, Klapczynski F, Ameri A. Association between ischemic stroke and Erdheim-Chester disease: a case report and review of literature. J Stroke Cerebrovasc Dis. 2017;26:e153–5.
2. Pires da Rosa G, Libanio D, Filipe Azevedo L. Analysis of the Cochrane Review: Fibrates for secondary prevention of cardiovascular disease and stroke. Rev Port Cardiol. 2017;36:55–8.
3. Stefanidis KB, Askew CD, Greaves K, Summers MJ. The effect of non-stroke cardiovascular disease states on risk for cognitive decline and dementia: a systematic and meta-analytic review. Neuropsychol Rev. 2018;28:1. https://doi.org/10.1007/s11065-017-9359-z.
4. Sterne JA, Bodalia PN, Bryden PA, Davies PA, Lopez-Lopez JA, Okoli GN, Thom HH, Caldwell DM, Dias S, Eaton D, et al. Oral anticoagulants for primary prevention, treatment and secondary prevention of venous thromboembolic disease, and for prevention of stroke in atrial fibrillation: systematic review, network meta-analysis and cost-effectiveness analysis. Health Technol Assess. 2017;21:1–386.
5. Yang H, Guo W, Li J, Cao S, Zhang J, Pan J, Wang Z, Wen P, Shi X, Zhang S. Leptin concentration and risk of coronary heart disease and stroke: a systematic review and meta-analysis. PLoS One. 2017;12:e0166360.
6. Feigin VL, Forouzanfar MH, Krishnamurthi R, Mensah GA, Connor M, Bennett DA, Moran AE, Sacco RL, Anderson L, Truelsen T, et al. Global and regional burden of stroke during 1990-2010: findings from the global burden of disease study 2010. Lancet. 2014;383:245–54.
7. Kim SY, Senatorov VV Jr, Morrissey CS, Lippmann K, Vazquez O, Milikovsky DZ, Gu F, Parada I, Prince DA, Becker AJ, et al. TGFbeta signaling is associated with changes in inflammatory gene expression and perineuronal net degradation around inhibitory neurons following various neurological insults. Sci Rep. 2017;7:7711.
8. Li Y, Zhang X, Cui L, Chen R, Zhang Y, Zhang C, Zhu X, He T, Shen Z, Dong L, et al. Salvianolic acids enhance cerebral angiogenesis and neurological recovery by activating JAK2/STAT3 signaling pathway after ischemic stroke in mice. J Neurochem. 2017;143:87–99.
9. Okabe N, Narita K, Miyamoto O. Axonal remodeling in the corticospinal tract after stroke: how does rehabilitative training modulate it? Neural Regen Res. 2017;12:185–92.
10. Tian X, Sun L, Feng D, Sun Q, Dou Y, Liu C, Zhou F, Li H, Shen H, Wang Z, Chen G. HMGB1 promotes neurovascular remodeling via rage in the late phase of subarachnoid hemorrhage. Brain Res. 2017;1670:135–45.
11. Mizuguchi Y, Takizawa T, Yoshida H, Uchida E. Dysregulated miRNA in progression of hepatocellular carcinoma: a systematic review. Hepatol Res. 2016;46:391–406.
12. Wen MM. Getting miRNA therapeutics into the target cells for neurodegenerative diseases: a mini-review. Front Mol Neurosci. 2016;9:129.
13. Ma H, Wu Y, Yang H, Liu J, Dan H, Zeng X, Zhou Y, Jiang L, Chen Q. MicroRNAs in oral lichen planus and potential miRNA-mRNA pathogenesis with essential cytokines: a review. Oral Surg Oral Med Oral Pathol Oral Radiol. 2016;122:164–73.

14. Gambari R, Brognara E, Spandidos DA, Fabbri E. Targeting oncomiRNAs and mimicking tumor suppressor miRNAs: Nuew trends in the development of miRNA therapeutic strategies in oncology (review). Int J Oncol. 2016;49:5–32.
15. Bartel DP. MicroRNAs: genomics, biogenesis, mechanism, and function. Cell. 2004;116:281–97.
16. Xiao S, Ma Y, Zhu H, Sun H, Yin Y, Feng G. miRNA functional synergistic network analysis of mice with ischemic stroke. Neurol Sci. 2015;36:143–8.
17. Chen Y, Song Y, Huang J, Qu M, Zhang Y, Geng J, Zhang Z, Liu J, Yang GY. Increased circulating Exosomal miRNA-223 is associated with acute ischemic stroke. Front Neurol. 2017;8:57.
18. Sabour S. The diagnostic value of serum miRNA-221-3p, miRNA-382-5p, and miRNA-4271 in ischemic stroke: methodological issue to avoid misinterpretation. J Stroke Cerebrovasc Dis. 2017;26:1161.
19. Wang Y, Ma Z, Kan P, Zhang B. The diagnostic value of serum miRNA-221-3p, miRNA-382-5p, and miRNA-4271 in ischemic stroke. J Stroke Cerebrovasc Dis. 2017;26:1055–60.
20. Madhavan B, Yue S, Galli U, Rana S, Gross W, Muller M, Giese NA, Kalthoff H, Becker T, Buchler MW, Zoller M. Combined evaluation of a panel of protein and miRNA serum-exosome biomarkers for pancreatic cancer diagnosis increases sensitivity and specificity. Int J Cancer. 2015;136:2616–27.
21. Valencia K, Luis-Ravelo D, Bovy N, Anton I, Martinez-Canarias S, Zandueta C, Ormazabal C, Struman I, Tabruyn S, Rebmann V, et al. miRNA cargo within exosome-like vesicle transfer influences metastatic bone colonization. Mol Oncol. 2014;8:689–703.
22. Ge Q, Zhou Y, Lu J, Bai Y, Xie X, Lu Z. miRNA in plasma exosome is stable under different storage conditions. Molecules. 2014;19:1568–75.
23. Yentrapalli R, Merl-Pham J, Azimzadeh O, Mutschelknaus L, Peters C, Hauck SM, Atkinson MJ, Tapio S, Moertl S. Quantitative changes in the protein and miRNA cargo of plasma exosome-like vesicles after exposure to ionizing radiation. Int J Radiat Biol. 2017;93:569–80.
24. Valadi H, Ekstrom K, Bossios A, Sjostrand M, Lee JJ, Lotvall JO. Exosome-mediated transfer of mRNAs and microRNAs is a novel mechanism of genetic exchange between cells. Nat Cell Biol. 2007;9:654–9.
25. Bam M, Yang X, Sen S, Zumbrun EE, Dennis L, Zhang J, Nagarkatti PS, Nagarkatti M. Characterization of dysregulated miRNA in peripheral blood mononuclear cells from ischemic stroke patients. Mol Neurobiol. 2018;55:1419–29.
26. Li DB, Liu JL, Wang W, Li RY, Yu DJ, Lan XY, Li JP. Plasma Exosomal miR-422a and miR-125b-2-3p serve as biomarkers for ischemic stroke. Curr Neurovasc Res. 2017;14:330–7.
27. Yang J, Zhang X, Chen X, Wang L, Yang G. Exosome mediated delivery of miR-124 promotes neurogenesis after ischemia. Mol Ther Nucleic Acids. 2017;7:278–87.
28. Schratt GM, Tuebing F, Nigh EA, Kane CG, Sabatini ME, Kiebler M, Greenberg ME. A brain-specific microRNA regulates dendritic spine development. Nature. 2006;439:283–9.
29. Huang W, Liu X, Cao J, Meng F, Li M, Chen B, Zhang J. miR-134 regulates ischemia/reperfusion injury-induced neuronal cell death by regulating CREB signaling. J Mol Neurosci. 2015;55:821–9.
30. Liu C, Peng Z, Zhang N, Yu L, Han S, Li D, Li J. Identification of differentially expressed microRNAs and their PKC-isoform specific gene network prediction during hypoxic pre-conditioning and focal cerebral ischemia of mice. J Neurochem. 2012;120:830–41.
31. Liu W, Wu J, Huang J, Zhuo P, Lin Y, Wang L, Lin R, Chen L, Tao J. Electroacupuncture regulates hippocampal synaptic plasticity via miR-134-mediated LIMK1 function in rats with ischemic stroke. Neural Plast. 2017; 2017:9545646.
32. Libby P. Fanning the flames: inflammation in cardiovascular diseases. Cardiovasc Res. 2015;107:307–9.
33. Gregersen I, Holm S, Dahl TB, Halvorsen B, Aukrust P. A focus on inflammation as a major risk factor for atherosclerotic cardiovascular diseases. Expert Rev Cardiovasc Ther. 2016;14:391–403.
34. Sallam N, Laher I. Exercise modulates oxidative stress and inflammation in aging and cardiovascular diseases. Oxidative Med Cell Longev. 2016;2016:7239639.
35. Waje-Andreassen U, Krakenes J, Ulvestad E, Thomassen L, Myhr KM, Aarseth J, Vedeler CA. IL-6: an early marker for outcome in acute ischemic stroke. Acta Neurol Scand. 2005;111:360–5.
36. Cojocaru IM, Cojocaru M, Tanasescu R, Iliescu I, Dumitrescu L, Silosi I. Expression of IL-6 activity in patients with acute ischemic stroke. Rom J Intern Med. 2009;47:393–6.
37. Kwan J, Horsfield G, Bryant T, Gawne-Cain M, Durward G, Byrne CD, Englyst NA. IL-6 is a predictive biomarker for stroke associated infection and future mortality in the elderly after an ischemic stroke. Exp Gerontol. 2013;48:960–5.
38. Sand PG. IL-6 variants in ischemic stroke. Ann Neurosci. 2016;23:60–1.
39. Zhang XF, Zou W, Yang Y. Effects of IL-6 and cortisol fluctuations in post-stroke depression. J Huazhong Univ Sci Technolog Med Sci. 2016;36:732–5.
40. Sun SL, Xie YM, Zhang Y, Wang ZF, Yang J, Wang DQ, Jiao Y, Chen J, Tao YH. Study on relationship between constitution and syndrome of MMP-9, IL-6 and MTHFR gene in patients with ischemic stroke. Zhongguo Zhong Yao Za Zhi. 2017;42:3602–12.
41. Chaudhuri JR, Mridula KR, Umamahesh M, Swathi A, Balaraju B, Bandaru VC. High sensitivity C-reactive protein levels in acute ischemic stroke and subtypes: a study from a tertiary care center. Iran J Neurol. 2013;12:92–7.
42. Hao S, Moyana T, Xiang J. Review: cancer immunotherapy by exosome-based vaccines. Cancer Biother Radiopharm. 2007;22:692–703.
43. Wan J, Yourshaw M, Mamsa H, Rudnik-Schoneborn S, Menezes MP, Hong JE, Leong DW, Senderek J, Salman MS, Chitayat D, et al. Mutations in the RNA exosome component gene EXOSC3 cause pontocerebellar hypoplasia and spinal motor neuron degeneration. Nat Genet. 2012;44:704–8.
44. Basso M, Pozzi S, Tortarolo M, Fiordaliso F, Bisighini C, Pasetto L, Spaltro G, Lidonnici D, Gensano F, Battaglia E, et al. Mutant copper-zinc superoxide dismutase (SOD1) induces protein secretion pathway alterations and exosome release in astrocytes: implications for disease spreading and motor neuron pathology in amyotrophic lateral sclerosis. J Biol Chem. 2013;288: 15699–711.
45. Richard P, Feng S, Manley JL. A SUMO-dependent interaction between Senataxin and the exosome, disrupted in the neurodegenerative disease AOA2, targets the exosome to sites of transcription-induced DNA damage. Genes Dev. 2013;27:2227–32.
46. Hamlett ED, Ledreux A, Potter H, Chial HJ, Patterson D, Espinosa JM, Bettcher BM, Granholm AC. Exosomal biomarkers in Down syndrome and Alzheimer's disease. Free Radic Biol Med. 2018;114:110–21.
47. Tofaris GK. A critical assessment of exosomes in the pathogenesis and stratification of Parkinson's disease. J Parkinsons Dis. 2017;7(4):569–76.
48. Huang S, Ge X, Yu J, Han Z, Yin Z, Li Y, Chen F, Wang H, Zhang J, Lei P. Increased miR-124-3p in microglial exosomes following traumatic brain injury inhibits neuronal inflammation and contributes to neurite outgrowth via their transfer into neurons. FASEB J. 2018;32(1):512–28.
49. Vicencio JM, Yellon DM, Sivaraman V, Das D, Boi-Doku C, Arjun S, Zheng Y, Riquelme JA, Kearney J, Sharma V, et al. Plasma exosomes protect the myocardium from ischemia-reperfusion injury. J Am Coll Cardiol. 2015;65:1525–36.
50. Simpson RJ, Lim JW, Moritz RL, Mathivanan S. Exosomes: proteomic insights and diagnostic potential. Expert Rev Proteomics. 2009;6:267–83.
51. Colombo E, Borgiani B, Verderio C, Furlan R. Microvesicles: novel biomarkers for neurological disorders. Front Physiol. 2012;3:63.
52. Ji Q, Ji Y, Peng J, Zhou X, Chen X, Zhao H, Xu T, Chen L, Xu Y. Increased brain-specific MiR-9 and MiR-124 in the serum exosomes of acute ischemic stroke patients. PLoS One. 2016;11:e0163645.
53. Jung KH, Chu K, Lee ST, Park HK, Bahn JJ, Kim DH, Kim JH, Kim M, Kun Lee S, Roh JK. Circulating endothelial microparticles as a marker of cerebrovascular disease. Ann Neurol. 2009;66:191–9.
54. Kuriyama N, Nagakane Y, Hosomi A, Ohara T, Kasai T, Harada S, Takeda K, Yamada K, Ozasa K, Tokuda T, et al. Evaluation of factors associated with elevated levels of platelet-derived microparticles in the acute phase of cerebral infarction. Clin Appl Thromb Hemost. 2010;16:26–32.
55. Nouraee N, Mowla SJ. miRNA therapeutics in cardiovascular diseases: promises and problems. Front Genet. 2015;6:232.
56. Chen Z, Wang K, Huang J, Zheng G, Lv Y, Luo N, Liang M, Huang L. Upregulated serum MiR-146b serves as a biomarker for acute ischemic stroke. Cell Physiol Biochem. 2018;45:397–405.
57. Xiang Y, Guo J, Peng YF, Tan T, Huang HT, Luo HC, Wei YS. Association of miR-21, miR-126 and miR-605 gene polymorphisms with ischemic stroke risk. Oncotarget. 2017;8:95755–63.
58. Wu J, Du K, Lu X. Elevated expressions of serum miR-15a, miR-16, and miR-17-5p are associated with acute ischemic stroke. Int J Clin Exp Med. 2015;8:21071–9.
59. Becker KJ. Inflammation and the silent sequelae of stroke. Neurotherapeutics. 2016;13:801–10.

Pre-stroke warfarin enhancement of collateralization in acute ischemic stroke

Jiaying Zhu[1,2†], Mengmeng Ma[1†], Yijia Guo[1], Muke Zhou[1], Jian Guo[1] and Li He[1*]

Abstract

Background: Warfarin therapies not only are used to prevent stroke in patients with high risk of cardioembolism such as patients with atrial fibrillation (AF) and rheumatic heart disease (RHD), but also was associated with lower stroke severity and more favorable functional outcomes in patients with acute ischemic stroke due to middle cerebral artery occlusion. It was speculated that pre-stroke warfarin may promote collateralization and result in reduced stroke severity. This study aimed to investigate the association between pre-stroke warfarin use and leptomeningeal collaterals in patients with acute ischemic stroke due to occlusion of the middle cerebral artery.

Methods: We enrolled consecutive acute ischemic stroke patients (occlusion of the middle cerebral artery within 24 h) with known history of AF and/or RHD at the neurology department of the West China Hospital from May 2011 to April 2017. Computed tomography angiography (CTA) before treatment was used to detect the thrombus. Regional leptomeningeal collateral (rLMC) score based on CTA images was used to assess collateral circulation. Prior use of warfarin was recorded. Univariate and multivariate analyses were performed to detect the association of prior warfarin use with the collateral circulation.

Results: A total of 120 patients were included; 29 (24.2%) were taking warfarin before stroke. The international normalized ratio (INR) in patients with prior warfarin use was 1.53 ± 1.00, compared with 1.02 ± 0.09 in patients without prior warfarin use ($P < 0.001$). Prior oral warfarin therapy was inversely associated with poor rLMC (OR = 0.07, 95%CI 0.01–0.44, $P = 0.005$). There were no associations between prior warfarin use and initial stroke severity or functional outcomes at 3 months.

Conclusion: Warfarin use seems improve collateralization in patients with acute stroke. However, clinical controlled studies should be used to verify this claim.

Keywords: Warfarin, Acute ischemic stroke, Collateral circulation

Background

Leptomeningeal collaterals are pre-existing anastomoses of distal regions of intracerebral small blood vessels [1, 2]. Collaterals provide the brain tissue with supplementary blood flow in the case of occlusion of primary intracranial arteries to protect brain tissue against irreversible damage [2]. Patients with good leptomeningeal collaterals usually have lower severity of stroke, better response to therapy, and better clinical outcome in acute ischemic stroke [3–6]. Collateral blood vessels could be a therapeutic target in acute ischemic stroke [2]. However, preexisting collaterals depend on cardiac and pulmonary illnesses, metabolic syndrome, hyperuricemia, aging, and genetic factors [2, 4, 7, 8]. Although there are no pharmacologic treatments proven to promote cerebral collateralization currently, some conventional stroke treatments may be available to enhance the collateral circulation [6]. Statins, which have modest antithrombotic pleiotropic effects, have been shown to be associated with the presence of better collaterals in patients with acute stroke [9].

* Correspondence: heli2003new@126.com
†Jia Ying Zhu and Mengmeng Ma contributed equally to this work.
1Department of Neurology, West China Hospital, Sichuan University, Chengdu, China
Full list of author information is available at the end of the article

In addition, numerous studies have demonstrated that oral anticoagulants (such as warfarin) reduced the risk of ischemic stroke [10]. Warfarin was also associated with lower stroke severity and more favorable functional outcomes when stroke occurs [11–13]. Although the mechanism for pre-stroke warfarin lowering stroke severity and improving functional outcomes was not very clear, two hypothesizes have been suggested. First, pre-stroke warfarin use may prevent thrombus formation and reduce the size of thrombi. Smaller thrombi cause distal infarctions and lower stroke severity and a more favorable clinical outcome [14, 15]. Secondly, pre-stroke warfarin use may promote collateralization since that the patients who used warfarin before stroke had lower stroke severity comparing with not using warfarin even though the patients of two groups had the similar thrombi and arterial occlusion site [16, 17]. Then it was speculated that pre-stroke warfarin may promote collateralization and result in reduced stroke severity. However, whether the association exit between pre-stroke warfarin use and collaterals still needs to be clarified. In this study, we aimed to evaluate the association between pre-stroke warfarin use and collaterals in acute ischemic stroke patients presenting with occlusion of the middle cerebral artery.

Methods

Study population

We performed a retrospective analysis of demographic, clinical, and radiographic data in consecutive patients at the Neurology Department of West China Hospital between May 2011 and April 2017. The inclusion criteria were: (1) ≥18 years of age; (2) history of AF and/or RHD; (3) available computed tomography angiography (CTA) images within 24 h of symptom onset; and (4) CTA detection of acute infarction due to occlusion of the M1 or M2 middle cerebral artery (MCA), with or without occlusion of the internal carotid artery (ICA). The exclusion criteria were: (1) pre-stroke modified Rankin Scale (mRS) score > 2; (2) severe extracranial vascular stenosis detected by CTA; or (3) < 90 days of follow-up.

Admission CT

All patients underwent non-contrast computed tomography (NCCT) and CTA. Imaging was conducted on a 128-slice Siemens SOMATOM Definition Flash double source CT scanner. NCCT helical scans were performed form the skull base to the vertex using the following parameters: 70 kV, 150 mA, and 5-mm collimation. CTA was performed using: 42 ml of contrast at 6 ml/s, 3 to 5 s delay from injection to scanning, 70 kV, 150 mA, 0.5 s/rotation, and 1.25-mm thick slice. The CTA scan covered the carotid bifurcation to the vertex. Maximum-intensity projection images (20 mm) were reconstructed in the axial, sagittal, and coronal planes.

Leptomeningeal collateral flow assessment

We assessed the degree of leptomeningeal collateral flow using the regional leptomeningeal collateral (rLMC) score (20 points) [3]. The rLMC score is based on scoring the pial and lenticulostriate arteries in six MCA regions (M1-M6) and in the anterior cerebral artery region and the basal ganglia (0 = no; 1 = less; 2 = equal or more prominent compared with a matching region in the pial artery of the contralateral hemisphere). The arteries in the Sylvian sulcus are given a higher score: 0 = not seen; 2 = less; 4 = same or more prominent compared with the opposite Sylvian sulcus. An rLMC score of 0–10 was defined as poor collateral flow, 11–16 was defined as moderate collateral flow, and 17–20 was defined as good collateral flow [3]. The assessment was performed by four radiologists with extensive experience in acute stroke imaging. The average score was used as the final score for the analyses.

Data collection

Clinical variables (age, gender, stroke risk factors, admission examinations, previous medications, thrombolytic therapy, and hemorrhagic transformation) were collected for each patient from the stroke database. All biochemical indexes were measured within 24 h of admission. The patient was considered to be using warfarin if they had been using it for at least 3 months prior to stroke and were still using warfarin when stroke occurred. Neurological severity was assessed by trained neurologists using the National Institutes of Health Stroke Scale (NIHSS, < 5 was defined as mild stroke, 5–14 as moderate stroke, and > 14 as severe stroke) [11, 18]. Intracerebral hemorrhage (ICH) was diagnosed according to the European Cooperative Acute Stroke Study (ECASS) criteria. All patients were managed optimally according to the current guidelines, physicians' experience, and patients' comorbidities. Follow-up mRS at 3-month after discharge was used to assess the functional outcome. All data collectors were blind to the baseline collateral status.

Statistical analysis

Statistical analysis was performed using SPSS 22.0 for Windows (IBM, Armonk, NY, USA). The patients were grouped as warfarin users vs. non-warfarin users. The potential determinants of collaterals evaluated based on previous reports in the literature were age, blood pressure, total cholesterol (treated as continuous variables), high-density lipoprotein cholesterol (HDL-C), and low-density lipoprotein cholesterol (LDL-C), and history of stroke, TIA, hypertension, diabetes, hypercholesterolemia, and pre-stroke statin use (treated as dichotomized variables). [19, 20] Continuous variables were expressed as means ± standard deviation or medians (interquartile range) and were analyzed using the Student's t test or the Mann-Whitney U test between two groups. When comparing percent distributions, the chi-square test was used but Fisher's exact test was used if the expected number in a category was < 5. Univariate logistic regression was used to determine the association between potential determinants and leptomeningeal collaterals and multivariate logistic regression was used to determine the association between pre-stroke warfarin use and collaterals. Model 1 was adjusted for age, gender, onset to door time; model 2 included model 1 and was additionally adjusted for stroke risk factors; model 3 included model 2 and was additionally adjusted for admission examinations, thrombus location, NIH stroke scale scores; model 4 included model 3 and was additionally adjusted for prior medications. Logistic regression was used to determine the clinical outcomes associated with pre-stroke warfarin use. P value < 0.05 was considered statistically significant.

Results

Baseline characteristics of the patients

A total of 120 participants were included in the study. Of them, 37 (30.8%) patients were male. Table 1 provided the characteristics of patients with pre-stroke warfarin use or not. Pre-stroke warfarin use was recorded in 29 (24.2%) patients. Compared to patients without warfarin use, those with warfarin use were more likely to be younger age ($P < 0.001$) and to have a higher international normalized ratio (INR) ($P < 0.001$).

Assessment of clinical factors associated with collateral status

Table 2 shows the association between clinical variables and rLMC scores (categorized as poor, moderate, and good). Previous coronary heart disease ($P = 0.023$), low-density lipoprotein cholesterol ($P = 0.008$), NIHSS ($P < 0.001$), thrombus location ($P < 0.001$), statin use ($P = 0.068$), and warfarin use ($P = 0.045$) were potential clinical factors associated with collateral flow. In the multivariate models (Table 3), prior warfarin use was inversely associated with poor rLMC (OR = 0.07, 95%CI 0.01–0.44, $P = 0.005$) after adjustment for confounding factors.

Association of Prior Warfarin use with stroke severity, Thrombus location, and clinical outcomes

Table 4 shows the association between prior warfarin use and initial stroke severity, thrombus location, and functional outcome. No significant difference was observed between prior warfarin use and stroke severity or follow-up mRS. Compared with patients without warfarin use exposure, thrombus location (M2 vs. ICA + M1/M1) was significantly different in warfarin users (OR = 0.38, 95%CI 0.16–0.91, $P = 0.03$). After adjustment for age, gender, previous antiplatelet and statins, warfarin users had a tendency to have distal vessel occlusion (OR = 0.37, 95%CI 0.13–1.03, $P = 0.056$).

Discussion

We performed a retrospective analysis of demographic, clinical, and radiographic data in consecutive patients with acute ischemic stroke presenting with the occlusion of middle cerebral artery to evaluate the association between pre-stroke warfarin use and collaterals by CTA images [21]. We found that pre-stroke oral warfarin use was inversely associated with poor leptomeningeal collaterals as identified. It showed that pre-stroke warfarin use may improve the poor cerebral collateral grade among acute ischemic stroke patients presenting with a major arterial occlusion by CTA images which is in accord with the hypothesis [10, 13].

This result also demonstrates a previously unidentified mechanism by which warfarin could lower the risks of poor collateral and reduce stroke severity. It was shown when intracranial artery occludes, secondary microthrombus may form in the distal small blood vessels of occluded artery [10, 15]. This will interfere with collateral circulations in the small vessels. Consequently, warfarin may enhance or facilitate collaterals by 1) preventing the secondary microthrombus formation in the distal small blood vessels of occluded artery, 2) promoting the lysis of thrombi in the distal small vessels and speeding up the resolution process of these thrombi at stroke onset.

The international normalized ratio (INR) value has confirmed an inverse association between admission INR and infarct size in acute ischemic stroke [11, 22–24]. In patients with higher INR (eg, an INR of 2–3), thrombus formation will be prevented and the resolution process of the new thrombus will be accelerated [25]. Indeed, one study conducted in Japan demonstrated that INR controlled between 1.60 and 1.99 is not effective for reducing the severity of ischemic stroke in patients with non-valvular atrial fibrillation [22]. Another study performed in the United States showed that therapeutic anticoagulation (INR ≥2) was associated with lower odds of moderate or severe stroke [11]. In this study, the INR values of the patients with pre-stroke warfarin were relatively lower. This may explain the result of this study that collateral enhancement was only in the patients with poor rLMC compared with other patients. Therefore, it may be needed to explore the underlying effect of the INR on collaterals and stroke severity in the future.

Table 1 Clinical characteristics of all participants ($n = 120$)

	All (n = 120)	Pre-stroke warfarin users		P value
		Yes (*n* = 29)	No (*n* = 91)	
Demographics, n (%)				
Age > 60 years	89 (74.2)	12 (41.4)	77 (84.6)	< 0.001
Male	37 (30.8)	8 (27.6)	29 (31.9)	0.664
Onset to door time < 6 h	80 (66.7)	17 (58.6)	63 (69.2)	0.291
Risk factors, n (%)				
Hypertension	60 (50.0)	10 (34.5)	50 (54.9)	0.055
Diabetes	16 (13.3)	3 (10.3)	13 (14.3)	0.759
Atrial fibrillation	112 (93.3)	22 (75.9)	90 (98.9)	< 0.001
Coronary heart disease	17 (14.2)	3 (10.3)	14 (15.4)	0.76
Previous stroke	16 (13.3)	2 (6.9)	14 (15.4)	0.352
Admission examinations, mean ± SD				
INR	1.15 ± 0.54	1.53 ± 1.00	1.02 ± 0.09	< 0.001
Systolic blood pressure	136.88 ± 20.08	133.86 ± 23.74	137.84 ± 18.81	0.356
Diastolic blood pressure	81.31 ± 15.03	82.93 ± 13.70	80.79 ± 15.47	0.507
Serum glucose	7.85 ± 2.40	7.45 ± 2.71	7.97 ± 2.29	0.311
Triglyceride	1.53 ± 1.60	1.90 ± 2.65	1.40 ± 1.08	0.72
Cholesterol	3.97 ± 0.99	3.91 ± 1.29	3.98 ± 0.88	0.325
HDL-C	1.38 ± 0.56	1.36 ± 0.79	1.39 ± 0.47	0.26
LDL-C	2.25 ± 0.72	2.16 ± 0.65	2.29 ± 0.74	0.402
Clinical factors, n (%)				
Thrombus location on CTA				0.078
ICA + M1	28 (23.3)	6 (20.7)	22 (24.2)	
M1	54 (45.0)	9 (31.0)	45 (49.5)	
M2	38 (31.7)	14 (48.3)	24 (26.3)	
NIHSS scores	13 (7–18)	12 (8–16)	13 (7–18)	
Thrombolysis	22 (18.3)	4 (13.8)	18 (19.8)	0.468
Intracranial hemorrhage	27 (22.5)	5 (17.2)	22 (24.2)	0.436
Pre-stroke medications, n (%)				
Antihypertensive drugs	49 (40.8)	10 (34.5)	39 (42.9)	0.424
Antidiabetics	14 (11.7)	3 (10.3)	11 (12.1)	0.549
Antiplatelet drugs	21 (17.5)	2 (6.90)	19 (20.9)	0.084
Statins	21 (17.5)	7 (24.1)	14 (15.4)	0.28

INR international normalized ratio, *HDL* high density lipoprotein, *LDL* high density lipoprotein, *CTA* computer tomography angiography; *ICA* internal carotid artery, *NIHSS* National Institutes of Health Stroke Scale

Previous studies have confirmed that vitamin K antagonists, such as warfarin, or non-vitamin antagonist oral anticoagulants (NOACs) reduce the risk of ischemic stroke [26]. Additionally, the current guidelines recommend warfarin or NOACs for stroke prevention in high-risk patients with AF or RHD. Nevertheless, many patients still fail to receive proper stroke prevention in the real world. A previous study showed that only 61.8% outpatients with AF (CHADS2 score ≥ 2) were treated with warfarin or NOACs [27]. In this study, we found that only 29 (31.9%) patients were treated with warfarin, and therefore the treatment rate is far below the rates observed in western countries. In addition, current guidelines suggest that a target INR between 2.0 to 3.0 is considered as effective [28]. Because of the high risk of intracranial hemorrhage in the Asian population, Japanese guidelines recommend that patients > 70 years of age should be controlled with a target INR of 1.60–2.60 [29]. In the United States, a large, nationwide and registry study indicated that in patients with acute ischemic stroke and a known history of AF, 30% were receiving some form of oral

Table 2 Associated factors with collateral circulation in acute ischemic stroke patients

	Poor (*n* = 43)	Moderate (*n* = 52)	Good (*n* = 25)	P value	Univariate logistic analysis	
					Poor vs. not poor rLMC	Good vs. not good rLMC
Age > 60 years	30 (69.8)	40 (76.9)	15 (60.0)	0.269	0.85 (0.36–1.97)	0.54 (0.21–1.38)
Hypertension history	24 (55.8)	25 (48.1)	11 (44.0)	0.601	1.36 (0.61–3.07)	0.85 (0.33–2.21)
Diabetes	6 (13.9)	8 (15.4)	2 (8.0)	0.664	0.89 (0.28–2.80)	0.48 (0.09–2.44)
Atrial fibrillation	42 (97.7)	48 (92.3)	22 (88.0)	0.282	3.50 (0.38–32.55)	0.61 (0.13–2.97)
Coronary heart disease	9 (20.9)	8 (15.4)	0 (0.0)	0.023	1.46 (0.51–4.17)	–
Previous stroke	5 (11.6)	10 (19.2)	1 (4.00)	0.168	0.55 (0.17–1.76)	0.18 (0.02–1.45)
Systolic blood pressure	34.98 ± 19.98	137.77 ± 21.91	38.28 ± 16.43	0.74	0.99 (0.95–1.02)	1.02 (0.97–1.07)
Diastolic blood pressure	82.67 ± 16.53	80.54 ± 14.04	80.56 ± 14.78	0.761	1.00 (0.96–1.05)	0.93 (0.87–0.99)
Serum glucose	8.33 ± 2.63	7.44 ± 2.17	7.84 ± 2.41	0.252	1.12 (0.98–1.40)	1.09 (0.88–1.34)
Triglyceride	1.51 ± 1.40	1.48 ± 1.99	1.63 ± 0.95	0.106	1.01 (0.69–1.47)	1.06 (0.79–1.39)
Cholesterol	3.92 ± 0.84	3.79 ± 1.09	4.43 ± 0.86	0.173	1.18 (0.75–1.85)	1.83 (1.16–3.40)
HDL-C	1.36 ± 0.44	1.38 ± 0.64	1.44 ± 0.57	0.864	0.91 (0.43–1.94)	1.17 (0.52–2.63)
LDL-C	2.35 ± 0.74	2.04 ± 0.68	2.54 ± 0.67	0.008	1.33 (0.79–2.24)	1.99 (1.07–3.72)
Antihypertensive drugs	17 (39.5)	22 (42.3)	10 (40.0)	0.959	0.89 (0.39–2.03)	0.91 (0.34–2.40)
Antidiabetics	6 (13.9)	7 (13.5)	1 (4.00)	0.44	1.04 (0.32–3.37)	0.27 (0.03–2.31)
Antiplatelet drugs	5 (11.6)	11 (21.2)	5 (20.0)	0.449	0.49 (0.16–1.54)	0.93 (0.29–3.05)
Statins	3 (6.9)	13 (25.0)	5 (20.0)	0.068	0.33 (0.06–0.85)	1.23 (0.40–3.77)
Warfarin	5 (11.6)	15 (28.9)	9 (36.0)	0.045	0.21 (0.10–0.83)	2.11 (0.81–5.48)

HDL high density lipoprotein, *LDL* high density lipoprotein, *CTA* computer tomography angiography, *ICA* internal carotid artery, *NIHSS* National Institutes of Health Stroke Scale, *LMC* leptomeningeal collateral

antithrombotic therapy before stroke onset, but that 64% of the warfarin-treated patients were receiving sub-therapeutic doses [11].

The presence of collateral cerebral circulation has been shown to be associated with better functional outcomes after stroke [3–6]. After acute ischemic stroke onset, collateral vessels provide the brain tissue with supplementary blood flow. Guidelines are available regarding the methods clinically available or under trial to promote collateral circulation after stroke (head position, induced hypertension, volume expansion, external counter pulsation, bypass surgery, albumin, nitric oxide, TNF-α inhibitors, statins [6]); but these methods are examined in the context of stroke management, not prevention. Nevertheless, some factors are known to be associated with collaterals. Previous studies have shown negative associations between hypertension and collaterals, and positive associations between statin use and collaterals [5, 9]. In addition, age, ischemic preconditioning, and cardiovascular risk factors are considered to be associated with collateral circulation patency [3, 30, 31]. Particularly, metabolic syndrome, high blood uric acid levels, and age have been associated with poor collaterals [4]. In the present study, the multivariable analysis showed that pre-stroke oral warfarin use was associated with collaterals, independently of age, gender, onset to door time, stroke risk factors, admission examinations, thrombus location, NIH stroke scale scores, and pre-stroke medications (model 4). This may be one reason why pre-stroke warfarin use affects stroke severity and clinical outcome. Nevertheless, additional studies in a larger population are necessary to corroborate our observations.

Table 3 Association between pre-stroke warfarin use and collaterals

	Poor rLMC vs. Not poor rLMC		Good rLMC vs. Not good rLMC	
	OR (95% CI)	P value	OR (95% CI)	P value
Unadjusted	0.21 (0.10–0.83)	0.021	2.11 (0.81–5.84)	0.125
Model 1	0.18 (0.05–0.61)	0.006	1.92 (0.66–5.62)	0.234
Model 2	0.17 (0.05–0.65)	0.009	2.12 (0.61–7.39)	0.239
Model 3	0.06 (0.01–0.37)	0.002	6.03 (0.94–38.71)	0.058
Model 4	0.07 (0.01–0.44)	0.005	4.80 (0.68–33.79)	0.115

Model 1: Adjusted for age, gender, onset to door time;
Model 2: Adjusted model 1 plus stroke risk factors;
Model 3: Adjusted model 2 plus admission examinations, thrombus location, NIH stroke scale scores;
Model 4: Adjusted model 3 plus prior medications

The major challenge for antithrombotic therapy among patients with AF or RHD is the risk of bleeding. In the present study, 22.5% of the patients with acute ischemic stroke were detected with ICH. A previous

Table 4 Association between pre-stroke warfarin use and clinical outcomes

	Univariate analysis		Multivariate analysis	
	OR (95% CI)	P value	OR (95% CI)	P value
NIHSS scores				
> 14 vs. 0–14	0.74 (0.31–1.76)	0.487	–	–
> 5 vs. 0–5	1.18 (0.39–3.53)	0.762	–	–
Thrombus location				
ICA + M1 vs. M1/M2	0.82 (0.29–2.27)	0.699	–	–
ICA + M1/M1 vs. M2	0.38 (0.16–0.91)	0.03	0.37 (0.13–1.03)	0.056*
Follow-up mRS scores				
0–3 vs. 4–6	1.43 (0.59–3.41)	0.425	–	–
0–2 vs. 3–6	1.49 (0.65–3.46)	0.348	–	–

*Adjusted age, gender, previous antiplatelet and statins, *NIHSS* National Institutes of Health Stroke Scale
ICA internal carotid artery, *mRS* modified Rankin Scale

report indicated that anticoagulant treatment after stroke onset was associated with significant increase in symptomatic intracranial bleeding [32], but we did not find that pre-stroke warfarin use was associated with ICH, which is supported by a previous study [13]. Nevertheless, due to the relatively small sample size in the present study, interpretation should be made with caution. There are several limitations to our study. First, the sample size was relatively small and we failed to perform subgroup analyses; hence, potential heterogeneity exists in the study population. Secondly, this study did not control for the use of previous antiplatelet therapy. Finally, based on the INR, most patients in the present study were found to receive inadequate antithrombotic therapy.

Conclusions

The results showed that prior warfarin use was inversely associated with the risk for poor collaterals in acute ischemic stroke patients presenting with occlusion of the middle cerebral artery, suggesting that warfarin use seems improve collateralization in patients with acute stroke. However, clinical controlled studies should be used to verify this claim.

Abbreviations

AF: Atrial fibrillation; CT: Computer tomography; CTA: Computer tomography angiography; ECASS: European Cooperative Acute Stroke Study; HDL: High density lipoprotein; ICA: Internal carotid artery; ICH: Intracerebral hemorrhage; INR: International normalized ratio; LDL: High density lipoprotein; MCA: Middle cerebral artery; MRI: Magnetic resonance imaging; mRS: Modified Rankin Scale; NCCT: Non-contrast computer tomography; NIHSS: National Institutes of Health Stroke Scale; NOACs: Non–vitamin antagonist oral anticoagulants; OR: Odds ratio; RHD: Rheumatic heart disease; rLMC: Regional leptomeningeal collateral; SD: Standard difference

Acknowledgments

We thank all the participants for their participation in this study.

Funding

This work was supported by National Comprehensive Demonstration Research on Prevention and Control of Chronic Diseases in Southwest China (2018YFC1311400 and 2018YFC1311401).

Authors' contributions

JZ and MM analyzed and interpreted the patient data and were the main contributors in writing the manuscript. They contributed equally to this work. YG performed the statistically analysis and was major contributor in writing the manuscript. MZ and JG collected the data and were the major contributors in writing the manuscript.
LH participated in the study design, data interpretation and revising the manuscript critically for important intellectual content. All authors read and approved the final manuscript.

Competing interests

The authors declare that they have no competing interests.

Author details

[1]Department of Neurology, West China Hospital, Sichuan University, Chengdu, China. [2]Department of Emergency, Gui Zhou provincial People's Hospital, Guiyang, China.

References

1. Liebeskind DS. Collateral circulation. Stroke. 2003;34(9):2279–84. https://doi.org/10.1161/01.str.0000086465.41263.06 Epub 2003/07/26. PubMed PMID: 12881609.
2. Shuaib A, Butcher K, Mohammad AA, Saqqur M, Liebeskind DS. Collateral blood vessels in acute ischaemic stroke: a potential therapeutic target. Lancet Neurol. 2011;10(10):909–21. https://doi.org/10.1016/s1474-4422(11)70195-8.
3. Menon BK, Smith EE, Modi J, Patel SK, Bhatia R, Watson TW, et al. Regional leptomeningeal score on CT angiography predicts clinical and imaging outcomes in patients with acute anterior circulation occlusions. AJNR Am J Neuroradiol. 2011;32(9):1640–5. https://doi.org/10.3174/ajnr.A2564 PubMed PMID: 21799045.
4. Menon BK, Smith EE, Coutts SB, Welsh DG, Faber JE, Goyal M, et al. Leptomeningeal collaterals are associated with modifiable metabolic risk factors. Ann Neurol. 2013;74(2):241–8. https://doi.org/10.1002/ana.23906 PubMed PMID: 23536377; PubMed Central PMCID: PMC3836863.
5. Lima FO, Furie KL, Silva GS, Lev MH, Camargo EC, Singhal AB, et al. The pattern of leptomeningeal collaterals on CT angiography is a strong predictor of long-term functional outcome in stroke patients with large vessel intracranial occlusion. Stroke. 2010;41(10):2316–22. https://doi.org/10.1161/STROKEAHA.110.592303 PubMed PMID: 20829514; PubMed Central PMCID: PMC4939434.
6. Bang OY, Goyal M, Liebeskind DS. Collateral circulation in ischemic stroke: assessment tools and therapeutic strategies. Stroke 2015;46(11):3302–3309. doi: https://doi.org/10.1161/STROKEAHA.115.010508. PubMed PMID: 26451027; PubMed Central PMCID: PMC4624512.
7. Teunissen PF, Horrevoets AJ, van Royen N. The coronary collateral circulation: genetic and environmental determinants in experimental models and humans. J Mol Cell Cardiol. 2012;52(4):897–904. https://doi.org/10.1016/j.yjmcc.2011.09.010 PubMed PMID: 21959171.
8. Epstein SE, Lassance-Soares RM, Faber JE, Burnett MS. Effects of aging on the collateral circulation, and therapeutic implications. Circulation. 2012; 125(25):3211–9. https://doi.org/10.1161/CIRCULATIONAHA.111.079038 PubMed PMID: 22733335.
9. Ovbiagele B, Saver JL, Starkman S, Kim D, Ali LK, Jahan R, et al. Statin enhancement of collateralization in acute stroke. Neurology. 2007;68(24): 2129–31. https://doi.org/10.1212/01.wnl.0000264931.34941.f0 PubMed PMID: 17562834.
10. Hylek EM, Skates SJ, Sheehan MA, Singer DE. An analysis of the lowest effective intensity of prophylactic anticoagulation for patients with nonrheumatic atrial fibrillation. N Engl J Med. 1996;335(8):540–6. https://doi.org/10.1056/nejm199608223350802 Epub 1996/08/22 PubMed PMID: 8678931.

11. Xian Y, O'Brien EC, Liang L, Xu H, Schwamm LH, Fonarow GC, et al. Association of Preceding Antithrombotic Treatment with Acute Ischemic Stroke Severity and in-Hospital Outcomes among Patients with Atrial Fibrillation. JAMA. 2017;317(10):1057–67. https://doi.org/10.1001/jama.2017.1371 PubMed PMID: 28291892.
12. Tziomalos K, Giampatzis V, Bouziana SD, Spanou M, Kostaki S, Papadopoulou M, et al. Adequacy of preadmission oral anticoagulation with vitamin K antagonists and ischemic stroke severity and outcome in patients with atrial fibrillation. J Thromb Thrombolysis. 2016;41(2):336–42. https://doi.org/10.1007/s11239-015-1262-y PubMed PMID: 26253707.
13. Audebert HJ, Schenk B, Schenkel J, Heuschmann PU. Impact of prestroke oral anticoagulation on severity and outcome of ischemic and hemorrhagic stroke in patients with atrial fibrillation. Cerebrovasc Dis. 2010;29(5):476–83. https://doi.org/10.1159/000297963 PubMed PMID: 20299787.
14. Miteff FLC, Bateman GA, Spratt N, McElduff P, Parsons MW. The independent predictive utility of computed tomography angiographic collateral status in acute ischaemic stroke. Brain. 2009;132(Pt 8):2231–8. https://doi.org/10.1093/brain/awp155.
15. YM WM, Minematsu K, Yamaguchi T. Effects of anticoagulation on infarct size and clinical outcome in acute cardioembolic stroke. Angiology. 2002;53(5):551–6.
16. DeFazio RALS, Morales CL, Levy RV, Dave KR, Lin HW, Abaffy T, Watson BD, Perez-Pinzon MA, Ohanna V. A protocol for characterizing the impact of collateral fl ow after middle cerebral artery occlusion. Transl Stroke Res. 2011;2(1):112–27.
17. Yuan FLX, Guan Y, Mu Z, Chen K, Wang Y, Yang GY. Collateral circulation prevents masticatory muscle impairment in rat middle cerebral artery occlusion model. J Synchrotron Radiat. 2014;21(6):1314–8. https://doi.org/10.1107/S1600577514016130 PubMed Central PMCID: PMCPMID: 25343800.
18. Kvistad CE, Logallo N, Oygarden H, Thomassen L, Waje-Andreassen U, Naess H. Elevated admission blood pressure and stroke severity in acute ischemic stroke: the Bergen NORSTROKE study. Cerebrovasc Dis. 2013;36(5–6):351–4. https://doi.org/10.1159/000355685 PubMed PMID: 24192488.
19. Pourati IKC, Rand W, Karas RH. Statin use is associated with enhanced collateralization of severely diseased coronary arteries. Am Heart J. 2003; 146(5):876–81.
20. Paciaroni M AG, Micheli S, Caso V. Efficacy and safety of anticoagulant treatment in acute cardioembolic stroke: a meta-analysis of randomized controlled trials. Stroke. 2007;38(2):423–430. Epub 430. doi: https://doi.org/10.1161/01.STR.0000254600.92975.1f. PubMed Central PMCID: PMC17204681.
21. Chalothorn DFJ. Formation and maturation of the native collateral circulation. J Mol Cell Cardiol. 2010;49:251–9.
22. Matsumoto M, Sakaguchi M, Okazaki S, Hashikawa K, Takahashi T, Matsumoto M, et al. Relationship between infarct volume and prothrombin time-international normalized ratio in ischemic stroke patients with Nonvalvular atrial fibrillation. Circ J. 2017;81(3):391–6. https://doi.org/10.1253/circj.CJ-16-0707 PubMed PMID: 28154247.
23. Ay H, Arsava EM, Gungor L, Greer D, Singhal AB, Furie KL, et al. Admission international normalized ratio and acute infarct volume in ischemic stroke. Ann Neurol. 2008;64(5):499–506. https://doi.org/10.1002/ana.21456 PubMed PMID: 18661516.
24. McDowell TYLJ, Florian J, Southworth MR, Grant S, Stockbridge N. Relationship between international normalized ratio and outcomes in modern trials with warfarin controls. Pharmacotherapy. 2018. https://doi.org/10.1002/phar.2161.
25. Yasaka MMK, Yamaguchi T. Optimal intensity of international normalized ratio in warfarin therapy for secondary prevention of stroke in patients with non-valvular atrial fibrillation. Intern Med. 2001;40(12):1183–8.
26. Penttilä TLM, Niiranen J, Mehtälä J, Khanfir H, Lassila R, Raatikainen P. Differences in the risk of stroke, bleeding events, and mortality between female and male patients with atrial fibrillation during warfarin therapy. Eur Heart J Cardiovasc Pharmacother. 2018. https://doi.org/10.1093/ehjcvp/pvy026 PubMed Central PMCID: PMCPMID: 30052822.
27. Hsu JC, Maddox TM, Kennedy K, Katz DF, Marzec LN, Lubitz SA, et al. Aspirin instead of Oral anticoagulant prescription in atrial fibrillation patients at risk for stroke. J Am Coll Cardiol 2016;67(25):2913–2923. Epub 2016/06/25. doi: https://doi.org/10.1016/j.jacc.2016.03.581. PubMed PMID: 27339487.
28. January CT, Wann LS, Alpert JS, Calkins H, Cigarroa JE, Cleveland JC, Jr., et al. 2014 AHA/ACC/HRS guideline for the management of patients with atrial fibrillation: executive summary: a report of the American College of Cardiology/American Heart Association task force on practice guidelines and the Heart Rhythm Society. Circulation 2014;130(23):2071–2104. Epub 2014/04/01. doi: https://doi.org/10.1161/cir.0000000000000040. PubMed PMID: 24682348.
29. Shinohara Y, Yamaguchi T. Outline of the Japanese guidelines for the Management of Stroke 2004 and subsequent revision. Int J Stroke 2008;3(1): 55–62. Epub 2008/08/19. doi: https://doi.org/10.1111/j.1747-4949.2008.00178.x. PubMed PMID: 18705916.
30. Faber JE, Zhang H, Lassance-Soares RM, Prabhakar P, Najafi AH, Burnett MS, et al. Aging causes collateral rarefaction and increased severity of ischemic injury in multiple tissues. Arterioscler Thromb Vasc Biol. 2011;31(8):1748–56. https://doi.org/10.1161/ATVBAHA.111.227314 PubMed PMID: 21617137; PubMed Central PMCID: PMC3141082.
31. Wang J, Peng X, Lassance-Soares RM, Najafi AH, Alderman LO, Sood S, et al. Aging-induced collateral dysfunction: impaired responsiveness of collaterals and susceptibility to apoptosis via dysfunctional eNOS signaling. J Cardiovasc Transl Res. 2011;4(6):779–89. https://doi.org/10.1007/s12265-011-9280-4 PubMed PMID: 21538183; PubMed Central PMCID: PMC3756560.
32. Paciaroni M, Agnelli G, Micheli S, Caso V. Efficacy and safety of anticoagulant treatment in acute cardioembolic stroke: a meta-analysis of randomized controlled trials. Stroke. 2007;38(2):423–30. https://doi.org/10.1161/01.STR.0000254600.92975.1f PubMed PMID: 17204681.

Permissions

All chapters in this book were first published in NEUROLOGY, by BioMed Central; hereby published with permission under the Creative Commons Attribution License or equivalent. Every chapter published in this book has been scrutinized by our experts. Their significance has been extensively debated. The topics covered herein carry significant findings which will fuel the growth of the discipline. They may even be implemented as practical applications or may be referred to as a beginning point for another development.

The contributors of this book come from diverse backgrounds, making this book a truly international effort. This book will bring forth new frontiers with its revolutionizing research information and detailed analysis of the nascent developments around the world.

We would like to thank all the contributing authors for lending their expertise to make the book truly unique. They have played a crucial role in the development of this book. Without their invaluable contributions this book wouldn't have been possible. They have made vital efforts to compile up to date information on the varied aspects of this subject to make this book a valuable addition to the collection of many professionals and students.

This book was conceptualized with the vision of imparting up-to-date information and advanced data in this field. To ensure the same, a matchless editorial board was set up. Every individual on the board went through rigorous rounds of assessment to prove their worth. After which they invested a large part of their time researching and compiling the most relevant data for our readers.

The editorial board has been involved in producing this book since its inception. They have spent rigorous hours researching and exploring the diverse topics which have resulted in the successful publishing of this book. They have passed on their knowledge of decades through this book. To expedite this challenging task, the publisher supported the team at every step. A small team of assistant editors was also appointed to further simplify the editing procedure and attain best results for the readers.

Apart from the editorial board, the designing team has also invested a significant amount of their time in understanding the subject and creating the most relevant covers. They scrutinized every image to scout for the most suitable representation of the subject and create an appropriate cover for the book.

The publishing team has been an ardent support to the editorial, designing and production team. Their endless efforts to recruit the best for this project, has resulted in the accomplishment of this book. They are a veteran in the field of academics and their pool of knowledge is as vast as their experience in printing. Their expertise and guidance has proved useful at every step. Their uncompromising quality standards have made this book an exceptional effort. Their encouragement from time to time has been an inspiration for everyone.

The publisher and the editorial board hope that this book will prove to be a valuable piece of knowledge for researchers, students, practitioners and scholars across the globe.

List of Contributors

Amytis Towfighi
Los Angeles County Department of Health Services, Los Angeles, California, USA
University of Southern California, Los Angeles, California, USA
Rancho Los Amigos National Rehabilitation Center, Downey, California, USA

Marilyn Corrales
Los Angeles County Department of Health Services, Los Angeles, California, USA
Rancho Los Amigos National Rehabilitation Center, Downey, California, USA

Theresa Sivers-Teixeira
University of Southern California, Los Angeles, California, USA
Rancho Los Amigos National Rehabilitation Center, Downey, California, USA

Valerie Hill
Rancho Los Amigos National Rehabilitation Center, Downey, California, USA

Monica Ayala-Rivera
Rancho Los Amigos National Rehabilitation Center, Downey, California, USA
University of California, Los Angeles (UCLA), Los Angeles, California, USA

Elizabeth Mojarro-Huang
Rancho Los Amigos National Rehabilitation Center, Downey, California, USA
Los Angeles County-University of Southern California (USC) Medical Center, Los Angeles, California, USA

Ana Montoya
Rancho Los Amigos National Rehabilitation Center, Downey, California, USA
Harbor-UCLA Medical Center, Torrance, California, USA
Olive View-UCLA Medical Center, Sylmar, California, USA

Beatrice Martinez
Rancho Los Amigos National Rehabilitation Center, Downey, California, USA
Harbor-UCLA Medical Center, Torrance, California, USA

Eric M. Cheng, Heather McCreath, Adam Richards, Frances Barry, William Cunningham and Honghu Liu
University of California, Los Angeles (UCLA), Los Angeles, California, USA

Bijal Mehta
University of California, Los Angeles (UCLA), Los Angeles, California, USA
Harbor-UCLA Medical Center, Torrance, California, USA

Nerses Sanossian
University of Southern California, Los Angeles, California, USA
Los Angeles County-University of Southern California (USC) Medical Center, Los Angeles, California, USA

Tara Dutta
Rancho Los Amigos National Rehabilitation Center, Downey, California, USA
Kaiser Permanente, Sacramento, California, USA

Jamie Tran
Harbor-UCLA Medical Center, Torrance, California, USA

Robert Bryg and Neal Rao
University of California, Los Angeles (UCLA), Los Angeles, California, USA
Olive View-UCLA Medical Center, Sylmar, California, USA

Shlee Song
Cedars Sinai Medical Center, Los Angeles, California, USA

Ali Razmara
Rancho Los Amigos National Rehabilitation Center, Downey, California, USA
Kaiser Permanente, Irvine, California, USA

Magaly Ramirez
Fielding School of Public Health, Department of Health Policy and Management, University of California, Los Angeles, Los Angeles, California, USA

Phyllis Willis
Watts Labor Community Action Committee, Watts, California, USA

Diane Factor and Mireya Macias
Worker Education and Resource Center, Los Angeles, California, USA

Nancy Ibrahim
Esperanza Community Housing, Los Angeles, California, USA

Shinyi Wu
School of Social Work, Edward R. Roybal Institute on Aging, and Daniel J. Epstein Department of Industrial and Systems Engineering, University of Southern California, Los Angeles, California, USA
RAND Corporation, Santa Monica, California, USA

David A. Ganz
University of California, Los Angeles (UCLA), Los Angeles, California, USA
RAND Corporation, Santa Monica, California, USA
Department of Veterans Affairs Greater Los Angeles Healthcare System, Los Angeles, California, USA

Jeremy Wacksman and Hilary Haber
Dimagi, Inc., Cambridge, Massachusetts, USA

Brian Mittman
Department of Veterans Affairs Greater Los Angeles Healthcare System, Los Angeles, California, USA

Barbara G. Vickrey
Icahn School of Medicine at Mount Sinai, New York, New York, USA

Pedro Castro and Elsa Azevedo
Department Neurology, São João Hospital Center, Faculty of Medicine of University of Porto, Alameda Professor Hernani Monteiro, 4200-319 Porto, Portugal

Isabel Rocha
Cardiovascular Autonomic Function Lab, Institute of Physiology, Faculty of Medicine of University of Lisbon, Lisbon, Portugal

Farzaneh Sorond
Department of Neurology, Division of Stroke and Neurocritical, Northwestern University Feinberg School of Medicine, Chicago, IL, USA

Jorge M. Serrador
Department of Pharmacology, Physiology and Neuroscience, Rutgers Biomedical Health Sciences, Newark, NJ, USA
Veterans Biomedical Research Institute and War Related Illness and Injury Study Center, Department of Veterans Affairs, East Orange, USA
Cardiovascular Electronics, National University of Ireland Galway, Galway, Ireland

Ann De Vos, Dirk Jacobs, Lien Van den Abbeele and Eugeen Vanmechelen
ADx NeuroSciences NV, Technologiepark 4, 9052 Ghent, Belgium

Maria Bjerke and Naomi De Roeck
Reference Center for Biological Markers of Dementia (BIODEM), Institute Born-Bunge, University of Antwerp, Antwerp, Belgium

Raf Brouns
Department of Neurology, Hospital ZorSaam, Terneuzen, The Netherlands

Kaat Guldolf and Sebastiaan Engelborghs
Reference Center for Biological Markers of Dementia (BIODEM), Institute Born-Bunge, University of Antwerp, Antwerp, Belgium
Department of Neurology and Memory Clinic, Hospital Network Antwerp (ZNA) Middelheim and Hoge Beuken, Antwerp, Belgium

Kaj Blennow
Clinical Neurochemistry Laboratory, Sahlgrenska University Hospital, Mölndal, Sweden
Institute of Neuroscience and Physiology, Department of Psychiatry and Neurochemistry, the Sahlgrenska Academy at the University of Gothenburg, Mölndal, Sweden

Henrik Zetterberg
Clinical Neurochemistry Laboratory, Sahlgrenska University Hospital, Mölndal, Sweden
Institute of Neuroscience and Physiology, Department of Psychiatry and Neurochemistry, the Sahlgrenska Academy at the University of Gothenburg, Mölndal, Sweden
Department of Molecular Neuroscience, UCL Institute of Neurology, London, UK

Sheamini Sivasampu
National Clinical Research Centre, Ministry of Health Malaysia, Kuala Lumpur, Malaysia

Wen Yea Hwong
National Clinical Research Centre, Ministry of Health Malaysia, Kuala Lumpur, Malaysia
Julius Center for Health Sciences and Primary Care, University Medical Center Utrecht, Utrecht, The Netherlands

Michiel L. Bots and Ilonca Vaartjes
Julius Center for Health Sciences and Primary Care, University Medical Center Utrecht, Utrecht, The Netherlands

Zariah Abdul Aziz
Department of Neurology, Hospital Sultanah Nur Zahirah, Kuala Terengganu, Terengganu, Malaysia

Norsima Nazifah Sidek
Clinical Research Centre, Hospital Sultanah Nur Zahirah, Kuala Terengganu, Terengganu, Malaysia

Sharmini Selvarajah
Julius Center for Health Sciences and Primary Care, University Medical Center Utrecht, Utrecht, The Netherlands
Sharmini Selvarajah Consulting, Selangor, Malaysia

L. Jaap Kappelle
Department of Neurology and Neurosurgery, Brain Center Rudolf Magnus, University Medical Center Utrecht, Utrecht, The Netherlands

Sonu Bhaskar
Western Sydney University (WSU), School of Medicine, South West Sydney Clinical School, Sydney, NSW 2170, Australia
Liverpool Hospital, Department of Neurology & Neurophysiology, Liverpool 2170, NSW, Australia
The Sydney Partnership for Health, Education, Research & Enterprise (SPHERE), Liverpool, NSW, Australia
Stroke & Neurology Research Group, Ingham Institute for Applied Medical Research, 1 Campbell Street, Liverpool, NSW 2170, Australia
Department of Neurology, John Hunter Hospital, Newcastle, NSW, Australia Priority Research Centre for Stroke & Brain Injury, Faculty of Health & Medicine, Hunter Medical Research institute (HMRI) and School of Medicine & Public Health, University of Newcastle, Newcastle, NSW, Australia

Dennis Cordato
Liverpool Hospital, Department of Neurology & Neurophysiology, Liverpool 2170, NSW, Australia
Stroke & Neurology Research Group, Ingham Institute for Applied Medical Research, 1 Campbell Street, Liverpool, NSW 2170, Australia
School of Medicine, University of New South Wales (UNSW), Sydney, NSW, Australia

Christopher Levi
Western Sydney University (WSU), School of Medicine, South West Sydney Clinical School, Sydney, NSW 2170, Australia
Liverpool Hospital, Department of Neurology & Neurophysiology, Liverpool 2170, NSW, Australia
The Sydney Partnership for Health, Education, Research & Enterprise (SPHERE), Liverpool, NSW, Australia
Stroke & Neurology Research Group, Ingham Institute for Applied Medical Research, 1 Campbell Street, Liverpool, NSW 2170, Australia
School of Medicine, University of New South Wales (UNSW), Sydney, NSW, Australia
Department of Neurology, John Hunter Hospital, Newcastle, NSW, Australia

Peter Stanwell
Priority Research Centre for Stroke & Brain Injury, Faculty of Health & Medicine, Hunter Medical Research institute (HMRI) and School of Medicine & Public Health, University of Newcastle, Newcastle, NSW, Australia

John Attia
Priority Research Centre for Stroke & Brain Injury, Faculty of Health & Medicine, Hunter Medical Research institute (HMRI) and School of Medicine & Public Health, University of Newcastle, Newcastle, NSW, Australia
Centre for Clinical Epidemiology & Biostatistics, Hunter Medical Research Institute, University of Newcastle, Newcastle, NSW, Australia

Seong-Joon Lee, Ji Man Hong, Sung Eun Lee and Jin Soo Lee
Department of Neurology, Ajou University School of Medicine, Ajou University Medical Center, San 5, Woncheon-dong, Yeongtong-gu, Suwon, Kyungki-do 443–721, South Korea

Dae Ryong Kang
Center of Biomedical Data Science/Institute of Genomic Cohort, Yonsei University Wonju College of Medicine, Wonju, South Korea

Bruce Ovbiagele
Department of Neurology, Medical University of South Carolina, Charleston, SC, USA

Andrew M. Demchuk
Calgary Stroke Program, Departments of Clinical Neurosciences and Radiology, Hotchkiss Brain Institute, University of Calgary, Calgary, AB, Canada

Nampet Jampathong, Malinee Laopaiboon, Siwanon Rattanakanokchai and Porjai Pattanittum
Department of Epidemiology and Biostatistics, Faculty of Public Health, Khon Kaen University, 123 Mittraphap Road, Nai-Muang, Muang District, Khon Kaen 40002, Thailand

Xiaomeng Yang
Vascular Neurology, Department of Neurology, Beijing Tiantan Hospital, Capital Medical University, No. 6 Tiantan Xili, Dongcheng District, Beijing 100050, China

Yongjun Wang
Vascular Neurology, Department of Neurology, Beijing Tiantan Hospital, Capital Medical University, No. 6 Tiantan Xili, Dongcheng District, Beijing 100050, China
Beijing Key Laboratory of Translational Medicine for Cerebrovascular Disease, No. 6 Tiantan Xili, Dongcheng District, Beijing 100050, China
China National Clinical Research Center for Neurological Diseases, No. 6 Tiantan Xili, Dongcheng District, Beijing 100050, China

Zixiao Li
Vascular Neurology, Department of Neurology, Beijing Tiantan Hospital, Capital Medical University, No. 6 Tiantan Xili, Dongcheng District, Beijing 100050, China
China National Clinical Research Center for Neurological Diseases, No. 6 Tiantan Xili, Dongcheng District, Beijing 100050, China

Shuya Li
Tiantan Clinical Trial and Research Center for Stroke, Department of Neurology, Beijing Tiantan Hospital, Capital Medical University, No.6 Tiantanxili, Dongcheng District, Beijing 100050, China

Deok-Soo Lee
Department of Neurology, College of Medicine, Dong-A University, 1, 3-ga Dongdaesin-dong, Seo-gu, Busan 602-715, Republic of Korea

Yong Jiang
Tiantan Clinical Trial and Research Center for Stroke, Department of Neurology, Beijing Tiantan Hospital, Capital Medical University, No.6 Tiantanxili, Dongcheng District, Beijing 100050, China
Center of Stroke, Beijing Institute for Brain Disorders, Beijing, China

Xingquan Zhao
Vascular Neurology, Department of Neurology, Beijing Tiantan Hospital, Capital Medical University, No. 6 Tiantan Xili, Dongcheng District, Beijing 100050, China
Center of Stroke, Beijing Institute for Brain Disorders, Beijing, China

Liping Liu
Neuro-intensive Care Unit, Department of Neurology, Beijing Tiantan Hospital, Capital Medical University, Beijing, China
Beijing Key Laboratory of Translational Medicine for Cerebrovascular Disease, No. 6 Tiantan Xili, Dongcheng District, Beijing 100050, China

Yilong Wang
Tiantan Clinical Trial and Research Center for Stroke, Department of Neurology, Beijing Tiantan Hospital, Capital Medical University, No.6 Tiantanxili, Dongcheng District, Beijing 100050, China
China National Clinical Research Center for Neurological Diseases, No. 6 Tiantan Xili, Dongcheng District, Beijing 100050, China

Dae-Hyun Kim, Hyun-Wook Nah and Jae-Kwan Cha
Busan-Ulsan Regional Cardiocerebrovascular Center, Dong-A University Hospital, Busan, Republic of Korea
Department of Neurology, College of Medicine, Dong-A University, 1, 3-ga Dongdaesin-dong, Seo-gu, Busan 602-715, Republic of Korea

Masahito Kawabori, Takeo Abumiya, Naoki Nakayama, Ken Kazumata, Shunsuke Terasaka and Kiyohiro Houkin
Department of Neurosurgery, Hokkaido University Graduate School of Medicine, Sapporo, Japan

Brenda Johnson
Department of Neurology, Johns Hopkins University School of Medicine, Baltimore, USA

Hideo Shichinohe
Department of Neurosurgery, Hokkaido University Graduate School of Medicine, Sapporo, Japan
Clinical Research and Medical Innovation Center, Hokkaido University Hospital, N14 W5, Kita ku, Sapporo 060-8648, Japan

Hiroaki Iijima, Tuyoshi Teramoto and Teruyo Arato
Clinical Research and Medical Innovation Center, Hokkaido University Hospital, N14 W5, Kita-ku, Sapporo 060-8648, Japan

Seung Hoon Song, Jeong Hee Kim, Joon Hwa Lee and Hahn Young Kim
Department of Neurology, Research Institute of Medical Science, Konkuk University School of Medicine, Konkuk University Medical Center, Seoul, Republic of Korea

Yeo-Min Yun
Department of Laboratory Medicine, Konkuk University School of Medicine, Konkuk University Medical Center, Seoul, Republic of Korea

Dong-Hee Choi
Department of Medical Science, Konkuk University School of Medicine, Seoul, Republic of Korea

Daniel J. Johnson and Steven M. Frank
Department of Anesthesiology and Critical Care Medicine, Johns Hopkins University School of Medicine, Baltimore, USA

Kartavya Sharma
Department of Anesthesiology and Critical Care Medicine, Johns Hopkins University School of Medicine, Baltimore, USA
Department of Neurology, Johns Hopkins University School of Medicine, Baltimore, USA
Department of Neurology, University of Kansas Medical Center, Mailstop 2012, 3901 Rainbow Blvd, Kansas City, KS 66160, USA

Robert D. Stevens
Department of Anesthesiology and Critical Care Medicine, Johns Hopkins University School of Medicine, Baltimore, USA
Department of Neurology, Johns Hopkins University School of Medicine, Baltimore, USA
Department of Neurosurgery, Johns Hopkins University School of Medicine, Baltimore, USA

Mikhail N. Kalinin and Dina R. Khasanova
Department of Neurology and Neurosurgery for Postgraduate Training, Kazan State Medical University, Kazan, Russia
Department of Neurology, Interregional Clinical Diagnostic Center, 12A Karbyshev St, Kazan 420101, Russia

Murat M. Ibatullin
Department of Neurology and Neurosurgery for Postgraduate Training, Kazan State Medical University, Kazan, Russia
Department of Radiology, Interregional Clinical Diagnostic Center, Kazan, Russia

Belma Doğan Güngen, Abdulkadir Tunç, Yeşim Güzey Aras, Aslı Aksoy Gündoğdu, Adil Can Güngen and Serdar Bal
Bezmialem Vakif Universitesi Tip Fakultesi Hastanesi, Istanbul, Turkey

Xiaoyu Zhang, Gaoting Ma, Zhangning Zhao and Meijia Zhu
Department of Neurology, Qianfoshan Hospital, Shandong University, Jinan 250014, China

Peter Kraft
Department of Neurology, University Hospital of Würzburg, Josef-Schneider-Str. 11, 97080 Würzburg, Germany

Daniel Mackenrodt
Department of Neurology, University Hospital of Würzburg, Josef-Schneider-Str. 11, 97080 Würzburg, Germany
Institute of Clinical Epidemiology and Biometry, University of Würzburg, Würzburg, Germany
Comprehensive Heart Failure Center, University of Würzburg, Würzburg, Germany

Anna Fleischer, Viktoria Rücker and Uwe Malzahn
Institute of Clinical Epidemiology and Biometry, University of Würzburg, Würzburg, Germany

Silke Wiedmann and Peter U. Heuschmann
Institute of Clinical Epidemiology and Biometry, University of Würzburg, Würzburg, Germany
Comprehensive Heart Failure Center, University of Würzburg, Würzburg, Germany

Christoph Kleinschnitz
Department of Neurology, University Hospital of Würzburg, Josef-Schneider-Str. 11, 97080 Würzburg, Germany
Comprehensive Heart Failure Center, University of Würzburg, Würzburg, Germany
Department of Neurology, University Hospital Essen, Essen, Germany

Stefan Störk and Caroline Morbach
Comprehensive Heart Failure Center, University of Würzburg, Würzburg, Germany
Department of Internal Medicine, University Hospital Würzburg, Würzburg, Germany

Lanying He and Jian Wang
Department of Neurology, The Second People's Hospital of Chengdu, Chengdu 400010, People's Republic of China

Weiwei Dong
Department of Neurology, First Affiliated Hospital, Chongqing Medical University, ChongqingChina, 400030, People's Republic of China

Shan shan Lu, Jun Xie, Chun qiu Su, Hai bin Shi and Xun ning Hong
Department of Radiology, The First Affiliated Hospital of Nanjing Medical University, No.300 Guangzhou Road, Gulou district, Nanjing 210029, Jiangsu Province, China

Song Ge
Department of Neurology, The First Affiliated Hospital of Nanjing Medical University, Nanjing 210029, Jiangsu Province, China

Thomas Toell, Christian Boehme, Lukas Mayer, Barbara Prantl, Michael Knoflach, Gudrun Schoenherr, Peter Willeit, Stefan Kiechl and Johann Willeit
Department of Neurology, Medical University of Innsbruck, Anichstraße 35, A-6020 Innsbruck, Austria

Stefan Krebs, Clemens Lang and Julia Ferrari
Department of Neurology, Hospital St. John of God, Johannes von Gott Platz 1, A-1020 Vienna, Austria

Karin Willeit
Department of Neurology, Medical University of Innsbruck, Anichstraße 35, A-6020 Innsbruck, Austria
Department of Neurology, Inselspital Bern, University Hospital, Freiburgstrasse, CH-3010 Bern, Switzerland

Gerhard Rumpold
Department of Medical Psychology, Medical University of Innsbruck, Schöpfstraße 23a, A-6020 Innsbruck, Austria

Andrea Griesmacher
Central Institute of Medical and Chemical Laboratory Diagnostics, University Hospital of Innsbruck, Anichstraße 35, A-6020 Innsbruck, Austria

Wilfried Lang
Department of Neurology, Hospital St. John of God, Johannes von Gott Platz 1, A-1020 Vienna, Austria
Sigmund Freud Private University, Medical Faculty, Campus Prater Freudplatz 1, A-1020 Vienna, Austria

Jingxia Zhou, Lin Chen, Bocan Chen, Shaozhu Huang, Chaosheng Zeng, Hairong Wu, Cong Chen and Faqing Long
Department of Neurology, The Second Affiliated Hospital of Hainan Medical University, Haikou 570311, Hainan Province, People's Republic of China

Mengmeng Ma, Yijia Guo, Muke Zhou, Jian Guo and Li He
Department of Neurology, West China Hospital, Sichuan University, Chengdu, China

Jiaying Zhu
Department of Neurology, West China Hospital, Sichuan University, Chengdu, China Department of Emergency, Gui Zhou provincial People's Hospital, Guiyang, China

Index

www.ingramcontent.com/pod-product-compliance
Lightning Source LLC
LaVergne TN
LVHW080649210926
848485LV00003B/354
9781639272891